NELSON

REVIEW

of

PEDIATRICS

NELSON

REVIEW

of

PEDIATRICS

RICHARD E. BEHRMAN, M.D.
Clinical Professor of Pediatrics
Stanford University School of Medicine
University of California, San Francisco
School of Medicine
Senior Vice President for Medical Affairs
The Lucile Packard Foundation for Children's Health
Palo Alto, California

ROBERT M. KLIEGMAN, M.D.
Professor and Chair
Department of Pediatrics
Medical College of Wisconsin
Pediatrician-in-Chief
Children's Hospital of Wisconsin
Milwaukee, Wisconsin

HAL B. JENSON, M.D.
Professor
Departments of Pediatrics and Microbiology
Chief, Pediatrics Infectious Diseases
The University of Texas Health Science Center at San Antonio
San Antonio, Texas

W.B. SAUNDERS COMPANY
A Division of Harcourt Brace & Company
Philadelphia   London   New York   St. Louis   Sydney   Toronto

W.B. SAUNDERS COMPANY
A Harcourt Health Sciences Company

The Curtis Center
Independence Square West
Philadelphia, Pennsylvania 19106

Library of Congress Cataloging-in-Publication Data

Behrman, Richard E.

Nelson review of pediatrics / Richard E. Behrman, Robert M. Kleigman,
Hal B. Jensen.—2nd ed.

p.   cm.

ISBN 0–7216–7785–1

1. Pediatrics—Examinations, questions, etc.   I. Title: Review of pediatrics.
  II. Kliegman, Robert M.   III. Jensen, Hal B.   IV. Title.   [DNLM:
  1. Pediatrics—Examination Questions.   WS 18.2 B421n 2000]

RJ48.2.N4 2000   618.92′00076—dc21   00–30060

NELSON REVIEW OF PEDIATRICS   ISBN 0–7216–7785–1

Printed in the United States of America.

Last digit is the print number: 9   8   7   6   5   4   3   2   1

Preface

The field of pediatrics has advanced at a phenomenal pace at the end of this millennium. The discovery of new diseases and new ways to classify diseases have been complemented by a better understanding of health and disease. New methodologies enhance our diagnostic skills and accuracy. These advances are reflected in the updated sixteenth edition of *Nelson Textbook of Pediatrics.*

The goal of this review is to help the reader continue to learn from the comprehensive, larger text, but in an active fashion. This work has been written in parallel with the sixteenth edition of *Nelson Textbook of Pediatrics* and is thus a self-assessment guide, which reinforces what was learned from the larger, parent text. Each question has been written to continue the education of the reader. Case-based questions and multiple-choice and matching questions and the corresponding explanations help to reinforce the knowledge of a broad spectrum of general pediatric facts.

Because learning occurs in many different settings, we anticipate that the questions in this review will help the reader benefit from the knowledge of the parent text. We believe that this learning activity will help the reader in career advancement and will contribute to the ability to care for children. Past experience of previous readers has suggested that this work will also aid in the preparation for important steps for progression within the field of pediatrics. This may include student final exams, resident inservice exams, and preparation for certification or recertification boards. The majority of the questions in this edition are new, but some questions from the previous review are repeated because of their excellent nature. Many questions are challenging, some are simple but of value as a review, and all are guaranteed to help the reader learn more pediatrics.

Finally, we encourage feedback from readers so that we may continue to create a reader-friendly study guide.

RICHARD E. BEHRMAN, M.D.
ROBERT M. KLEIGMAN, M.D.
HAL B. JENSON, M.D.

Contents

PART 1

The Field of Pediatrics

The broad field of pediatrics encompasses the art and science of medicine across the wide age range of 24-weeks' gestation, immature neonates to 6-foot 8-inch adolescent athletes. This part of the *Nelson Textbook of Pediatrics* covers the history of pediatrics in addition to providing information about the epidemiology and lives of children both in the United States and abroad. It addresses the importance of understanding the cultural background of families in the context of disease prevention and therapy in an international setting. Furthermore, it informs us about important ethical approaches to patient care that enable us, as physicians, and our patients' families to make good medical decisions. In addition, this part emphasizes an essential aspect that distinguishes pediatrics as a specialty—that is, preventive pediatrics. Finally, an excellent detailed approach to the well child is developed for readers.

The questions for this part reinforce readers' learning on these basic topics. An understanding of these concepts creates an excellent foundation for practicing pediatricians, child advocates, and epidemiologists.

1. Injuries, congenital anomalies, and malignancy are the three leading causes of death for which age group?
   A. 0–1 year
   B. 1–4 years
   C. 5–9 years
   D. 10–14 years
   E. 15–24 years

2. The three leading causes of death for 15- to 24-year-olds are
   A. injuries, malignancy, suicide
   B. injuries, malignancy, homicide
   C. injuries, anomalies, malignancy
   D. injuries, homicide, suicide
   E. injuries, malignancy, diseases of the heart

3. In ethical principles, withholding futile medical treatment is no different from
   A. homicide
   B. battery
   C. beneficence
   D. withdrawing treatment
   E. paternalism

4. Of the following parts of a physical examination, which portion should usually be performed first on an infant or toddler?
   A. Abdominal examination
   B. Ear examination
   C. Extremity examination
   D. Cardiac examination
   E. Pharyngeal examination

5. Global improvements in child mortality are primarily the result of
   A. antibiotics and improved distribution of essential drugs
   B. smallpox eradication and control of other vaccine-preventable illnesses
   C. oral rehydration therapy
   D. basic public health programs

6. In order to prevent malnutrition in infants younger than 1 year, the best advice you should give a nursing mother who discovers that she is pregnant again and lives in a developing country is to
   A. continue nursing as long as possible and begin adding appropriate weaning food after 6 months of age
   B. consider an alternative to breast milk and wean as soon as possible to an appropriate weaning food
   C. discontinue the pregnancy and use family planning until the nursing child is 2 years old

D. wean as soon as possible to an appropriate weaning food

7. Which of the following statements about diarrheal disease programs in developing countries are true?
   A. Such programs have been most successful when pursued as selective initiatives.
   B. U.S. health programs are being modeled after the successes of diarrheal disease programs abroad.
   C. Oral rehydration therapy (ORT) solutions are standardized to include specific carbohydrates.
   D. Nurses are the appropriate personnel to provide education about diarrheal disease prevention and treatment.

8. The ranking for infant mortality according to race, from highest to lowest, is best described as
   A. black > white > Hispanic > Native American
   B. black > Hispanic > white > Native American
   C. black > Native American > white = Hispanic
   D. Native American > black > Hispanic > white
   E. Native American > black > white = Hispanic

9. Congenital anomalies are the second greatest categorized cause of death in which age groups?
   A. 0–1 year
   B. 1–4 years
   C. 5–14 years
   D. 15–24 years
   E. *A* and *B*
   F. None of the above

10. *Autonomy* is best described as
    A. based on rational decisions
    B. an absolute right
    C. a religious doctrine
    D. not applicable to children
    E. making decisions based on your values

11. *Competence* is best described as
    A. not being present in teens
    B. the ability to understand possible consequences of actions
    C. not being related to autonomy
    D. needed to be determined by a psychiatrist
    E. being culturally determined

12. *Beneficence* is best described as
    A. a good feeling
    B. being secondary to autonomy in competent patients
    C. being secondary to autonomy in neonates
    D. doing harm
    E. none of the above

13. *Distributive justice* is best defined as
    A. rationing according to insurance status
    B. euthanasia (active or passive) by court order
    C. inequality in access to care
    D. limiting access based on need
    E. treatment of all patients with the same disease with equally beneficial therapies

14. All of the following are statements of the Declaration of Alma Ata related to child health in developing countries EXCEPT
    A. health care is independent of social and economic forces
    B. health is a state of complete well-being
    C. Health is not the absence of disease
    D. People have a right to partake in their health care
    E. Diversion of resources such as from the military should be used to meet primary care goals

15. GOBI-FFF recognizes the importance of all of the following to improve global child health EXCEPT
    A. female education
    B. food
    C. growth monitoring
    D. family planning

E. oral rehydration

F. immunization

G. formula from commercial sources

H. breast-feeding

16. Pneumonia in children living in developing countries is characterized by all of the following EXCEPT
   A. unusual pathogens
   B. similar bacterial profile to the United States
   C. similar viral profile to the United States
   D. high rates of secondary infections
   E. vitamin A sufficiency

17. Parasite infestation in third-world countries is best characterized as
   A. responsive to vitamin A
   B. a common cause of diarrhea
   C. a common cause of nutritional deficiencies
   D. preventable by immunization
   E. responding to oral rehydration prevention

18. All are true about scheduled health supervision visits EXCEPT
   A. infants should be seen at 1 week of age
   B. between 1 and 4 years of age, there should be five visits
   C. adolescents (11 years or older) should be seen every other year
   D. middle childhood age children (5–10 years) should be seen at 5, 6, 8, and 10 years
   E. a prenatal visit is optimal

19. All are true about diaper dermatitis EXCEPT
   A. it is the most common skin disorder in infants
   B. its incidence peaks at 1–2 months
   C. it responds to frequent diaper changes
   D. barrier creams may be helpful
   E. hyperabsorbent diapers reduce the risk

20. Teething is associated with all of the following EXCEPT

A. drooling

B. gingival swelling

C. irritability

D. rash

E. relief with acetaminophen

21. The best approach to successful child sleeping includes all of the following EXCEPT
   A. permitting the child to settle
   B. transition objects
   C. a bottle of apple juice
   D. a consistent routine
   E. recognizing that arousal doesn't always produce awakening

22. In the United States, the average age for toilet training is
   A. 12 months
   B. 15 months
   C. 20 months
   D. 27 months
   E. 36 months

23. Time out for discipline is one recommended approach for young children. The recommended duration is
   A. as long as needed
   B. 1 minute per age in years
   C. 5 minutes per age in years
   D. depends on the punishment
   E. depends on the behavior

24. Developmental dimensions of value in understanding the assessment of a child's illness include all of the following EXCEPT
   A. decreased respiratory rate with increased age
   B. nonpulmonary influences on respirations (gastric filling)
   C. nearsightedness in newborns
   D. absence of fever in infected neonates
   E. inability to assess infants with the Glasgow coma score

25. The presence of the rooting reflex in a 2-year-old obtunded child indicates
   A. normal age-related reflex

B. hypoglycemia

C. hunger

D. time to wean

E. abnormal frontal cortex

26. Growth and development should be assessed at
    A. yearly intervals
    B. times of stress
    C. times of abnormalities
    D. each well child visit

E. entry to primary, middle, and high school

27. Warning the parents of a child who can now grasp and bring small objects to the mouth about the risk of foreign-body aspiration is
    A. part of CPR
    B. anticipatory guidance
    C. readiness for preschool
    D. part of Head Start training
    E. basic first aid

PART 2

Growth and Development

This part of the *Nelson Textbook* is a broad but specific guide through the multiple developmental stages and normal physical and mental progression of a maturing child. The physical, emotional, social, neurodevelopmental, language, and intellectual aspects of normal and abnormal behavior are highlighted for each stage of development: the fetus, newborn, first year, second year, preschool, early school, and adolescent periods. Even more importly, this part helps readers assess normal and abnormal patterns of growth and development. Understanding the range of human biologic variation is also emphasized.

The study of growth and development is distinctive for pediatricians. Understanding the progression of organ system maturity is critical for the care of patients and for communication with them. Questions in this part focus on learning these skills in the context of patients and factual information.

---

1. **Matching:** Erikson stages of development

   1. 0–1 year of age
   2. 2–3 years of age
   3. 3–6 years of age
   4. 6–12 years of age
   5. 12–20 years of age

   A. Industry vs. inferiority
   B. Identity vs. identity diffusion
   C. Basic trust
   D. Initiative vs. guilt
   E. Autonomy vs. shame and doubt

2. Behavioral states in the newborn period include

   A. quite and active sleep
   B. drowsy and alert
   C. fussy and crying
   D. all of the above
   E. none of the above

3. The best formula to approximate average weight (kg) for a 4-year-old is

   A. $\dfrac{\text{age (years)} \times 7 - 5}{2}$
   B. age [years] $\times$ 2 + 8
   C. $\dfrac{\text{age (months)} + 9}{2}$
   D. (age [years] $\times$ 5 + 17)
   E. (age [years] $\times$ 7 + 5)

4. A normal infant may cry for up to 3 hours a day during the development peak time of this behavior. The peak of crying is at about what age?

   A. 2 weeks
   B. 4 weeks
   C. 6 months
   D. 6 weeks
   E. 4 months

5. The best feeding protocol for a temperamentally irregular infant is

   A. a fixed schedule
   B. based on the parents' schedule
   C. every 1–2 hours
   D. on demand
   E. 60 minutes for each feeding

6. Object permanence is not present in a 2-month-old, whose response to dropping a ball is

   A. staring momentarily at the spot the ball was dropped from
   B. eyes descending as the ball descends
   C. crying when the ball hits the ground
   D. smiling at the game of hide-and-seek
   E. none of the above

7. The ability to manipulate small objects with the pincer grasp is usually noted at what age?

A. 0–2 months

B. 3–5 months

C. 6–7 months

D. 8–9 months

E. 10–12 months

8. A developmentally normal child, who is just able to sit without support, transfer objects from hand to hand, and speaks in a monosyllabic babble, is probably what age?

A. 3 months

B. 4 months

C. 9 months

D. 6 months

E. 11 months

9. Transitional objects are

A. training underwear

B. shoes without laces

C. cups with a special drinking spout

D. blankets and teddy bears

E. none of the above

10. Handedness is usually determined by what age?

A. 2–4 months

B. 6–12 months

C. 15–18 months

D. 20–24 months

E. 36–48 months

11. The best approach for parents to help a preschool child overcome monster fears is

A. to rationalize that monsters don't exist

B. to read books that do not have monsters in them

C. to have the pediatrician explain that monsters are make-believe

D. to use "great power" like monster spray to keep monsters away

E. none of the above

12. A mother brings her 6 1/2 month-old circumcised boy to you for a "sick" visit. You saw the child 2 weeks earlier for health maintenance, including a DTP immunization, and the child appeared well. The mother's complaint is that the baby is waking up every night and is fussy during the day, especially when she leaves him. The child's history is otherwise normal, and physical examination reveals no problems. Which one of the following is most appropriate?

A. Perform urinalysis and obtain a complete blood count to rule out urinary tract infection.

B. Request that the mother feed the infant more.

C. Reassure the mother that the behavior is normal and will pass in time.

D. Reassure the mother that the behavior will pass because it is a reaction to the DTP shot.

13. The biopsychosocial model of development, when applied to the child's height, includes all of the following EXCEPT

A. the child's genetic endowment

B. personal eating habits

C. access to food

D. parents' beliefs

E. differences between breast milk and formula

14. All of the following are true about a child's temperament EXCEPT

A. temperament is absolute and stable throughout one's life

B. biology influences temperament

C. it is a pattern of the child's responses

D. it is relatively resistant to parents' attempts of modification

E. it helps parents understand the child's behavior without guilt

15. A 3-year-old is described as "she ran before she walked" and "she is never hungry at the same time" and "she goes from toy to toy" is best described as

A. autistic

B. having a specific temperament

C. attention deficit hyperactivity disorder

D. developmental pervasive disorder

E. deaf

16. **Matching:** Freud vs. Erikson

Freud	*Erikson*
1. Oral	A. Initiative vs. guilt
2. Anal	B. Basic trust
3. Oedipal	C. Identity vs. identity diffusion
4. Latency	D. Autonomy vs. shame and doubt
5. Adolescence	E. Industry vs. inferiority

17. The visual activity of a newborn permits recognition of an object held at
    A. 1–2 inches
    B. 8–12 inches
    C. 15–24 inches
    D. 24–30 inches
    E. 30–36 inches

18. A just-born neonate spends about 40 minutes with the mother but then falls asleep and does not respond to the mother's voice. This lack of activity is
    A. suggestive of sepsis
    B. suggestive of sedation
    C. normal
    D. a seizure
    E. apnea

19. The six behaviors of the neonate include all of the following EXCEPT
    A. quiet sleep
    B. active sleep
    C. drowsy
    D. alert
    E. colic
    F. fussy
    G. crying

20. The best formula for approximating average weight for a 9-month-old in kilograms is
    A. $\dfrac{age\ (mo)\ +\ 9}{2}$
    B. age (mo) + 11
    C. age (yr) $\times$ 2 + 8
    D. age (yr) $\times$ 5 + 17
    E. age (yr) $\times$ 7 + 5

21. The best formula for approximating average height in centimeters for a 4-year-old is
    A. age (yr) $\times$ 2.5 + 30
    B. age (yr) $\times$ 6 + 77
    C. age (yr) $\times$ 7 + 5
    D. age (yr) $\times$ 5 + 7
    E. age (yr) $\times$ 2.5 − 6

22. All of the following is true about growth in the first month of life EXCEPT
    A. weight may decrease 10% in the first week
    B. weight should equal or exceed birthweight by 2 weeks
    C. once gaining weight, the infant should gain 30 g/day
    D. preterm infants take longer to regain birthweight
    E. the high fat content of colostrum enhances weight gain in the first week of life

23. Crying in the first 2 months of life is characterized by all of the following EXCEPT
    A. teething
    B. peaking at 6 weeks
    C. at peak time, crying is for a total of 3 hours day
    D. crying occurs in response to obvious stimuli
    E. crying occurs when no stimulus is obvious

24. A child who scribbles, walks alone, speaks one real word, and pretends to drink from a cup is how old?
    A. 8 months
    B. 13 months
    C. 16 months
    D. 20 months
    E. 24 months

25. A child who rolls back to front, has a thumb-finger grasp, inhibits to no, and bangs two cubes is how old?
    A. 7–8 months
    B. 10–12 months
    C. 12–15 months

D. 3–4 months

E. 15–18 months

26. Growth between 3 and 4 months of age is best characterized by
    A. accelerating to a rate of 45 g/day
    B. slowing to a rate of 10 g/day
    C. slowing to a rate of 20 g/day
    D. accelerating to a rate of 20 g/day
    E. no change compared with that between 0 and 2 months

27. Feeding between 6 and 12 months of age is best characterized by all of the following EXCEPT
    A. willingness to be fed by a stranger
    B. the appearance of autonomy
    C. finger foods
    D. turning away from the spoon
    E. holding a spoon

28. A child who skips, names four colors, and dresses and undresses is how old?
    A. 15 months
    B. 24 months
    C. 30 months
    D. 18 months
    E. 60 months

29. Early walking suggests
    A. preoccupation with objects
    B. advanced social development
    C. advanced language development
    D. high activity type
    E. spasticity

30. Between 2 and 5 years of age, language increases; as a rule, the number of words in a sentence is
    A. based on knowledge of numbers
    B. equal to the age of the child in years
    C. independent of the environment
    D. independent of the number of questions asked the child by adults
    E. based on the ABC's

31. All of the following are true about language development EXCEPT
    A. deaf children may create their own language
    B. the basics for language may be "hard wired" in the brain
    C. language has no role in behavior regulation
    D. delayed language may signify deafness
    E. delayed language may signify mental retardation

32. Growth during the years between 6 and 12 years is characterized by annual weight and height increments of
    A. 3.5 kg: 6 cm
    B. 6 kg: 3.5 cm
    C. 5 kg: 10 cm
    D. 10 kg: 5 cm
    E. 1.5 kg: 5 cm

33. Word-finding difficulties may result in all of the following EXCEPT
    A. difficulty in expressing feelings
    B. difficulty in verbal self-defense
    C. frustration
    D. success in English class
    E. physical acting out

34. **Matching:** Adolescents
    1. Dehydroepi-androsterone sulfate
    2. Female: first sign of puberty
    3. Female: mid-puberty
    4. Male: late puberty
    5. Male: early puberty

    A. Axillary hair
    B. Underarm odor
    C. Voice change
    D. Breast bud
    E. Testicular enlargement

PART 3

Psychologic Disorders

Mental health problems are common concerns of parents and result in multiple symptoms in childhood and adolescence. This part of the *Nelson Textbook* includes an extensive series of chapters that discuss the assessment and interviewing process in addition to psychosomatic illness; vegetative, habit, mood, and anxiety disorders; suicide; disruptive behavioral and attention deficit hyperactivity disorders; sexual behavior; psychoses; and treatment approaches to the many common mental health symptoms of children. This part of the book is a logical continuum from normal growth and development and helps the reader gain a better understanding of what is a normal or an abnormal or pathologic manifestation of an underlying disorder related to personality or mental health. Common issues such as enuresis, encopresis, sleep problems, and attention deficit hyperactivity disorder have definite biologic-organic substrates and are also included here.

The questions in this part do not prepare you for a psychiatry residency but do reinforce the important mental health principles that are discussed in greater detail in the *Nelson Textbook*. Because mental health issues directly or indirectly affect children so greatly, this part of the *Nelson Textbook* is critical to all pediatricians.

1. Neuroleptic antipsychotic agents produce all of the following unwanted side effects EXCEPT
   A. bradykinesia
   B. hyperthermia
   C. tardive dyskinesia
   D. inappropriate ADH
   E. sedation

2. A 4-year-old boy is noted to have stereotypic body movements, poor verbal and nonverbal communication, and absent empathy. At daycare, he has not made any friends. The most likely diagnosis is
   A. attention deficit hyperactivity disorder
   B. dysthymic syndrome
   C. deaf-mutism
   D. autism
   E. cerebral palsy

3. Matching:
   1. Belief that one is a member of the opposite gender
   2. Sense of self as either male or female
   3. Comfort with cultural expectations
   4. Cross-dressing

      A. Gender role
      B. Gender identity
      C. Transsexualism
      D. Transvestism

4. Head banging, hair twirling, rocking, thumb sucking, teeth grinding, and nail biting all are
   A. habit disorders that probably relieve tension
   B. easy to cure in children
   C. evidence of insecurity in the majority of children and poor parenting by their parents
   D. tics

5. Which of the following statements about Gilles de la Tourette syndrome is true?
   A. It is characterized by tics and coprolalia.
   B. It is characterized by tics and encopresis.
   C. It is treated with haloperidol and methylphenidate.
   D. It is a common disorder of childhood.
   E. It affects girls more often than boys.

6. Night terrors are associated with
   A. REM sleep
   B. overeating after 7:00 p.m.

C. the use of antipsychotic medication

D. inception in preschool years and sometimes somnambulism

E. anger within the family

7. Conduct disorder in childhood and adolescence is associated with all of the following EXCEPT

   A. antisocial behavior

   B. criminality in the father

   C. physical abuse

   D. marital discord within the home

   E. mental retardation

8. Completed suicides in childhood and adolescence can be associated with all of the following EXCEPT

   A. previous suicide attempts

   B. alcohol or drug abuse

   C. a history of depression and suicide within the family

   D. easy access to firearms

   E. perfectionism within the classroom

9. A child in the third grade has problems with spelling and reading. She appears very quiet and confused in class. Her teacher has noticed that this girl has trouble following directions. Her mind seems to wander whenever the teacher tells a story or explains something complicated. She is skilled in art and so far has performed well in arithmetic. Which of the following diagnostic procedures is most likely to yield useful findings in this child?

   A. An attention deficit questionnaire

   B. An intelligence test

   C. A language evaluation

   D. A psychiatric assessment to rule out depression

   E. A neurologic examination

10. An 11-year-old child has excellent ideas in a class discussion, but what she records on paper is primitive and unsophisticated. She can spell well in isolation and understands rules of punctuation and capitalization, but in her own writing she makes multiple errors and mistakes in punctuation and capitalization. Her

handwriting is legible, but writing is painfully slow. This girl most likely is having problems with

   A. expressive language

   B. graphomotor production

   C. ideation

   D. attention

   E. simultaneous retrieval memory

11. Somatoform disorders, as part of psychosomatic illness, include all of the following EXCEPT

   A. conversion reaction

   B. asthma

   C. hypochondriasis

   D. pain disorders

   E. none of the above

12. Munchausen by proxy syndrome is characterized by all of the following EXCEPT

   A. recurrent illness that cannot be explained

   B. experienced pediatricians' stating that they have never seen such a case

   C. symptoms that disappear with the parent present

   D. an attentive parent caregiver who never goes home

   E. an unworried parent caregiver

   F. poor response to therapy

   G. doctor shopping

13. **Matching:**

   1. Chronic stealing
   2. Continuous arguing
   3. Fire setting
   4. Obscene language
   5. Rape
   6. Property destruction
   7. Poor school performance
   8. Sibling rivalry as the cause

   A. Conduct disorder
   B. Oppositional defiant disorder
   C. Neither
   D. Both

14. When a 7-year-old child fails to cooperate with care in the hospital, one should suspect
    A. immaturity
    B. embarrassment
    C. negativism
    D. fearfulness
    E. oppositionism

15. If a parent does not appear readily reassured by the diagnosis or treatment plan, one should suspect
    A. hidden anxiety
    B. mistrust
    C. negativism
    D. oppositionism
    E. aggression

16. Noncompliance may be due to
    A. misunderstanding
    B. language barriers
    C. reservation of diagnosis
    D. unanswered questions about the ramifications of not treating
    E. contrary advice (grandparent, Internet)
    F. all of the above

17. **Matching:** Test of cognition
    1. Bayley scales
    2. Stanford-Binet
    3. Wechsler Adult Intelligence Scale
    4. Wechsler Intelligence Scale for Children
    5. Kaufman assessment battery for children

    A. 16 yr–adult
    B. 0–42 months
    C. 2 yr–adult
    D. 2.5–12.5 years
    E. 6–16 years

18. **Matching:** Testing
    1. Auditory perception

    A. Boston naming test

    2. Language
    3. Verbal memory
    4. Abstract reasoning
    5. Nonverbal memory
    6. Motor proficiency

    B. Seashore rhythms test
    C. Wisconsin card sorting test
    D. Rey complex figure test
    E. Purdue peg board test
    F. California verbal learning test

19. Psychosocial problems may manifest as disturbances in
    A. feelings
    B. body function
    C. behavior
    D. performance
    E. all of the above

20. Psychiatric disorders are more common than in the general population of children in all of the following EXCEPT
    A. smart students
    B. head trauma
    C. mental retardation
    D. epilepsy
    E. prematurity
    F. encephalitis

21. Conversion reactions are best characterized by
    A. sudden onset
    B. traceable to a precipitating event
    C. involvement of special senses
    D. pseudoseizures
    E. end abruptly
    F. all of the above

22. *Enuresis* is defined as
    A. wetting 2 times per week for 3 consecutive months
    B. wetting 2 times per week for any 3 months in a year
    C. not being dry at 3 years of age
    D. not being dry at 4 years of age
    E. wetting at 5 years of age on two occasions

23. *Nocturnal enuresis* is described by all of the following EXCEPT

A. being primary or secondary
B. having a strong genetic component
C. occurring at all stages of sleep
D. when primary, being associated with emotional disorders
E. being more common in males

24. Treatment of enuresis should include all of the following EXCEPT
   A. enlisting the cooperation of the child
   B. having the child void before retiring
   C. using alarms
   D. having the child launder the soiled sheets
   E. waking the child repeatedly

25. A 5-year-old is noted by the parents to snore at night. The child has also had problems staying awake in preschool and has had behavioral problems. The father also snores. Physical examination of the child reveals large, pink, nonexudative tonsils. The most appropriate next step is
   A. laryngoscopy
   B. polysomnography
   C. ambulatory apnea monitor
   D. telemetry
   E. arterial blood gas

26. The most likely diagnosis of the patient in Question 25 is
   A. tonsillitis
   B. peritonsillar abscess
   C. obstructive sleep apnea syndrome
   D. Tangier disease
   E. narcolepsy

27. The appropriate therapy of severe obstructive sleep apnea syndrome is
   A. adenotonsillectomy
   B. tracheostomy
   C. parapharyngeal muscle surgery
   D. theophylline
   E. bilevel positive airway pressure

28. Risk factors for obstructive sleep apnea syndrome include all of the following EXCEPT
   A. retroposition of the mandible

B. small triangular chin
C. long oval face
D. long or soft palate
E. all of the above

29. All of the following are considered a habit disorder EXCEPT
   A. tics
   B. bruxism
   C. trichotillomania
   D. stuttering
   E. thumb sucking

30. Tics are characterized by all of the following EXCEPT
   A. difficulty in controlling behavior
   B. a brief transient amnesia after the tic
   C. disappears in sleep
   D. may follow encephalitis
   E. EEG is normal

31. All are true about Gilles de la Tourette syndrome EXCEPT
   A. drugs that increase dopaminergic action worsen it
   B. some patients have pediatric autoimmune neuropsychiatric disorder
   C. some patients have oppositional defiant disorder
   D. Lyme disease may sometimes mimic Tourette syndrome
   E. management with haloperidol or pimozide is often unsuccessful

32. A third-grade student refuses to go back to school after the winter break. She now needs her mother to go to sleep with her and complains of headache, bellyache, and muscle pain. The physical exam is totally normal, but you notice the child is very clingy to the mother. The most likely diagnosis is
   A. stranger anxiety
   B. school anxiety
   C. stranger reaction
   D. separation anxiety disorder
   E. narcolepsy

33. Obsessive compulsive disorder may be associated with all of the following EXCEPT
   A. overconcern with body wastes

B. prior group A streptococcal infection

C. excessive fears

D. a need for sameness

E. increased metabolic activity in the corpus callosum

F. excessive checking of locks

34. Major depression is characterized by
    A. weight loss
    B. weight gain
    C. insomnia
    D. hypersomnia
    E. dysphoria
    F. all of the above

35. Major depression in children may be characterized by
    A. a strong genetic component
    B. never beginning before adolescence
    C. absence of hallucinations
    D. no risk of depression in adulthood
    E. none of the above

36. The treatment of choice for childhood onset of major depression is
    A. monoamine oxidase inhibitors
    B. tricyclic antidepressants
    C. serotonin reuptake inhibitors
    D. benzodiazepines
    E. none of the above

37. All of the following are true about suicide EXCEPT
    A. 15–40% of completed suicides are preceded by attempts
    B. there are 5–45 attempts for each suicide
    C. access to guns increases the risk
    D. alcohol use is unrelated to suicide
    E. depression is related to suicide

38. Important things to consider after an attempted suicide include all of the following EXCEPT
    A. is the patient less depressed?
    B. is the patient physiologically stable?
    C. does the patient still want to die?
    D. are precipitating events still active?

E. does the patient have a future view or orientation?

F. have the shame and guilt been moderated?

G. all of the above

39. A 2-year-old doesn't get his way in a crowded toy store. He starts to cry and hit and roll on the floor. The parent should do all of the following EXCEPT
    A. yell and punish him
    B. acknowledge the child's frustration
    C. quietly explain that his response is not acceptable
    D. give him time and space to recover
    E. nonemotionally place him on a time out

40. A 4-year-old is seen hitting his sister. When asked what he has done, he lies. This is most likely
    A. pathologic and needs punishment
    B. displacement
    C. reaction formation
    D. avoidance of an unpleasant punishment
    E. none of the above

41. All of the following are true about minor stealing EXCEPT
    A. all (almost) children steal at least once
    B. it must be overemphasized to avoid a second episode
    C. they should return the stolen item
    D. it may be learned from parents
    E. it may be impulsive

42. A 26-month-old male has a history of poor speech development, tantrum-like rages, and rocking repetitive ritualistic behavior. He attends day care but spends most of his time in solitary play. The most likely diagnosis is
    A. encephalitis
    B. latent slow virus infection
    C. Rasmussen disease
    D. autism
    E. Prader-Willi syndrome

43. Additional features of the disease of the patient in Question 42 include all of the following EXCEPT
    A. empathy
    B. preoccupation with body parts
    C. prevalence of 3–4/1000
    D. association with fragile X
    E. visual scanning of the fingers

44. **Matching:**
    1. Asperger disorder
    2. Heller dementia
    3. Rett disorder
    4. Schizophrenia

    A. Childhood disintegrative disorder
    B. X-linked dominant
    C. Delusions
    D. Obsessional idiosyncratic interests

45. **Matching:** Psychopharmacology
    1. Clozapine
    2. Dextroam-phetamine
    3. Pemoline
    4. Fluoxetine

    A. Narcolepsy
    B. Metabolized by cytochrome P-450 system
    C. Aggression

    5. Guanfacine

    D. Seizures
    E. Hepatitis

46. All of the following are true about attention deficit hyperactivity disorder EXCEPT
    A. males exceed affected females
    B. tic disorders may coexist with ADHD
    C. patients dislike or avoid sustained mental efforts
    D. oppositional defiant disorders never coexist with ADHD
    E. substance abuse occurs in adolescents

47. Possible complications of stimulant drug therapy of attention deficit hyperactivity disorder include all of the following EXCEPT
    A. jitteriness
    B. difficulty sleeping
    C. abdominal pain
    D. tics
    E. increased appetite

PART 4

Social Issues

In an ever-changing socioeconomic climate, social issues have direct or indirect effects on the mental and physical health of children. Societal and personal issues such as adoption, foster care, a mobile family, childcare, separation from and death of loved ones, violence, and neglect and abuse of children all create problems for the children we care for and thus require physicians to be aware of the adverse circumstances associated with these issues. In addition, it is important for physicians to help children and families to adjust and to cope with these issues. It is the physician's obligation to accurately prevent, detect, treat, and counsel families involved with social problems.

Questions related to this part of the *Nelson Textbook* help build on the basic principles discussed in the individual chapters on each topic. This reinforcement is essential as more and more of our children encounter challenging social issues each day.

---

1. A 6-month-old boy is brought to the emergency room and is afebrile but responds poorly to tactile and auditory stimuli. He becomes apneic and unresponsive after a generalized seizure. The parents state that he was perfectly well in the car on the way to the hospital and that they only brought him to the emergency room because of constipation. He requires 10 minutes of cardiopulmonary resuscitation, after which he is noticed to have a bulging fontanel and bilateral retinal hemorrhages. A chest x-ray reveals two posterior rib fractures. The most likely diagnosis is
   A. CPR-induced retinal hemorrhages and rib fractures
   B. hemorrhagic shock and encephalopathy
   C. hemophilia
   D. status epilepticus
   E. child abuse—shaken baby syndrome

2. **Matching:** Differential diagnosis of child abuse
   1. Multiple fractures
   2. Ecchymosis
   3. Perineal burns
   4. Bruises (old)
   5. Cigarette burn

   A. *Candida* diaper rash
   B. Osteogenesis imperfecta
   C. Thrombocytopenia
   D. Impetigo
   E. Mongolian spots

3. A young child's response to the death of a parent often is characterized by
   A. depression and weight loss
   B. denial and magical wishing
   C. anger and crying
   D. wishes of death for himself or herself
   E. none of the above

4. The effect that statements such as "stop it or you'll give me a headache" have on young children is to
   A. teach a child to behave
   B. give children a pattern of headaches
   C. create guilt and unrealistic fault
   D. provide parents with a way to cope
   E. prepare children for separation

5. All of the following are true about adoption EXCEPT
   A. 42% are step-parent or relative adoptions
   B. most adopted children are from foreign countries
   C. 1 million children are adopted in the United States each year
   D. 15% are adopted through foster care
   E. 2–4% of American families have adopted children

6. All of the following are true about foster care EXCEPT
   A. chronic medical illness is present in 35% of children

B. 60% of preschool children have developmental delay

C. 42% are white children

D. the majority of foster children receive EPSDT services

E. children frequently stay at more than one foster care home

7. High-quality childcare can influence all of the following EXCEPT
   A. child cognition
   B. future academic achievement
   C. social development
   D. sibling rivalry
   E. scores on standardized tests

8. A 3-year-old missing from his mother's house approximately 1 month after a divorce. The most likely explanation is
   A. sleep walking
   B. drug reaction
   C. running away from his mother
   D. looking for his father
   E. anxiety reaction

9. After divorce, children may demonstrate all of the following EXCEPT
   A. being overburdened by maintaining two homes
   B. withdrawal
   C. indifference at times of reunions
   D. academic deterioration
   E. expectations that the parents will never get back together

10. All of the following are age-related behavioral responses to experiencing violence EXCEPT
    A. *infants*—poor sleep
    B. *adolescents*—short-fuse responses
    C. *toddlers*—excessive appetite
    D. *toddlers*—clingy
    E. *school age*—post-traumatic stress syndrome

11. Munchausen syndrome by proxy is characterized by all of the following EXCEPT
    A. 10% mortality
    B. multiple hospitalizations

C. induced manifestations by caregiver

D. parents who readily admit their abuse

E. use of medications or toxins

12. Which of the following is associated with an increased risk of child abuse?
    A. Poverty
    B. Military base residence
    C. Spouse abuse
    D. Unplanned pregnancy
    E. All of the above

13. A 2-month-old is admitted with a fracture of the right femur. The mother states that the baby fell off a low couch onto a plush carpeted floor and did not cry. Thereafter, the baby appeared fine. Three days later, the grandmother noted that the baby cried when she changed the diaper and that the leg was swollen. In the emergency room, there was also a bruise noted over the sternum that was also said to have occurred during the fall 3 days ago. The mother states that she bleeds easily, but the father of the baby is well. An x-ray reveals a spiral fracture of the femur. Features of this case suggestive of abuse include all of the following EXCEPT
    A. multiple sites of injury
    B. implausible explanation for injury
    C. grandmother's deep concern
    D. injury incompatible with the nature of the fall
    E. delayed seeking of medical attention

14. Cardiopulmonary resuscitation in a child with head trauma from child abuse commonly results in all of the following EXCEPT
    A. recovery of a pulse
    B. retinal hemorrhages and broken ribs
    C. recovery of respirations
    D. normal sinus rhythm
    E. recovery from cyanosis

15. Sexual abuse includes all of the following EXCEPT
    A. exposure of sexual anatomy
    B. touching of genitals by two preadolescents

C. showing pornography to a child

D. using a child to create pornography

E. incest

16. Pedophiles are best described as
    A. being female
    B. never having repeated experiences
    C. seeking positions to be in contact with children
    D. preferring females
    E. being highly violent

17. A 4-year-old is admitted to the hospital for her third evaluation of vaginal bleeding. The mother noted bright-red blood on the child's underwear. Previous examinations revealed a normal Tanner stage 1, 4-year-old female with normal external genitalia. Pelvic ultrasound results were normal, as was the serum estradiol. The hemoglobin and platelet counts were normal, as was the bleeding time and coagulation studies. The pelvic examination results under anesthesia also were normal. The next step in the examination is to
    A. determine the blood type of the blood on the underwear
    B. interrogate the father
    C. isolate the parents and child
    D. determine von Willebrand factor levels
    E. measure fibronectin in the vagina

18. The most likely diagnosis for the child in Question 17 is
    A. precious puberty
    B. sexual abuse
    C. vaginitis
    D. coagulopathy
    E. Munchausen syndrome by proxy

PART 5

Children with Special Health Needs

It is stated that at least 10% of all children may have a chronic illness. Furthermore, a small percentage of children use the majority of our health care resources. In addition, although chronic illness or disability may interfere with some function, it is important to recognize the positive aspects of the child and to focus on strengths and ways to maximize these strengths as well as to reduce dysfunction or disability. Many curriculums have weaknesses in this area of pediatrics; this is an unfortunate circumstance for trainees and their future patients. A new chapter on the rapidly growing field of pediatric palliative care has been added to help the pediatrician relieve pain and suffering in children with acute and chronic illnesses or those at the end of their lives.

1. A mentally retarded child with microphthalmia, microcephaly, chorioretinitis, and a history of a neonatal petechial rash most likely has
   A. chromosomal syndrome
   B. TORCH infection
   C. fetal alcohol syndrome
   D. galactosemia
   E. hyperammonemia

2. Frequent problems of children with common chronic illnesses include all of the following EXCEPT
   A. unpredictability
   B. pain
   C. expense
   D. multiple providers
   E. failure to graduate high school
   F. isolation
   G. psychologic or behavioral problems

3. An infant with multiple grotesque congenital anomalies dies on the third day of life. Her mother has not had an opportunity to see her before death owing to postpartum complications. When informed of the baby's death, she says she wants to see her. She cannot be moved from where she is receiving intensive care. The best response to her request is to
   A. tell her that she is too sick to see the baby
   B. tell her that she will be able to see the baby later
   C. take the baby to her bedside
   D. tell her she won't want to see the baby
   E. tell her that it is too late for her to see the baby

4. The parents of a 10-year-old girl with mental retardation are seeking information on what to expect for her future. The youngster is in a mainstreamed educational program, is just beginning to master simple reading skills, and has one close friend. Recognizing the difficulty of long-term prognostication, which of the following is a possible life goal for this child?
   A. holding a regular job
   B. getting married
   C. having children
   D. all of the above

5. A preschooler with Down syndrome is seen for a routine health supervision visit. A knowledgeable clinician will pay

particular attention to screening for problems that are known to occur with increased frequency in children with this condition. Which of the following conditions would be LEAST likely to be found?

A. atlantoaxial instability

B. neurogenic bladder

C. hypothyroidism

D. conductive hearing loss

6. A 3-year-old boy with a limited vocabulary is referred for formal psychometric testing and is found to have an IQ of 60. Physical examination is essentially unremarkable except for mild hypotonia. Appropriate initial laboratory studies would include all of the following EXCEPT

A. karyotype, including test for fragile X

B. audiologic evaluation

C. cranial CT scans

D. formal speech and language evaluation

7. The general approach to psychosocial failure to thrive includes all of the following EXCEPT

A. keeping meal time brief

B. offering solid foods before liquids

C. forcing the child to eat

D. minimizing environmental distractions

E. minimizing the intake of water and juice

8. The most appropriate way to assess growth in premature infants to diagnose failure to thrive includes (may pick more than one)

A. use corrected age (subtract weeks premature) until the patient reaches 1–2 years of age

B. determine whether two major growth percentiles are crossed

C. add additional weight as if the child were born at term

D. determine the weight: length ratio

E. don't use head circumference until 24 months

9. Major causes of failure to thrive include all of the following EXCEPT

A. formula feeding

B. failure to provide sufficient calories

C. failure to ingest sufficient calories

D. failure to retain sufficient calories

E. malabsorption

10. The leading cause of failure to thrive between 0 and 3 months is

A. TORCH infection

B. psychosocial

C. gastrointestinal reflux

D. cystic fibrosis

E. inborn errors of metabolism

11. Snoring and mouth breathing as a cause of failure to thrive suggests

A. streptococcal pharyngitis

B. mononucleosis

C. obstructive sleep apnea

D. anterior meningocele

E. cerebral palsy

12. An 8-month-old presents with failure to thrive. The past medical history includes severe thrush and *Candida* diaper rash and recurrent otitis media with perforation. On physical examinations the patient has generalized lymphadenopathy and hepatosplenomegaly; there is also bilateral parotitis. The most likely diagnosis is

A. mononucleosis

B. familial histiocytosis

C. X-linked combined immunodeficiency

D. AIDS

E. psychosocial failure to thrive

13. All of the following are true about children with chronic illness EXCEPT

A. children with disabilities rarely survive to adulthood

B. 6–7% of children has some limitation of activity

C. 1–2% of children meet the definition of severe disability

D. of disabled children, 40% have learning and developmental disorders

E. of disabled children, 35% have chronic physical conditions

14. Principles of care for children with chronic diseases include all of the following EXCEPT
    A. early detection
    B. amelioration of functional consequences
    C. calling children with asthma "asthmatics"
    D. prevention of secondary psychosocial handicaps
    E. treatment in the context of the family

15. The Individuals with Disabilities Education Act includes all of the following EXCEPT
    A. support of state programs of early intervention
    B. providing cash assistance for children with disabilities
    C. education in the least restrictive manner
    D. support of the state programs of special education

16. **Matching:**

Disease	Rate per 1,000
1. Asthma	A. 10
2. Congenital heart disease	B. 3
3. Seizure disorder	C. 0.2
4. Diabetes mellitus	D. 15
5. Cystic fibrosis	E. 1.4
6. Hemophilia	F. 0.06
7. Muscular dystrophy	G. 0.15

17. A sixth-grade child with chronic arthritis views the cause of chronic illness typically as due to
    A. germ theory
    B. punishment for bad behavior
    C. physiologic mechanisms
    D. not following rules
    E. not taking medicines

18. Mental retardation is best classified by
    A. mild, moderate, severe, profound

B. imbecile, retarded, functional
C. IQ percentiles
D. support needs (intermittent, limited, extensive, pervasive)
E. none of the above

19. Common identifiable causes of mental retardation include all of the following EXCEPT
    A. trisomy 21
    B. hypothyroidism
    C. fetal alcohol syndrome
    D. fragile X syndrome
    E. cystic fibrosis

20. All are true about mental retardation EXCEPT
    A. 3% of the population have an IQ less than 2 standard deviations below the mean
    B. severe retardation is inversely related to socioeconomic status
    C. 5% of children with mental retardation are profoundly affected
    D. the reported incidence increases at entry to school
    E. language development is a first clue to mild retardation

21. The 10 adaptive skill areas to assess children with mental retardation include all of the following EXCEPT
    A. communication
    B. sports
    C. self-care
    D. home living
    E. social skills
    F. community use
    G. self-direction
    H. health and safety
    I. functional academics
    J. leisure
    K. work

22. All males with mental retardation without an obvious etiology should next be tested with
    A. plasma ammonia
    B. blood lead

C. EEG

D. chromosomes

E. cranial CT

23. A 3-year-old presents with microcephaly and mental retardation. Her mother had a flu-like illness during the second month of pregnancy. At birth, the baby had petechia and hepatosplenomegaly, which have resolved. The most likely diagnosis is

A. congenital HIV

B. congenital rubella

C. congenital parvovirus

D. isoimmune neonatal thrombocytopenia

E. subacute sclerosing panencephalitis

24. **Matching:** Palliative care groupings

1. Cure possible but uncertain
2. Chronic course with intermittent exacerbations, death likely
3. Palliative care needed from time of diagnosis
4. Unpredictable course, nonprogressive CNS injury, death likely

A. Cystic fibrosis

B. Inborn errors of metabolism

C. Cancer

D. Cerebral palsy

25. A 4-year-old's concept of death may include all of the following EXCEPT

A. it may be reversible

B. it is like sleep

C. dead people still eat and breathe

D. they understand causality

E. it is a functional state

26. The fear of dying in young children is best described as fear of

A. the afterlife

B. the unknown

C. separation

D. transcendentalism

E. existentialism

27. Perpetuating the myth of "everything is going to be all right" with a dying child will

A. help reassure the child

B. hide "bad things" from the child

C. enhance an awareness of eventual death

D. alleviate fears

E. prevent exploration of fears

28. Giving an estimate of how long a child with a serious condition will survive will

A. be inaccurate

B. help accept the diagnosis

C. avoid unnecessary expenses

D. provide time to remove the child from school

E. enhance communication between siblings and the child

PART 6

Nutrition

Nutrition, once a major component of medical education, unfortunately is often an undertaught topic. Students and residents may not be able to identify a specific "nutrition department" or curriculum in their formal education and often have difficulty in recognizing nutritional disorders. Nutrition is an essential topic, not just because of the occasional patient (in the United States) with an identifiable nutritional deficiency (much more common in developing countries) but because of the great influence that appropriate nutrition has on supporting normal growth and development. In addition, parents are increasingly aware of nutritional issues and constantly bring nutrition questions to the pediatrician. Nutritional support of children with chronic diseases (diabetes, cancer, inflammatory bowel disease) is an important component in the care of these children.

Questions in this part address normal and abnormal states of water, energy, nutrient, and vitamin intake. Normal feeding practices are addressed as well.

---

1. The breast-fed infant of a strict vegan may experience which vitamin deficiency if the mother is not receiving supplements of this vitamin?
   A. K
   B. B_6
   C. B_{12}
   D. Folate
   E. Biotin

2. **Matching:** Vitamin deficiencies
   1. Xerosis conjunctivae
   2. Tender nerves
   3. Photosensitivity
   4. Seizures
   5. Bitot spots
   6. Diarrhea
   7. Cheilosis
   8. Alopecia
   9. Subperiosteal hemorrhage
   10. Craniotabes
   11. Cerebellar ataxia

   A. B_1 (thiamine)
   B. Riboflavin
   C. A
   D. Niacin
   E. B_6
   F. Biotin
   G. C (ascorbic acid)
   H. D
   I. E

3. **Matching:** Mineral deficiencies
   1. Zinc
   2. Selenium

   A. Rickets
   B. Dwarfism

   3. Phosphorus
   4. Iron
   5. Iodine
   6. Calcium
   7. Fluoride
   8. Manganese
   9. Chloride

   C. Microcytic anemia
   D. Cardiomyopathy
   E. Caries
   F. Goiter
   G. Metabolic alkalosis
   H. None known

4. **Matching:** Vitamin excess
   1. D
   2. C
   3. B_6
   4. A
   5. B_{12}

   A. Neuropathy
   B. Hypercalcemia
   C. Pseudotumor cerebri
   D. Oxaluria
   E. Unknown

5. **Matching**
   1. Contains approximately 20 calories per ounce
   2. Gastrointestinal allergy less common
   3. Free of bacterial contamination
   4. Contains secretory IgA antibodies

   A. Breast milk only
   B. Formula only
   C. Both breast milk and formula
   D. Neither breast milk or formula

5. Associated with increased mortality rates in underdeveloped countries

6. Associated with decreased incidence of colic and eczema

7. Associated with prolonged unconjugated hyperbilirubinemia

8. Higher carbohydrate concentration but lower protein concentration

6. The best source of iron for 1-month-old infants is
   A. iron-fortified cereals
   B. yellow vegetables
   C. fruits
   D. breast milk
   E. 2% low-fat cow's milk

7. A 4-month-old with vitamin D–deficient rickets would be expected to show all of the following EXCEPT
   A. craniotabes
   B. bowlegs
   C. rosary
   D. low serum phosphate levels
   E. high alkaline phosphatase levels

8. The estimated average requirement (EAR) of a nutrient is best defined as
   A. a dietary reference index
   B. the recommended dietary allowance
   C. being age and gender specific to meet the needs of 50% of persons
   D. encompassing the range of the lower and upper limits of a nutrient
   E. a daily average performed once each year

9. The AI (adequate intake) in infants is estimated from

A. bomb calorimetry
B. the EAR
C. the RDA
D. the intake of nutrients from human milk
E. intakes that will prevent deferrable nutrient deficiencies

10. **Matching:** Mineral deficiencies
    1. Fluorine   A. Goiter
    2. Iodine   B. Rickets
    3. Phosphorus   C. Caries
    4. Zinc   D. Cardiomyopathy
    5. Selenium   E. Dwarfism
    6. Copper   F. Anemia

11. **Matching:** Mineral excess
    1. Calcium   A. Cardiomyopathy
    2. Cobalt   B. Hemolysis
    3. Selenium   C. Alopecia
    4. Zinc   D. Hemosiderosis
    5. Copper   E. Renal stones
    6. Iron   F. Copper deficiency

12. All of the following are advantages of breast-feeding EXCEPT
    A. reduced incidence of allergy
    B. reduced incidence of otitis media
    C. reduced incidence of colic
    D. increased psychologic comfort
    E. vitamin K content
    F. utility for preterm infants > 2000 g

13. Problems associated with breast-feeding include all of the following EXCEPT
    A. less than optimal nutrients for infants < 1000 g
    B. vitamin K content
    C. transmission of live viruses
    D. hyperbilirubinemia
    E. contraindicated in erythroblastosis fetalis

14. Atypical features about infant colic include all of the following EXCEPT
    A. fever
    B. onset in the first week of life
    C. onset at age 6 months

D. sudden onset

E. crying mainly in the early morning

15. True observations about infant feeding include all of the following EXCEPT
    A. self-feeding with a spoon at age 12 months should be encouraged
    B. infants will select a balanced diet
    C. consistent rejection of one food group should suggest food allergy
    D. infants should be put to bed with a bottle of milk
    E. one should respect the likes and dislikes of infant tastes

16. All of the following are true about the clinical manifestations of kwashiorkor EXCEPT
    A. the presence of edema
    B. rash in sun-exposed areas
    C. hypochromotrichia
    D. weak muscles
    E. an increased susceptibility to infection

17. All of the following are true about the laboratory manifestations of kwashiorkor EXCEPT
    A. persistent ketonuria
    B. hypoalbuminemia
    C. hypoglycemia
    D. potassium deficiency
    E. low serum amylase levels

18. All of the following are true about obesity in children EXCEPT
    A. obese children eat more junk food
    B. single gene disorders are rare causes of obesity
    C. obesity may be associated with insulin resistance

D. the highest prevalence of obesity in the United States is in the Northeast

E. Menarche may be earlier in obese girls

19. Complications of obesity in childhood include all of the following EXCEPT
    A. angina
    B. Blount disease
    C. slipped capital femoral epiphysis
    D. sleep apnea
    E. glucose intolerance

20. **Matching:** Vitamin dependency states
    1. Vitamin A
    2. Riboflavin
    3. Vitamin B$_{12}$
    4. Vitamin C
    5. Niacin

    A. Methylmalonic acidemia
    B. Hyperkeratosis follicularis
    C. Chédiak-Higashi
    D. Hartnup disease
    E. Pyruvate kinase deficiency

21. Physical features of vitamin D–deficient rickets include all of the following EXCEPT
    A. Bitot spots
    B. craniotabes
    C. enlargement of the costochondral junctions
    D. thickening of the ankles and wrists
    E. large anterior fontanel
    F. bowed legs

22. Clinical features of vitamin E deficiency include all of the following EXCEPT
    A. cerebellar ataxia
    B. muscle weakness
    C. peripheral neuropathy
    D. hemolysis
    E. hepatosplenomegaly

PART 7

Pathophysiology of Body Fluids and Fluid Therapy

A "Peanuts" cartoon once depicted a dehydrated Charlie Brown being graciously treated by Sally with a statement that all he needed was a little salt and water. If only this were as easy in all of our nonfictional patients. Normal and abnormal states of water, minerals, and acid-base balance often perplex the most intelligent pediatrician. Formulas for calculating replacement, maintenance, ongoing losses, and insensible losses have baffled the most astute nephrologist who hopes that the kidneys are smarter than we are. This part covers the various states of fluid, electrolyte, and acid-base disturbances. In addition, specific diseases are addressed in more detail.

Questions in this part help readers better understand the issues of acid-base abnormalities, dehydration, and electrolyte disturbances. As is always needed in this topic, the questions reinforce the basic principles of pathophysiology, diagnosis, and therapy.

1. Diabetes insipidus may be due to all of the following EXCEPT
   A. pituitary adenoma
   B. renal epithelial ADH reception defect
   C. hypokalemia
   D. hypercalcemia
   E. adrenal deficiency

2. A 1-month-old boy presents with severe failure to thrive, emesis, and a temperature of 41°C. Serum electrolyte measurements reveal a sodium level of 185 mEq/L, and the urine specific gravity is 1001. The most likely diagnosis is
   A. adrenal insufficiency
   B. salt poisoning
   C. hypernatremic dehydration
   D. malignant hyperthermia
   E. nephrogenic diabetes insipidus

3. A well-grown 6-month-old presents with a tonic-clonic seizure lasting 30 minutes. The child is found to be hypothermic and remains lethargic. The diet history reveals that the mother is a participant in the WIC program but, because it is the end of the month, she has begun to dilute the remaining formula with water because there is not enough to last until she receives her next allotment of formula next week. The most likely diagnosis is
   A. hypocalcemia
   B. hyponatremia
   C. hypoglycemia
   D. hypernatremia
   E. hypokalemia

4. Hyperkalemia may be associated with all of the following EXCEPT
   A. succinylcholine use
   B. burns
   C. trauma
   D. chemotherapy
   E. metabolic alkalosis
   F. digitalis toxicity
   G. uremia

5. A normal anion gap acidosis is most likely due to
   A. diabetes mellitus
   B. renal tubular acidosis
   C. nephrotic syndrome
   D. uremia
   E. shock

6. A 10-month-old patient with vomiting and diarrhea, tachycardia, normal blood pressure, dry mucous membranes, a

capillary refill time of 2 seconds, deep respirations, and irritability is what percent dehydrated?

A. 0–3%

B. 3–5%

C. 6–9%

D. 10–12%

E. 12–15%

7. A serious complication of the treatment of hypernatremic dehydration is

A. cerebral thrombosis

B. cerebral edema

C. hyperchloremia

D. hypoglycemia

E. none of the above

8. The best method to reduce the potassium level during hyperkalemia, by reducing the body burden of potassium, is

A. sodium bicarbonate infusion

B. glucose and insulin infusion

C. calcium infusion

D. albuterol aerosol

E. Kayexalate enema

9. The finding of marked metabolic alkalosis with acidic urine indicates

A. marked sodium depletion

B. marked potassium depletion

C. hyperventilation

D. diabetes mellitus

E. laboratory error

10. Insensible water loss includes which of the following (may choose more than one)?

A. Sweat

B. Fecal loss

C. Evaporative loss from skin

D. Respiratory water loss

E. Obligate water for urinary solute excretion

11. Which drug or agent may inhibit antidiuretic hormone release?

A. Demerol

B. Barbiturates

C. Alcohol

D. Nicotine

E. α-Adrenergic drugs

12. Hypernatremia may be induced by all of the following EXCEPT

A. hyperglycemia

B. adipsia

C. insufficient breast-feeding

D. gastroenteritis

E. nephrogenic diabetes insipidus

13. The most common cause of nutritional hyponatremia is

A. salt substitutes

B. low-salt diets

C. the WIC syndrome

D. Lasix therapy

E. vegan diets

14. **Matching**: Hyponatremia etiologies

1. Renal loss
2. Extrarenal loss
3. Nutrition
4. Water excess and gain
5. Excess of sodium and water

A. Burns
B. Nephrosis
C. Osmotic load
D. WIC syndrome
E. Syndrome of inappropriate ADH

15. Manifestations of hyperkalemia include all of the following EXCEPT

A. paresthesias

B. weakness

C. paralysis

D. wide QRS complex

E. tetany

16. Potential causes of hyperkalemia include all of the following EXCEPT

A. succinylcholine

B. digitalis toxicity

C. acute renal failure

D. albuterol overdose

E. captopril overdose

17. An increased anion gap occurs in all of the following EXCEPT

A. diabetic ketoacidosis

B. renal tubular acidosis

C. salicylate poisoning

D. methylmalonic acidemia

E. ethylene glycol poisoning

18. A preterm infant born to a mother with severe pre-eclampsia is noted to be hypotonic and apneic in the delivery room. After resuscitation and stabilization, she remains hypotonic with decreased deep tendon reflexes in the arms and knees. The mother's treatment included hydralazine, magnesium sulfate, and indomethacin. The laboratory evaluation of this patient should include (may choose more than one)

A. serum calcium

B. arterial blood gas

C. serum magnesium

D. CBC

E. anion gap

19. The serum magnesium level in the patient in Question 18 is 6.5 mg/dL. The next step in the treatment should include (may choose more than one)

A. continue mechanical ventilation

B. infuse normal saline

C. add calcium to the intravenous solution

D. begin chelation therapy

E. administer KCl

20. Possible consequences of hypophosphatemia include all of the following EXCEPT

A. hypocalcemia

B. hemolysis

C. rhabdomyolysis

D. paresthesias

E. confusion

PART 8

The Acutely Ill Child

Nowhere else in pediatrics are the basic physiologic principles that are taught in the first 2 years of medical school more important to apply than in the care of acutely ill children. In addition, the principles of prevention, acute stabilization, and pharmacology all apply to these children. Discussion of acutely ill children includes topics such as injury control, evaluation, emergency services, critical care medicine, coma, resuscitation, shock, drowning, burns, hypothermia, acute respiratory distress syndrome, and principles of drug therapy. Pain management is especially critical in the care of an acutely ill pediatric patient who has a medical or surgical disease. In addition, the medical and ethical issues surrounding organ transplantation and procurement are integrally related to the care of neurologically injured (brain dead) patients.

Questions in this part work closely with the related chapters in the *Nelson Textbook* to help readers identify, prioritize, stabilize, and treat acutely ill children. Specific diseases are discussed in other parts of the *Nelson Textbook*, but the basic principles of multiple system organ dysfunction such as that occurring in shock are included in this part.

1. Indications for admission to the hospital after a burn injury may include all of the following EXCEPT
   A. suspected child abuse
   B. electric burns through an extremity
   C. perineum burns
   D. poor follow-up
   E. unimmunized for tetanus
   F. inhalation injury

2. Which of the following statements about the neonatal pain experience (compared with the adult) is true?
   A. Neonates have a higher pain threshold.
   B. Perception is reduced because of immaturity.
   C. Unmyelinated C fibers transmit nociceptive signals.
   D. Narcotics are dangerous and produce addiction.
   E. The stress hormone response is markedly attenuated.

3. A poor prognosis after a near drowning is associated with all of the following EXCEPT
   A. initial Glasgow Coma Scale score of less than 5

   B. no brain-stem activity at 24 hours
   C. no purposeful movement at 24 hours
   D. submersion greater than 10 minutes
   E. age

4. A 10-year-old boy has a Glasgow Coma Scale score of 4 and experiences irregular respirations after head trauma. The next important step in the care of this patient is to
   A. perform endotracheal intubation
   B. administer 20 mL/kg of lactated Ringer's solution
   C. administer naloxone
   D. administer mannitol
   E. obtain a head CT scan

5. The patient described in Question 4 is successfully intubated but then is shown to have a blood pressure of 150/100 and a pulse of 50. The next step should be to
   A. induce hyperventilation
   B. administer dexamethasone
   C. obtain a head CT scan
   D. administer furosemide
   E. increase the PEEP

6. After hyperventilation, the vital signs of the patient described in Question 4 normalize. The next step is to perform
   A. lumbar puncture

B. head CT scan

C. skeletal survey

D. coagulation profile

E. type and cross-match

7. **Matching:** Cold injuries
   1. Persistent sweating, pain hypersensitivity
   2. Stinging, aching skin
   3. Erythematous, vesicular, ulcerative lesions
   4. Clumsiness, confusion
   5. Purple, papular-nodular lesions

   A. Frostbite
   B. Chilblain
   C. Hypothermia
   D. Panniculitis
   E. Trench foot

8. Epinephrine is useful in cardiopulmonary arrest for all of the following EXCEPT
   A. bradycardia
   B. asystole
   C. apnea
   D. hypotension
   E. anaphylaxis

9. The leading cause of death among children between 4 and 15 years of age is
   A. malignancy
   B. AIDS
   C. motor vehicle accidents
   D. burns
   E. drowning

10. A 10-year-old boy sustained significant trauma and hemorrhage in a motor vehicle accident. After 15 minutes of resuscitation, you are unable to find a peripheral vein for cannulation. You should now
    A. place a Swan-Ganz catheter
    B. perform a femoral cutdown
    C. administer fluid by nasogastric tube
    D. place an intraosseous line
    E. give intratracheal medications

11. **Matching:**
    1. Pulmonary aspiration
    2. Inactivates surfactant
    3. Washes out surfactant
    4. Ventilation-perfusions mismatch
    5. Tracheitis
    6. Hypothermia
    7. Hemolysis

    A. Seawater drowning
    B. Freshwater drowning
    C. Both
    D. Neither

12. Which of the following statements about home ownership of firearms is true?
    A. It has not been shown to appreciably increase the risk of suicide in teens.
    B. It does not increase the risk of homicide.
    C. It poses a risk to adolescents even if guns are kept unloaded and locked.
    D. It has been shown to be safe if children are properly educated about gun safety.
    E. It is inappropriate to bring up in a discussion during well child visits.

13. The most common burn injury resulting in hospitalization in young children is due to
    A. house fires
    B. clothing ignition
    C. hot food or drinks
    D. hot tap water
    E. fireworks

14. Adequate fluid resuscitation in a burn patient is best monitored by which of the following?
    A. Serial hematocrit determinations during the first 24 hours
    B. Direct (Swan-Ganz catheter) measurement of cardiac filling pressure
    C. Serial measurements of serum albumin levels
    D. Hourly urine volume determination
    E. Serial serum sodium levels

15. Which of the following burn patterns is suggestive of child abuse?
    A. Scald burn on side of face, neck, and shoulder
    B. Burn on palm of hand
    C. Glove distribution burns on both hands and wrists
    D. Burn on calf and thigh of one leg

16. Indications for immobilization of the cervical spine in a pediatric trauma patient include all of the following EXCEPT
    A. head injury
    B. first rib fracture
    C. neck pain
    D. multiple system injury
    E. midface fractures
    F. fall from 15 feet
    G. bathtub drowning

17. In the first 2 months of life, a febrile, previously full-term infant is more likely than an older febrile child is to have
    A. Sepsis caused by *Streptococcus pyogenes*
    B. Pharyngitis caused by group A streptococci
    C. Meningitis caused by *Neisseria meningitidis*
    D. Urinary tract infection caused by *Staphylococcus epidermidis*
    E. Sepsis caused by group B streptococci

18. A 3-month-old, former 29-week-premature infant has been scheduled for repair of bilateral inguinal hernias. The infant had received mechanical ventilation for the first 6 days of life and had apnea of prematurity that resolved 5 weeks ago. The infant is feeding well and gaining weight and has no requirement for supplemental oxygen. The hematocrit is 28. The HMO clerk approves the surgery on an outpatient basis. All of the following are true EXCEPT
    A. risk of postoperative apnea is increased by anemia
    B. accepted standard of care includes overnight inpatient apnea monitoring for this infant after general anesthesia because of a significant risk of postoperative apnea
    C. postponing the surgery incurs a small but real risk of incarceration, with complications that may include bowel obstruction and infarction of testes or ovaries
    D. after a spinal anesthetic, monitoring for apnea is not required, and the infant can be sent home from the postanesthetic care unit on the day of surgery

19. A 5-year-old underwent a tonsillectomy and an adenoidectomy under general anesthesia. The parents tell you that the anesthesiologist said that she "fought the mask and cried a lot" on induction. You are the pediatrician for this child, and 8 days after surgery, the parents call to report that the child, who previously slept well at night, now awakens nightly screaming with bad dreams. She is more irritable and cranky than before surgery and has angry outbursts. She is more "clingy" and wants her parents to cuddle her frequently. She reports that in her dreams, she can't move, there is a tube in her throat, and she feels the surgeon cutting her throat. A review of her anesthetic record suggests an uneventful intraoperative course, with stable vital signs. All of the following statements about this situation are true EXCEPT
    A. this is an extreme reaction and suggests a severe underlying tendency toward psychiatric illness
    B. traumatic induction of anesthesia can commonly produce behavioral changes for several weeks—in the majority of cases, these resolve within 4–6 weeks
    C. parental presence for mask induction of anesthesia may reduce the distress of induction for some children and may reduce the incidence of some postoperative behavioral changes
    D. intraoperative awareness can occur during general anesthesia and could possibly account for the content of her dreams and some of the severity of these behavioral changes

20. A 12-year-old, 45-kg, previously healthy child is now on the pediatric ward 2 hours after repair of a forearm fracture under general anesthesia. You are called because of a fever of 40.6°C, a respiratory rate of 60 breaths per minute, a heart rate of 140 beats per minute, and "the child's color looks a bit off." Over the phone, the nurse reviews for you the anesthetic record and reports that general anesthesia' was administered after a "rapid sequence induction" because the child had eaten a large meal just before the injury. The nurse notes from the record that anesthetic induction was performed with Pentothal and succinylcholine. Anesthesia was maintained with halothane in a mixture of nitrous oxide and oxygen, and the child received morphine 3 mg IV before awakening. The anesthesia record notes stable vital signs during surgery, which lasted 30 minutes. All of the following are true EXCEPT

    A. prior to your examining the patient, from this history, your two primary differential diagnoses are aspiration pneumonitis and malignant hyperthermia

    B. because a rapid sequence induction was successful and the intraoperative vital signs were stable, aspiration pneumonitis was prevented and is very low in the differential diagnosis

    C. atelectasis is a more common cause of postoperative fever than either malignant hyperthermia or aspiration pneumonitis; this child's severity of fever, tachypnea, and "color looks a bit off" are typical for the diagnosis of atelectasis

    D. untreated pain increases respiratory rates, but rarely to this degree

21. The clinical history is the same as in Question 20. An arterial blood sample while the child was breathing room air is Po_2 78, Pco_2 58, pH 7.20; serum potassium 7.1. The urine appears somewhat dark. The child is alert and appears moderately anxious and uncomfortable. Immediate interventions should include all of the following EXCEPT

    A. IV sodium bicarbonate

    B. IV calcium gluconate or calcium chloride

    C. IV dantrolene

    D. An IV bolus of 20 mL/kg of normal saline and administration of IV mannitol and furosemide

    E. endotracheal intubation and positive pressure ventilation

22. A 4-year-old child is scheduled for elective branchial cleft cyst excision. One week prior to the procedure, the mother noticed that the child had a new productive cough, rhinorrhea, and low-grade fever. On the day of the scheduled procedure, the fever is gone and the chest examination is normal except for the persistent cough and scattered end-expiratory wheezes. The mother is a heavy smoker. All of the following are true EXCEPT

    A. the presence of a recent upper and/or lower respiratory infection increases the incidence of both intraoperative and postoperative complications such as hypoxia, laryngospasm, cough, or bronchospasm

    B. the risk of significant airway problems is greatest in younger children

    C. environmental exposure to cigarette smoke increases the risk of airway problems during anesthesia in children

    D. the increased risk of airway problems subsides within 4 days after rhinorrhea subsides

23. All of the following statements regarding drowning or near drowning in childhood are correct EXCEPT

    A. drowning is the leading cause of injury death for children less than 5 years old in the United States

    B. residential swimming pools are the most common drowning site for children less than 5 years old, accounting for 60–90% of all childhood drowning in this age group

    C. up to 80% of residential swimming

pool drowning in toddlers could be prevented if pools were fenced on all four sides, with a self-latching gate, and pool owners knew basic CPR
D. approximately 50% of all drowning events involve alcohol or illicit drug use as contributing factors
E. most bathtub drowning occurs in 15- to 30-month-old children

24. A comatose 3-year-old child is admitted to the pediatric intensive care unit after warm water near drowning. His Glasgow Coma Score on admission was 5. Which of the following prognostic indicators is most reassuring that the child will have a good neurologic recovery?
A. Spontaneous purposeful movement and normal brain stem function on neurologic examination at 24 hours, even though the child is not awake
B. Normal intracranial pressure
C. Normal CT scan of the brain
D. Submersion duration of 10 minutes
E. Initial blood glucose of 360 mg/dL

25. Which of the following statements about the management of drowning or near-drowning victims is most correct?
A. Careful monitoring and control of intracranial pressure is the mainstay of neurologic management.
B. Positive end-expiratory pressure is frequently needed to reverse hypoxemia.
C. Intravenous fluids should initially be withheld to minimize the risk of exacerbating cerebral edema.
D. Insulin is used to correct hyperglycemia after hypoxic-ischemic injury.
E. Most victims aspirate large quantities of fluid (>20 mL/kg) and require manual pulmonary drainage.

26. Which of the following measures is least likely to be effective as part of preventive strategies aimed at decreasing the number of children who drown?
A. Swimming pool covers and alarms
B. Swimming lessons for children older than 4 years

C. Water safety instruction in the schools
D. Counseling teenagers and adults about alcohol and drug use
E. Fencing swimming pools on all four sides with a self-latching gate

27. Children who have a high risk of drowning include each of the following groups EXCEPT
A. toddlers
B. minorities
C. males
D. otherwise healthy children who have a seizure disorder
E. young teenagers

28. A 14-month-old, 10-kg boy undergoes a major elective hip operation with a stable intraoperative course noteworthy for a 600-mL blood loss. Past medical history is significant for a myelomeningocele, repaired shortly after birth, with paraparesis and a sensory level at L1. He has chronic renal failure, with a preoperative BUN of 88 and a creatinine of 2.2. Postoperatively, he was begun on a continuous intravenous morphine infusion of 0.3 mg/hour (0.03 mg/kg/hour), which is a typical starting infusion rate. On the evening after surgery, he was sleepy but rousable and appeared to have minimal discomfort. At 6 a.m. the next morning, he was obtunded, with pinpoint pupils and a respiratory rate of 6 breaths/minute. Which of the following factors is least likely to be contributing to his obtundation?
A. Delayed renal excretion of active metabolites of morphine
B. Minimal painful stimulus from the surgery because of his sensory level
C. The CNS depressant effects of uremia and electrolyte disturbances
D. Diminished respiratory responses to hypoxemia and hypercarbia in patients with myelomeningocele
E. The increased sensitivity of infants to opioid-induced respiratory depression

29. A 9-year-old, 40-kg boy with widely metastatic osteogenic sarcoma has been at home for the past 2 weeks with his

family for palliative care. He has received oral morphine elixir for his pain, 6 mg every 6 hours. When you call the house, the family reports that the child has had ongoing severe pain and that he is withdrawn and immobile in bed. Which of the following reasons is most likely to account for his lack of pain relief?

A. He has become addicted to morphine, so this dose is no longer sufficient.

B. This dose is too small and the dosing interval is too long to maintain analgesic plasma concentrations for the majority of patients with widespread cancer pain.

C. Morphine is ineffective for most metastatic bone pain.

D. Because he is curled up in bed, he is probably more depressed than experiencing pain, and morphine would not be expected to improve depressed mood.

30. A 12-year-old girl comes to your office with a complaint of recurrent, severe throbbing headaches. They have occurred monthly for the past 4 years but are now happening about once every 1–2 weeks. They occur more frequently on school days than during weekends. The headaches are often accompanied by nausea and a "stomachache," though she never vomits. She never awakens with a headache in the morning. When the headaches occur, the patient lies down and takes a nap in a dark room, and they generally improve within 2–5 hours. Family history is noteworthy for migraine in her mother and paternal grandfather. Her school performance and attendance is excellent, and she reports no recent changes in mood, cognition, balance, or motor function. She is growing and gaining weight appropriately. Results of thorough physical examination, including neurologic examination and funduscopic examination, are normal. Which one of the following statements about her headaches is true?

A. Because the girl has nausea and headaches of increasing frequency, an immediate head MRI scan is mandatory to rule out a brain tumor.

B. Cognitive-behavioral techniques, including relaxation and biofeedback training, are ineffective in this situation because they work for tension/muscle contraction headaches but not for migraine.

C. Nonsteroidal anti-inflammatory drugs such as ibuprofen, are of no benefit for treating migraine episodes because migraine does not involve inflammation but rather involves constriction and dilatation of dural blood vessels, and NSAIDs do not alter vascular tone.

D. The serotonin receptor agonist sumatriptan often causes an acute sensation of chest tightness.

31. In response to social overtures (being held, hugged, kissed, talked to), a febrile infant demonstrates no smile with a dull, expressionless face without alerting to stimuli. The most appropriate response to this situation is

A. administer ceftriaxone IM after a blood culture and have the parent and child return to the office in the morning

B. if the child is over 6 months of age, obtain a blood culture and have the parents return to the office if the patient remains febrile

C. administer acetaminophen and reassess after the infant is no longer febrile

D. administer ceftriaxone after obtaining a blood, urine, and CSF culture and admit the child to the hospital

E. administer a normal saline bolus of 20 mL/kg and reevaluate in 1 hour

32. Paradoxical irritability may be present with all of the following EXCEPT

A. osteomyelitis

B. appendicitis

C. extremity cellulitis

D. meningitis

E. pneumonia

33. Homicide is the leading cause of death among which age group?

A. 0–1 year

B. 5–6 years

C. 9–10 years

D. 12–15 years

E. 15–18 years

34. Injury prevention is best approached by

A. education of parents

B. persuasion of families

C. changes in product design

D. environmental modifications

E. none of the above

35. Pupillary responses and AVPU are alternatives to what test during a trauma code?

A. Head CT

B. Funduscopic examination

C. Cold calorics

D. Apneic testing

E. Glasgow coma score

36. A previously healthy 7-month-old white male presents one summer day with a temperature of 41.1°C, a pulse of 190, a respiratory rate of 70, and a blood pressure of 65/20. He has a 1-day history of diarrhea (five stools in 24 hours) and is now unresponsive to verbal commands or painful stimuli. The most appropriate initial therapy is

A. cooling blankets

B. aspirin (100 mg/kg)

C. ceftriaxone (150 mg/kg)

D. dantrolene (10 mg/kg)

E. normal saline (20–40 mL/kg)

37. After receiving normal saline pushes, the patient in Question 36 remains unconscious. A lumbar puncture reveals 3 WBC, 10 RBC, a protein of 30 mg/dL, and a glucose of 75 mg/dL. After the lumbar puncture, he is noted to be bleeding at venipuncture sites. The most likely diagnosis is

A. herpes simplex encephalitis

B. meningococcemia

C. salicylate poisoning

D. hemorrhagic shock encephalopathy syndrome

E. malignant hyperthermia

38. A 5-year-old patient with near drowning in icy water presents with fixed dilated pupils and deep coma. He is apneic and pulseless with a temperature of 25°C. The most appropriate approach to his care is

A. do nothing because he is already dead

B. begin rewarming and initiate CPR when the core temperature is above 32°C

C. administer epinephrine and then atropine followed by defibrillation if the pulse doesn't increase to over 60 beats/minute

D. begin resuscitation with rescue breaths and chest compressions

E. apply a heating blanket after drying the patient and reassess in 10 minutes

39. Acute first aid of burns include all of the following EXCEPT

A. apply vegetable oil or butter

B. wash off chemicals with copious water irrigation

C. roll not run, then cover with blanket

D. cut rings off potentially involved fingers

E. prevent cooling

40. A burn wound characterized by the absence of painful sensation that doesn't bleed or have capillary refilling is best classified as

A. first degree

B. moderate to severe

C. second degree

D. midlevel

E. full thickness

41. The outpatient management of a minor burn (first or second degree) involving less than 10% body surface area could include all of the following EXCEPT

A. apply silver sulfadiazine (Silvadene)

B. apply bacitracin

C. begin prophylactic penicillin

D. leave blisters intact

E. use acetaminophen for pain

42. All of the following about high-tension electric burns are true EXCEPT

A. rhabdomyolysis may produce renal failure

B. multiple exit wounds suggest extensive visceral injury

C. if stable in the emergency room, the patient may be observed at home

D. limb amputations are possible

E. clothing may catch fire from arcing

43. A 5-year-old comes to your office with 4 nontender, 2-cm, blue-red discolored nodules over both cheeks on the face. The day before, she was sledding down the local snow covered hill. The most likely diagnosis is

A. child abuse

B. facial cellulitis

C. thrombocytopenia purpura

D. Henoch-Schönlein purpura

E. panniculitis

44. **Matching:** Anesthetic risks

1. Retroviral agents
2. Cocaine
3. Succinylcholine
4. Oxygen
5. Anthracyclines

A. Interacts with meperidine to produce seizures

B. Avoid with bleomycin

C. Increased risk of myocardial depression with volatile agents

D. Inhibits benzodiazepine clearance

E. Avoid in the presence of hyperkalemia

45. A 12-year-old with spina bifida experiences respiratory distress during induction of anesthesia for an orthopedic procedure. He has been otherwise well prior to this hospital admission. Past medical history reveals surgery for closure of the spina bifida at age 3 days, placement of a ventricular peritoneal shunt at 1 month of life, and release of contractures at 6 years of life. He is on ampicillin prophylaxis for recurrent urinary tract infections since birth and

has to be catheterized for urination. The most likely diagnosis is

A. ampicillin hypersensitivity

B. urosepsis

C. reactive airway disease

D. status epilepticus

E. latex anaphylaxis

46. **Matching:** Anesthesia drugs

1. Succinylcholine
2. Pancuronium
3. Ketamine
4. Propofol
5. Fentanyl

A. Endogenous catecholamine release

B. Associated with malignant hyperthermia

C. Vagolytic

D. Chest rigidity

E. May produce hypotension

47. A red-haired, blue-eyed, Caucasian 15-year-old with a small congenital nevus undergoes a biopsy to rule out melanoma. For pain control, naproxen (Naprosyn) 15 mg/kg TID is given. Two days after surgery, blood is noted to be oozing from the wound, which won't stop bleeding. All of the following are correct EXCEPT

A. the dose of naproxen is high

B. bleeding is a complication of naproxen

C. bleeding would have been avoided by using ibuprofen

D. Naproxen is preferred over aspirin because naproxen is not associated with Reye syndrome

E. acetaminophen has no direct antiplatelet affect

48. Neuropathic pain is best described as

A. dull and nonlocalized

B. responding well to opioids

C. never demonstrating allodynia

D. burning or stabbing

E. never producing local atrophy

49. The concept of accident-prone children can best be stated to have

A. created a way to identify at risk children

B. prevented many injuries

C. developed safe preschool environments

D. eliminated the need for bike helmets in low-risk children

E. taken attention away from more modifiable approaches to injury protection

50. All of the following are true about scald burns EXCEPT

A. water at a temperature of 150°F produces a full-thickness burn in 2 seconds

B. scald burns generally are not lethal

C. new water heaters should be set at 125°F

D. scald burns in a splash pattern suggest child abuse

E. scald burns on the palms, soles, and buttocks suggest abuse

51. A 10-year-old child with a history of asthma presents to your office sleepy, with a respiratory rate of 40, marked intercostal retractions, and few wheezes. Of the following, which is the best mode of transport to the local emergency department, which is 10 minutes away?

A. BLS ambulance

B. ALS ambulance

C. The mother's car

D. Your car

E. Aeromedical helicopter transport

52. A child with a seizure disorder is having recurrent seizures. She is currently arousable and is spontaneously breathing but has gurgling upper airway sounds. Appropriate measures would include all of the following EXCEPT

A. insertion of an oropharyngeal airway

B. providing oxygen with a face mask

C. positioning of the airway with the chin-lift maneuver

D. suctioning of the oropharynx

E. monitoring of oxygen saturation

53. Which of the following statements about basic life support measures is FALSE?

A. Chest compressions are performed a fingerbreadth below the intermamillary line in infants.

B. The ratio of compressions to ventilations during CPR is 5:1 for infants and children.

C. The chin lift is the desired method for opening the airway in traumatized children.

D. Effective chest compressions should result in a palpable central pulse.

E. Efficacy of ventilation is determined by watching for adequate chest rise.

PART 9

Human Genetics

Recent years have seen a massive expansion in our understanding of human genetics. Indeed, inheritance patterns such as mitochondrial inheritance or parental disomy are now identified. Furthermore, our ability to locate genes on human chromosomes and then clone the actual gene and identify the gene's product has greatly enhanced our knowledge of diseases and is leading to the development of specific and novel forms of diagnosis and therapy.

Questions in this part are directed at clinical physicians and not at molecular biologists. Nonetheless, a basic understanding of this wonderful science is essential for all pediatricians. Because genetic disturbances of all kinds are common in children and influence development, growth, and susceptibility to diseases such as cancer, readers should pay particular attention to this growing area of pediatrics.

1. A mentally retarded 15-year-old boy is found to have macroorchidism and large, prominent ears. He most likely has
   A. cerebral giantism
   B. acromegaly
   C. hypothyroidism
   D. trisomy 21
   E. fragile X syndrome

2. Patients with Turner syndrome should undergo careful analysis of their chromosomes for Y chromosome material because they may
   A. become masculinized
   B. grow tall
   C. become pregnant
   D. experience gonadoblastoma
   E. none of the above

3. **Matching:** Trisomies
   1. Cleft lip
   2. Rocker-bottom feet
   3. Hypoplastic ribs
   4. Risk of abortion
   5. Brushfield spots
   6. Meiotic nondysjunction
   7. Duodenal atresia

   A. Trisomy 13
   B. Trisomy 18
   C. Trisomy 21
   D. All of the above
   E. None of the above

8. Normal intelligence
9. Epicanthal folds
10. Hypotonia

4. Kearns-Sayre syndrome and Leber hereditary optic neuropathy are noted in both males and females but are inherited only through the mother. These are examples of
   A. uniparental disomy
   B. mitochondrial inheritance
   C. anticipation
   D. X-linked recessive inheritance
   E. X-linked dominant inheritance

5. **Matching:** For each of the following diseases, select the appropriate pattern of inheritance.
   1. Achondroplasia
   2. Sickle cell disease
   3. Phenylketonuria
   4. Bruton hypo-gammaglobu-linemia
   5. Color blindness
   6. Polycystic kidney (adult type)

   A. Autosomal recessive
   B. Autosomal dominant
   C. X-linked recessive
   D. X-linked dominant

7. Vitamin
   D–resistant
   rickets
8. Tuberous
   sclerosis
9. Hurler
   syndrome
10. Hemophilia A
    (factor VIII
    deficiency)
11. Hemophilia B
    (factor IX
    deficiency)
12. Duchenne
    muscular
    dystrophy

6. Strictly speaking, maternal inheritance is best defined as
   A. X-linked recessive
   B. only females are afflicted
   C. only males are afflicted
   D. involvement of mitochondrial DNA
   E. monoparental disomy

7. Tay-Sachs disease is best described by
   A. only affecting Ashkenazi Jews
   B. having a single genetic defect
   C. producing disease in only males
   D. having genetic heterogenicity
   E. having an adult-onset variety

8. All are true about homeobox genes EXCEPT
   A. they determine the eventual fate of embryonic tissue
   B. they are master switches controlling other developmental genes
   C. they regulate transcription during development
   D. once affected by a homeobox gene, the tissue may revert to a more primitive undifferentiated state
   E. homeobox gene mutations produce aniridia

9. Homeobox gene mutations have been associated with all of the following EXCEPT
   A. hand-foot-uterus syndrome
   B. hypodontia

C. Waardenburg syndrome
D. pituitary hormone deficiency
E. type 1 diabetes mellitus

10. FISH in genetic testing is best described as
    A. a way to prepare RNA
    B. an enzyme assay to detect mutations
    C. scraping of the buccal cells
    D. a test to identify the chromosomal location of an affected gene
    E. fibroblast inhibition selective histology

11. The polymerase chain reaction is best described as
    A. a method to produce many antigenic epitopes
    B. a method to amplify small quantities of DNA or RNA
    C. a Southern blot
    D. a Northern blot
    E. a Western blot

12. Trinucleotide repeats are implicated in the etiology of all of the following EXCEPT
    A. fragile X syndrome
    B. neurofibromatosis
    C. Friedreich ataxia
    D. spinocerebellar ataxia type I
    E. myotonic dystrophy

13. Genetic anticipation is best described as
    A. increased severity in subsequent generations
    B. a neuromuscular disorder with anxiety
    C. reduced penetrance in females
    D. enhanced expressivity in males
    E. imprinting

14. The pedigree in Figure 9–1 best depicts
    A. imprinting
    B. autosomal dominant inheritance
    C. X-linked recessive inheritance
    D. parental disomy
    E. anticipation

15. The pedigree in Figure 9–2 best depicts what pattern of inheritance?
    A. Autosomal dominant
    B. Autosomal recessive

GENERATION

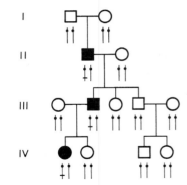

Figure 9-1

C. X-linked dominant

D. Mitochondrial

E. X-linked recessive

16. Multifactorial inheritance is characterized by all of the following EXCEPT
   A. some disorders having a sex predilection
   B. recurrence rates of 2–10% in first-degree relatives
   C. symptomatic carriers
   D. concordance rates in identical twins of 20–63%
   E. more severe symptoms in an affected infant predicts a greater recurrence risk

GENERATION

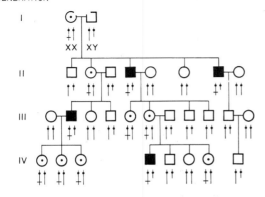

† X Chromosome   † Y Chromosome   ⊙ Carrier Female

Figure 9-2

17. Down syndrome due to translocation of a third chromosome 21 is best described by all of the following EXCEPT
   A. it accounts for 4% of patients with Down syndrome
   B. translocation occurs most often to chromosomes 13, 14, 15, or 21
   C. patients with translocation 21 have a milder phenotype
   D. the recurrence risk is about 30%
   E. carriers have a normal phenotype

18. **Matching:** Deletion syndrome
   1. 5p −
   2. 21q −
   3. 18p −
   4. 4p −
   5. 13q −

   A. Hypertonia, microcephaly, downward-slanting palpebral fissures
   B. Greek helmet "facies"
   C. Most patients (80%) have mild mental retardation and minor malformations
   D. Low birthweight, failure to thrive, severe mental retardation
   E. Cri-du-chat syndrome

19. **Matching:** Microdeletions
   1. 7q23 −
   2. 22q11 −
   3. 20p12 −
   4. 15q11 − 13 paternal
   5. 15q11 − 13 maternal

   A. DiGeorge—velocardiofacial syndrome
   B. Alagille syndrome
   C. Prader-Willi syndrome
   D. Williams syndrome
   E. Angelman syndrome

20. The most important reason to carefully screen for Y chromosome material in patients with Turner syndrome is to
   A. avoid masculinization
   B. provide birth control
   C. provide androgen therapy
   D. screen for gonadoblastoma
   E. screen for prostate cancer

21. Hypomelanosis of Ito is characterized by all of the following EXCEPT
   A. macular hypopigmented whorls and streaks
   B. ocular and CNS abnormalities

C. mosaic autosomal chromosome anomalies

D. mosaic sex chromosome anomalies

E. normal chromosome studies in skin fibroblasts

22. A 1-year-old presents with a disease that is classically an autosomal recessive trait (such as cystic fibrosis). The father is tested and, with 99% confidence, he is demonstrated to be negative for the carrier state. The most likely explanation is

A. mutation to an autosomal dominant trait

B. uniparental isodisomy transmission from the mother

C. uniparental isodisomy transmission from the father

D. imprinting of the missing recessive gene

E. mitochondrial recombination

23. Prader-Willi syndrome may occur from a uniparental maternal disomy of chromosome 15. There is no parental chromosome 15. The expressed phenotype is an example of

A. decreased penetrance

B. increased expressivity

C. imprinting

D. mitochondrial inheritance

E. nondisjunction

24. A newborn infant is noted to have dysmorphic features. The pregnancy was complicated by breech presentation, decreased fetal movements, and polyhydramnios. The child demonstrates hypotonia, a flat face, flattened occiput, epicanthal folds, and abdominal distention. The most likely cause of this child's dysmorphology is

A. trisomy 13

B. trisomy 18

C. Edwards syndrome

D. trisomy 8

E. trisomy 21

25. To evaluate abdominal distention, a KUB reveals a "double bubble" sign. The best explanation for the neonate's abdominal distention is

A. Hirschsprung disease

B. meconium ileus

C. meconium plug

D. duodenal atresia

E. pyloric atresia

PART 10

Metabolic Diseases

Welcome back to biochemistry, metabolic pathways, and unusual odors in urine samples, and now the potential for cure, successful management, or palliation of what is traditionally called inborn errors of metabolism. This part of the *Nelson Textbook* includes chapters on defects in the metabolism of amino acids, carbohydrates, lipids, mucopolysaccharides, purines, pyrimidines, and porphyrins. The new area of inborn errors of glycoprotein degradation is also covered in detail. It also includes excellent chapters on hypoglycemia and on the approach to inborn errors of metabolism. Individually, each inborn error of metabolism is relatively rare, but together all of these disorders at one time or another can keep a house office busy and up all night when an affected patient becomes ill or presents in a metabolic crisis.

Questions in this part may jog your biochemistry memory but are more likely to help reinforce important aspects about the recognition and management of inborn errors of metabolism.

---

1. **Matching:** For each inborn error of amino acid metabolism, select the correct urine odor.

   1. Glutaric acidemia (type II)
   2. Phenylketonuria
   3. Methionine malabsorption
   4. Trimethylaminuria
   5. Oasthouse disease
   6. Hawkinsinuria

   A. Cabbage
   B. Hoplike
   C. Sweaty feet
   D. Rotting fish
   E. Mousy
   F. Swimming pool
   G. Maple syrup

2. Self-destructive behavior is a component of
   A. xanthinuria
   B. Lesch-Nyhan syndrome
   C. orotic aciduria
   D. adenosine deaminase deficiency

3. A 9-day-old full-term infant is admitted to the hospital with lethargy, fever, and increasing jaundice. Physical examination also reveals hepatomegaly. Laboratory results reveal a blood glucose value of 10 mg/dL, total and direct bilirubin values of 15 and 7 mg/dL, respectively, and liver enzyme test results of AST = 700 and ALT = 650. The next day, the blood culture is positive for a gram-negative rod. The most likely diagnosis is
   A. necrotizing enterocolitis
   B. galactosemia
   C. neonatal hepatitis
   D. glycogen storage disease
   E. biliary atresia

4. A previously healthy 6-month-old presents with hepatomegaly, lethargy, increasing jaundice, and severe emesis. The child appears dehydrated; the urine also has a positive reaction for reducing substances. The child's diet has been solely breast milk until 5 months of age, when fruit juices and baby food were added to the diet. The most likely diagnosis is
   A. galactosemia
   B. glycogen storage disease
   C. benign fructosuria
   D. hereditary fructose intolerance
   E. pyruvate carboxylase deficiency

5. A 2-month-old presents with failure to thrive, emesis, alopecia, skin rash, and chronic metabolic acidosis. An older sibling died at 3 months of age with hypotonia and chronic lactic acidosis. One important diagnostic study should be determination of

A. blood galactose level

B. serum lactate dehydrogenase level

C. serum biotinidase level

D. plasma triglyceride levels

E. serum calcium and magnesium levels

6. A previously healthy 4-month-old now manifests increasing hypotonia and poor feeding. Physical examination reveals macroglossia, a gallop rhythm and tachycardia, marked flaccidity, but normal mental status. Laboratory studies reveal a blood glucose level of 85 mg/dL and sinus tachycardia with a shortened PR interval on an electrocardiogram. The most helpful diagnostic study would be

A. MRI of the spine

B. glucagon infusion test

C. muscle biopsy

D. lumbar puncture

7. **Matching:** Match the disease with its enzyme.

1.	α-Galactosidase	A.	Hurler
2.	Iduronidase	B.	Gaucher
3.	Sphingomyelinase	C.	Tay-Sachs
4.	β-Hexosaminidase A	D.	Niemann-Pick A
5.	β-Glucosidase	E.	Fabry

8. A 15-year-old Ashkenazi Jewish girl is seen because of chronic fatigue. On examination, she seems pale and thin and has a somewhat large abdomen. Her spleen is felt in the iliac fossa. She is mentally alert and has a history of normal development and normal school performance. Her blood count shows hemoglobin of 9.0 g/dL and a white blood cell count of 3000 with normal differential and no abnormal cells. Platelet count is 60,000. The likely diagnosis is

A. Tay-Sachs disease

B. Niemann-Pick A disease

C. Gaucher type I disease

D. Mucolipidosis IV

E. Canavan disease

9. A 13-month-old infant is found comatose in bed after sleeping later than usual. On physical examination, the infant is afebrile and of normal size, and the liver is palpated 4 cm below the costal margin. The plasma glucose level is 15 mg/dL, the bicarbonate level is 20 mEq/L, BUN is 35 mg/dL, ammonia is 295 μmol/L, AST is 320 U/L, ALT is 425 U/L, and bilirubin is normal. Urinalysis is negative for glucose, ketones, protein, and reducing substances. Which of the following is the most likely diagnosis?

A. Medium-chain acyl-CoA dehydrogenase deficiency

B. Glucose-6-phosphatase deficiency (type I glycogenosis)

C. Congenital hyperinsulinism

D. Growth hormone deficiency

E. Isovaleric acidemia

10. Which of the following porphyrias is NOT associated with cutaneous manifestations?

A. Porphyria cutanea tarda

B. Erythropoietic protoporphyria

C. Acute intermittent porphyria

D. Variegate porphyria

E. Congenital erythropoietic porphyria

11. Peroxisomal disorders in the neonatal period are most commonly manifested by

A. hypotonia and seizures

B. adrenal insufficiency

C. renal cysts

D. multiple congenital malformations

E. enlarged liver

12. Plasma very-long-chain fatty acids are elevated in all of the following peroxisomal disorders EXCEPT

A. Zellweger syndrome

B. rhizomelic chondrodysplasia punctata

C. pseudo-Zellweger syndrome

D. neonatal adrenoleukodystrophy

E. infantile Refsum disease

13. Of the following physical findings found in some patients with hyperlipidemia, which one is most likely to be found in a 17-year-old boy with heterozygous familial hypercholesterolemia?

A. Arcus corneae

B. Xanthelasma

C. Cutaneous xanthomas over the buttocks

D. Tuberous xanthomas causing Achilles tendinitis

E. Tuberous xanthomas over the elbow

14. The glycoproteinoses are a class of disorders that result from the deficiency of specific lysosomal enzymes that are required for the degradation of glycoproteins. Each statement about the glycoproteinoses is true EXCEPT

A. Most are inherited as autosomal recessive traits

B. The disease course is usually progressive

C. Enzyme replacement therapy is available for most of the disorders

D. Prenatal diagnosis of affected fetuses is possible

E. The clinical phenotype tends to vary among affected individuals

15. The mucolipidoses result from the abnormal targeting of lysosomal enzymes to the lysosome. Each statement about the mucolipidoses is correct EXCEPT

A. cellular levels of the lysosomal enzymes are low

B. clinical features are similar to those in Hurler syndrome

C. prenatal diagnosis is possible

D. no specific therapy is available

E. all affected patients die in early childhood

16. The parents of a 2-year-old boy with Tay-Sachs disease ask you about the availability of prenatal testing in their pregnancy. When counseling this couple about prenatal diagnosis, it would be most appropriate to include which one of the following statements:

A. Testing can be performed on chorionic villus cells obtained as early as 10 weeks of pregnancy.

B. Results of prenatal diagnosis testing for Tay-Sachs disease are considered investigational.

C. Testing is only possible if the parents' mutations in the hexosaminidase gene are known.

D. The risk that they could have a similarly affected child in their next pregnancy is no greater than that of any other couple.

E. Prenatal diagnosis should only be considered after testing has been conducted on each parent to prove carrier status.

17. A 7-month-old boy has been healthy and developing normally since birth. His mother now reports that he has decreased eye contact with her, even during feedings. The infant also startles very easily when there is a loud noise in the house. Of the following, the most appropriate diagnostic test to confirm the etiology of these findings is the measurement of

A. leukocyte β-hexosaminidase A activity

B. serum concentration of amino acids

C. serum concentration of ammonia

D. urinary mucopolysaccharides

E. urinary organic acids

18. A 10-year-old girl is noted on a routine physical examination to have splenomegaly. Laboratory testing reveals thrombocytopenia and moderate edema, and she is referred to a hematologist for further evaluation. Bone marrow aspiration is performed and reveals the presence of Gaucher cells. When discussing therapeutic options with the parents of this child, it would be most appropriate to include which of the following statements?

A. If a compatible donor can be found, bone marrow transplantation is recommended.

B. No treatment is available other than supportive care.

C. Many children with Gaucher disease require periodic blood transfusions.

D. It is likely that the patient will someday require splenectomy.

E. Enzyme replacement therapy has been shown to reverse the hematologic abnormalities.

19. The lipid storage diseases are a group of disorders that result from specific enzymatic deficiencies. Each statement about these disorders is true EXCEPT
    A. prenatal diagnosis is available for most of the lipidoses
    B. diagnosis of these disorders usually requires liver biopsy
    C. the genes encoding most of the enzymes have been cloned
    D. progressive disease with neurologic involvement is common
    E. the clinical manifestations can be predicted from the site of the substrate storage

20. A 7-month-old white female presents with severe developmental delay and episodes of vomiting. Physical examination reveals blue eyes, light skin with an eczematoid rash, and hyperactive deep tendon reflexes. There is failure to thrive and microcephaly. The most likely diagnosis is
    A. child neglect
    B. TORCH infection
    C. VATER syndrome
    D. phenylketonuria
    E. galactosemia

21. Appropriate treatment of the child in Question 20 before the onset of serious symptoms is helpful in preventing severe retardation. Overtreatment may result in
    A. obesity and striae
    B. a musty, mousy odor
    C. headache and pseudotumor cerebri
    D. rectal prolapse and colitis
    E. anorexia, lethargy, and rash

22. Dietary restriction of phenylalanine during pregnancy to serum levels of 10 mg/dL prevents all of the following EXCEPT
    A. spontaneous abortion
    B. preeclampsia
    C. fetal microcephaly
    D. fetal congenital heart disease
    E. mental retardation in the child

23. A 2-month-old male of French Canadian heritage presents with fever, irritability, vomiting, and jaundice. Physical examination reveals an obtunded infant with hepatomegaly and jaundice. Laboratory studies reveal a blood glucose level of 10 mg/dL and elevated liver transaminases. The most likely diagnosis is
    A. tyrosinemia
    B. hepatitis D
    C. SIDS
    D. herpes simplex hepatitis
    E. nesidioblastosis

24. The best approach to the diagnosis of the patient in Question 23 is
    A. serum amino acids
    B. assay fumarylacetoacetate hydrolyase
    C. urine reducing substances
    D. liver scan
    E. serum organic acids

25. The most useful therapeutic approach to the patient in Questions 23 and 24 is
    A. restriction of dietary phenylalanine
    B. restriction of dietary methionine
    C. 2(nitro-4-trifluoromethylbenzoyl) 1–3 cyclohexanedione
    D. phenylacetic acid plus benzoic acid
    E. succinylacetoacetate

26. Complications of tyrosinemia include all of the following EXCEPT
    A. cataracts
    B. renal tubular acidosis
    C. peripheral neuropathy
    D. cirrhosis
    E. hepatic carcinoma

27. In general, albinism is characterized by all of the following EXCEPT
    A. hypopigmented skin and hair
    B. photophobia
    C. late-onset blindness
    D. skin cancer
    E. nail hypoplasia

28. **Matching:**

    1. Platelet dysfunction
    2. Sensorineural deafness
    3. Hemizygotic male has complete syndrome
    4. Mutation in KIT gene
    5. Giant granules in granulocytes

    A. Chédiak-Higashi syndrome
    B. Hermansky-Pudlak syndrome
    C. Waardenburg syndrome
    D. Piebaldism
    E. Nettleship full type ocular albinism

29. A 4-year-old blue-eyed white female manifests a malar flush, mild mental retardation, subluxation of the ocular lens, iridodonesis, and Marfanoid-like features (tall, thin, arachnodactyly). The most likely diagnosis is
    A. Hawkinsinuria
    B. alcaptonuria
    C. piebaldism
    D. homocystinuria
    E. Angelman syndrome

30. Additional complications that may occur in the patient in Question 29 include all of the following EXCEPT
    A. seizures
    B. thromboembolism
    C. osteoporosis
    D. scoliosis
    E. cardiomyopathy

31. Treatment is initiated with high-dose vitamin B_6 but no response is observed. The most likely explanation is
    A. folate deficiency
    B. malabsorption
    C. gastric hypersecretion
    D. vitamin B_1 deficiency
    E. vitamin C deficiency

32. A 1-week-old infant presents with poor feeding, vomiting, lethargy, and opisthotonus posturing. The critical impression is meningitis, but all cultures are negative. Seizures occur and hypoglycemia is documented; however, the seizures do not stop after the hypoglycemia is corrected with intravenous glucose. The arterial blood gas is 7.10 P_{CO_2} 23, P_{O_2} 90, with an anion gap of 35. A CT scan demonstrates cerebral edema. The most likely etiology is
    A. kernicterus
    B. Reye syndrome
    C. nesidioblastosis
    D. viral encephalitis
    E. organic acidemia

33. To evaluate the patient in question 32, all of the following are appropriate EXCEPT
    A. serum organic acids
    B. urine carnitine
    C. serum amino acids
    D. serum 17-hydroxyprogesterone
    E. serum ammonia

34. The plasma amino acids in the patient in Questions 32 and 33 reveal a marked elevation of leucine, isoleucine, and valine. The most likely diagnosis is
    A. maple syrup urine disease
    B. galactosemia
    C. Fanconi syndrome
    D. carnitine deficiency
    E. Hartnup disease

35. **Matching:**

    1. Isovaleric acidemia
    2. Infantile multiple carboxylase deficiency
    3. Juvenile multiple carboxylase deficiency
    4. Dietary biotin deficiency
    5. 3-Methylglutaconic aciduria type II
    6. 3-Methylglutaconic aciduria type III

    A. Alopecia
    B. Seborrheic dermatitis
    C. Consumption of raw eggs
    D. X-linked cardiomyopathy
    E. Pancytopenia
    F. Choreoathetoid movements

36. A 10-day-old manifests profound coma one day after an illness characterized by emesis, poor oral intake, and hypotonia. Laboratory findings reveal 4+ ketonuria,

an arterial blood gas of 6.9, P_{CO_2} 19, P_{O_2} 95, an anion gap of 37, and an absolute neutrophil of 400. The most likely diagnosis is

A. galactosemia
B. glycogen storage disease type II
C. methylmalonic acidemia
D. phenylketonuria
E. primary carnitine deficiency

37. In addition to routine supportive care, what additional therapy would be most appropriate for the child in Question 36?
A. Vitamin B_{12}
B. Vitamin B_1
C. Biotin
D. Vitamin C
E. Folate

38. A 1-day-old presents with failure to suck, hypotonia, lethargy, and refractile myoclonic seizures. The infant is normocephalic and laboratory studies reveal normal serum pH and glucose, calcium, ammonia, and electrolyte levels. The birth history is unremarkable, and the Apgar score was 9 and 9. Hyperglycinemia is present in a mild to moderate range. The next most appropriate test is
A. urine glycine
B. serum carnitine
C. cerebrospinal fluid glycine
D. cerebrospinal fluid glucose
E. urine ketones

39. Deficiency of trimethylamine oxidase results in what symptoms?
A. Seizures
B. Body odor of rotten fish
C. Alopecia
D. Edema
E. Hepatomegaly

40. A 5-day-old infant manifests tachypnea, poor feeding, vomiting, and decreased responsiveness. A sepsis workup is performed, and the child is started on a D10W infusion and receives ampicillin and cefotaxime. The condition worsens,

and the child becomes unresponsive to stimuli. All cultures are negative after 48 hours. The arterial blood gas is 7.45, P_{CO_2} 36, P_{O_2} 100, the anion gap is normal, the blood glucose is 75 mg/dL, and serum ammonia is 500 μM. The most likely diagnosis is
A. congenital hyperinsulinism with hyperammonemia
B. urea cycle defect
C. methylmalonic acidemia
D. maple syrup urine disease
E. lysinuric protein intolerance

41. Serum amino acids are normal and the urine orotic acid is elevated in the patient in Question 40. The most likely diagnosis is
A. carbamyl phosphate synthetase deficiency
B. transient neonatal hyperammonemia
C. N-acetylglutamate synthase deficiency
D. argininosuccinic acidemia
E. ornithine transcarbamylase deficiency

42. During acute metabolic decompensation, all of the following are appropriate therapy EXCEPT
A. 10% glucose infusion
B. albumin infusion
C. sodium benzoate
D. sodium phenylacetate
E. arginine hydrochloride

43. Lysinuric protein intolerance is characterized by all of the following EXCEPT
A. severe and universal mental retardation
B. pulmonary fibrosis
C. hyperammonemia
D. failure to thrive
E. symptoms beginning after weaning from breast milk

44. A 10-month-old Ashkenazi Jewish female manifests hypotonia and macrocephaly. By 18 months of age, she has hyper-reflexia and optic atrophy. Additional problems include failure to thrive and swallowing difficulties. MRI demonstrates diffuse white matter degeneration of the cerebral cortex. The most likely diagnosis is

A. adrenal insufficiency

B. cerebral palsy

C. encephalomyelitis

D. Alexander disease

E. Canavan disease

45. A 14-month-old male of Northern European ancestry experienced an upper respiratory tract infection and anorexia. On the second day of the illness, he began to vomit, and by that evening he was unresponsive. On the way to the hospital, he had a generalized seizure lasting 10 minutes. At the hospital, he had a blood glucose of 10 mg/dL; his urinalysis showed no ketones. Liver function tests, anion gap, and serum ammonia were all normal. The most likely diagnosis is

A. medium-chain acyl CoA dehydrogenase deficiency

B. maple syrup urine disease

C. glutaric aciduria type I

D. glutamate formiminotransferase deficiency

E. galactosemia

46. Chronic therapy for the patient in Question 45 is best characterized by

A. avoiding fasts for longer than 10–12 hours

B. high-fat diet

C. low-carnitine diet

D. galactose-free diet

E. nasogastric drip feedings overnight

47. **Matching:**

1. Peroxisomal disorder
2. Disorder of peroxisomal import
3. X-linked
4. Primarily African-American
5. Most severe
6. Least severe
7. Neonatal dysmorphism

A. Zellweger
B. Neonatal adre-noleukodystro-phy
C. Infantile Refsum disease
D. All
E. None

8. Pigmentary retinal degeneration
9. Hirschsprung disease
10. Restriction of phytanic acid in diet

48. A 7-year-old male previously "A" student demonstrates progressive hyperactivity is diagnosed with attention deficit hyperactivity disorder. Despite therapy, his school performance deteriorates. He has difficulty understanding people when spoken to on the telephone. Seizures developed 6 months later. Physical examination reveals slight diffuse hyperpigmentation, spasticity, and reduced deep tendon reflexes. The most likely diagnosis is

A. acute demyelinating encephalitis

B. Guillain-Barré syndrome

C. Zellweger disease

D. X-linked adrenoleukodystrophy

E. Charcot-Marie tooth neuropathy

49. The best diagnostic test for the patient in Question 48 is

A. serum amino acids

B. nerve conduction studies

C. serum very-long-chain fatty acids

D. MRI angiography

E. cerebrospinal fluid myelin basic protein

50. Patients with heterozygous familial hypercholesterolemia have xanthomas. The best site to look for xanthomas is

A. eyelids

B. helix of ear

C. flexor tendon of the elbow

D. patella tendon

E. Achilles tendon

51. All of the following are present in children with homozygous familial hypercholesterolemia EXCEPT

A. hypertriglyceridemia

B. arcus cornea

C. xanthomas on tendons

D. xanthomas on the buttocks

E. myocardial infarction in teens

52. The best approach to therapy for patients with homozygous familial hypercholesteremia is

A. liver transplantation

B. LDL apheresis

C. atorvastatin

D. gene therapy

E. none of the above

53. **Matching:** Lipidosis

1. Tay-Sachs	A. Cherry red spot
2. Sandhoff	B. Hepatospleno-megaly
3. Niemann-Pick	
4. GM₁-gangliosidosis	C. Both *A* and *B*
5. Mucolipidosis I	D. Neither *A* nor *B*

54. A 16-year-old presents with easy bruisability and chronic fatigue. He has a 3-year history of bone pain and poor growth. Physical examination reveals hepatosplenomegaly. Laboratory studies reveal normal liver enzymes but a hematocrit of 25% and a platelet count of 25,000. X-rays of the skeleton reveal long bone lytic lesions and osteosclerosis. The most likely diagnosis is

A. leukemia

B. sickle cell anemia

C. Tay-Sachs disease

D. Hunter syndrome

E. Gaucher disease

55. The best diagnostic test for the patient in Question 54 is

A. bone marrow

B. assay acid β-glucosidase in leukocytes

C. ophthalmoscopy for cherry red spot

D. urine long-chain amino acids

E. urine long-chain fatty acids

56. Treatment of the patient in Questions 54 and 55 is best achieved with

A. liver transplantation

B. purified placental acid β-glucosidase

C. lovastatin

D. plasmapheresis

E. sphingomyelinase of lysosomal origin

57. Metachromatic leukodystrophy, an autosomal recessive white matter disease, is characterized by all of the following EXCEPT

A. presentation between 12 and 18 months of age

B. genu recurvatum

C. cherry red spot on retina

D. myoclonic seizures

E. absent deep tendon reflexes and hypotonia

58. **Matching:** Glycogen storage diseases

1. Von Gierke	A. Muscle cramps, exercise intolerance
2. Pompe	
3. McArdle	
4. Fanconi-Bickel	B. Severe hypoglycemia, hepatomegaly
5. Anderson	
	C. Cardiomegaly, hypotonia
	D. Progressive early cirrhosis, failure to thrive
	E. Renal tubular dysfunction, rickets

59. Disorder of carbohydrate-deficient glycoprotein structure are characterized by all of the following EXCEPT

A. autosomal recessive inheritance

B. thrombocytopenia

C. facial dysmorphism

D. hypotonia

E. stroke-like episodes

F. diminished deep tendon reflexes

PART 11

The Fetus and Neonatal Infant

The good news is that the infant mortality rate is falling. The bad news is that the low-birthweight rate has not declined in more than two decades. This means that past readers of this part of the *Nelson Textbook* have learned their lessons well and have mastered technology, physiology, science, and the art of neonatal intensive care. We are increasingly called on to care for less mature infants; many of these immature neonates develop the diseases or complications discussed in the chapters in this part of the *Nelson Textbook*. Dysmorphology, prenatal diagnosis, and therapy, as well as fetal disorders and specific neonatal infections, are also covered here. Other neonatal problems are discussed in the organ system–specific parts of the *Nelson Textbook* or in the infectious disease part.

You do not need to be a neonatologist to correctly identify the answers to these questions. The questions are directed at what a general pediatrician needs to know about fetal disorders and high-risk neonates, as well as their stabilization, initial management, and short and long-term prognosis.

---

1. **Matching:** Malformations

   1. Deletion of elastin allele
   2. Microdeletion 16p13.3
   3. Deletion of band q11–12
   4. Endocardial Cushing effects
   5. Mandibular hypoplasia
   6. Tracheoesophageal fistula
   7. Anal atresia
   8. Radial hypoplasia

   A. Rubinstein-Taybi syndrome
   B. Trisomy 21
   C. Williams syndrome
   D. Pierre Robin syndrome
   E. Prader-Willi syndrome
   F. VATER syndrome
   G. None of the above

2. An infant has the following findings at 5 minutes of life: pulse 130 per minute, cyanotic hands and feet, good muscle tone, and a strong cry and grimace. This infant's Apgar score is
   A. 7
   B. 8
   C. 9
   D. 10

3. Jaundice is most likely to be physiologic in a term infant in which of the following situations?

   A. Jaundice at 12 hours of age
   B. Serum bilirubin level increasing less than 5 mg/dL/24 hours in the first 2–4 days
   C. Direct (conjugated) serum bilirubin greater than 1 mg/dL
   D. Jaundice at 12 days of age

4. Which of the following is most appropriate for treating hyperbilirubinemia (11.2 mg/dL) in a 3-week-old, breast-fed infant with normal growth and development?
   A. Phototherapy
   B. Exchange transfusion
   C. Phenobarbital
   D. None of the above

5. A 2-week-old infant is brought to the emergency room in coma with retinal hemorrhages and severe pallor. He was born at home and was first seen by a physician at 10 days of age and placed on amoxicillin for otitis media. His diet is breast milk. The day before admission, his parents took him in a four-wheel-drive vehicle on a hot day over a rough road in the mountains. Seizures began 8 hours later, and he steadily deteriorated for the next 16 hours. He oozes blood from all

venipuncture sites. Diagnostic tests should include all of the following EXCEPT

A. coagulation studies

B. skeletal survey

C. CT scan

D. complete blood count

E. lumbar puncture

6. Immediate therapy for the infant described in Question 5 should include administration of vitamin

A. A

B. B₆ (pyridoxine)

C. C

D. E

E. K

7. The diagnosis for the child described in Question 5 is most likely

A. pyridoxine deficiency

B. severe scurvy

C. hemorrhagic disease of the newborn

D. child abuse

E. hypervitaminosis A

8. The death of the infant described in Question 5 could have been prevented by which one of the following measures?

A. AquaMEPHYTON (vitamin K) at birth

B. Home-visitor services

C. Discontinuance of antibiotics

D. Proper use of an infant seat

E. An air conditioner

9. You are called to the delivery of a boy at 42 weeks' gestational age with thick meconium-stained fluid and type II decelerations. The obstetrician rapidly delivers the infant and hands him to you for care. The boy is hypotonic, cyanotic, apneic, and bradycardic. The most appropriate step is to

A. stimulate the infant to breathe

B. administer epinephrine

C. provide positive-pressure bag-and-mask ventilation

D. intubate the trachea and provide positive-pressure ventilation

E. intubate the trachea and apply negative-pressure suction

10. A 1700-g infant is born at 36 weeks' gestation complicated by severe oligohydramnios. The Apgar scores are 3 at 1 minute and 5 at 5 minutes. The infant requires endotracheal tube placement as part of the resuscitation and continued mechanical ventilation to improve the arterial blood gases. At 1 hour of age, the infant shows acute deterioration with cyanosis, bradycardia, and hypotension. The most likely diagnosis for this acute change is

A. patent ductus arteriosus

B. intraventricular hemorrhage

C. hypoglycemia

D. pneumothorax

E. respiratory distress syndrome

11. A 3600-g, breast-fed white female, 42 weeks' gestational age, is noted to have persistent hyperbilirubinemia at 2 weeks of age. On physical examination, the infant has not gained weight since birth and has decreased tone, an umbilical hernia, and an anterior fontanel measuring 4 × 6 cm. The most likely diagnosis is

A. Crigler-Najjar syndrome

B. Gilbert disease

C. biliary atresia

D. hypothyroidism

E. galactosemia

12. A 4-week-old, A-positive, African-American former 40-week's-gestational-age infant was born to an O-positive mother and experienced hyperbilirubinemia requiring 2 days of phototherapy on the newborn nursery after birth. The infant appears apathetic and demonstrates pallor, a grade 2/6 systolic ejection murmur, and a heart rate of 175. The most likely diagnosis is

A. anemia of chronic disease

B. cholestasis secondary to neonatal hepatitis

C. hereditary spherocytosis

D. sickle cell anemia hemolytic crisis

E. ABO incompatibility with continued hemolysis

13. A term infant is born with Apgar scores
of 5 at 1 minute and 7 at 5 minutes. The
infant has a heart rate of 170 and
demonstrates pallor with
hepatosplenomegaly. A Kleihauer-Betke
test on maternal blood yields positive
results. The most likely diagnosis is
   A. erythroblastosis fetalis
   B. hereditary spherocytosis
   C. chronic fetal-maternal hemorrhage
   D. ABO incompatibility
   E. Blackfan-Diamond syndrome

14. A newborn female has a ventricular
septal defect, cleft lip and palate, and
imperforate anus. All of the following
laboratory tests would be appropriate
EXCEPT
   A. a karyotype analysis
   B. TORCH titer
   C. renal ultrasonography
   D. ultrasonography of the brain

15. **Matching:** Congenital infections
   1. Megaesophagus
   2. Patent ductus
   arteriosus
   3. Cerebral
   periventricular
   calcifications
   4. Limb
   hypoplasia
   5. Myocarditis
   6. Fetal anemia
   7. Hydrocephalus

   A. CMV
   B. Varicella
   C. Enteroviruses
   D. Rubella
   E. Parvovirus
   F. Toxoplasmosis
   G. *Trypanosoma cruzi*

16. A 2700-g, 36-week's-gestational-age
white male is born after 22 hours of
premature rupture of the amniotic
membranes. The Apgar scores are 3 and
5. He immediately experiences respiratory
distress and cyanosis requiring
endotracheal intubation and mechanical
ventilation with 100% oxygen. Vital signs
are temperature 35.7°C, heart rate 195,
and mean blood pressure of 22 mm Hg.
Laboratory tests reveal a white blood cell
count of 1500 and 59,000 platelets. The
next most appropriate treatment for this
child is to administer
   A. surfactant by aerosol

   B. intravenous ampicillin and gentamicin
   C. intravenous steroids
   D. intravenous acyclovir
   E. oscillator ventilation

17. The patient described in Question 16 is
most likely suffering from
   A. respiratory distress syndrome
   B. diaphragmatic hernia
   C. congenital pneumonia with sepsis
   D. pneumothorax
   E. TORCH infection

18. The blueberry muffin appearance in
infants with TORCH infections most likely
represents
   A. palpable purpura
   B. dermal erythropoiesis
   C. metastatic hepatic tissue
   D. viral lesions
   E. none of the above

19. The predominant cause of low-
birthweight births in America is
   A. intrauterine growth retardation
   B. prematurity
   C. multiple gestations
   D. uterine bleeding
   E. teenage pregnancy

20. Harlequin color change is a sign of
   A. congenital ichthyosis
   B. TORCH infections
   C. erythroderma
   D. normal physiology
   E. spinal cord trauma

21. A 2-day-old is noted to have conjunctival
and retinal hemorrhages. The most likely
etiology is
   A. child abuse
   B. maternal isoimmune
   thrombocytopenia
   C. maternal idiopathic thrombocytopenia
   purpura
   D. force of birthing process
   E. forceps delivery

22. The Apgar score is
    A. a predictor of future development quotients
    B. a predictor of cerebral palsy
    C. a systematic method to assess the newborn at birth
    D. a predictor of neonatal survival
    E. none of the above

23. Reasons to avoid the early discharge of a normal term infant include all of the following EXCEPT
    A. jaundice evident on day 1
    B. positive VDRL
    C. bleeding after circumcision
    D. two successful feedings
    E. no stools

24. **Matching:** Maternal serum α-fetoprotein levels
    1. Multifetal gestation   A. High
    2. Trisomy 21   B. Low
    3. Congenital nephrosis
    4. Trisomy 18
    5. Neural tube defects

25. **Matching:** Maternal drugs and the fetus and newborn
    1. Accutane   A. Neonatal heart failure
    2. Blue cohosh herbal tea   B. Oligohydramnios
    3. Iodide   C. Spina bifida
    4. Ibuprofen   D. Arthrogryposis
    5. Valproate   E. Facial-ear anomalies
    6. Misoprostol   F. Goiter

26. **Matching:** Fetal ultrasonography (may choose more than one)
    1. Nuchal pad thickening   A. Trisomies
    2. Choroid plexus cysts   B. Cystic fibrosis
    3. Echogenic bowel   C. Dandy-Walker cyst
                                D. Renal obstruction

    4. Pyelectasis
    5. Dilated cerebral ventricles

27. **Matching:** Drugs and the neonate
    1. Chloramphenicol   A. Pyloric stenosis
    2. Prostaglandins   B. Goiter
    3. Dexamethasone   C. Gray baby syndrome
    4. Iodine antiseptics D. Cardiomyopathy
    5. Pancuronium   E. Contractures

28. A term baby of an uncomplicated pregnancy is born limp, cyanotic, and apneic after a difficult vaginal delivery. Possible considerations for this state include all of the following EXCEPT
    A. prolapsed umbilical cord
    B. central nervous system trauma
    C. administration of morphine to the mother
    D. Klumpke paralysis
    E. administration of local anesthetic into the fetal scalp

29. After intubation and resuscitation, the patient in Question 28 remains limp but appears aware and looks around, although the baby does not cry when the toes are pinched. This most likely diagnosis is
    A. congenital botulism
    B. narcotic overdose
    C. transection of the spinal cord
    D. congenital myasthenia gravis
    E. neurosyphilis

30. A patient with Apgar scores of 1 and 2 at 1 and 5 minutes, respectively, appears hyperalert and has hyperactive deep tendon reflexes and mydriasis. The most likely diagnosis is
    A. stage I hypoxic ischemic encephalopathy
    B. stage II hypoxic ischemic encephalopathy
    C. stage III hypoxic ischemic encephalopathy

D. kernicterus

E. intraventricular hemorrhage

31. A 750-g black female experienced respiratory distress after a preterm delivery at 27 weeks' gestation. Pregnancy was uncomplicated, but labor was abrupt and therefore the mother did not receive betamethasone or penicillin therapy. After birth, the infant experienced respiratory distress and required intubation and ventilation with 100% O_2. The possible causes of the respiratory distress include (may choose more than one)

A. pneumothorax

B. respiratory distress syndrome

C. patent ductus arterious

D. group B streptococcal sepsis

E. transient tachypnea

32. The patient in Question 31 was also treated with the endotracheal instillation of exogenous surfactant. This is likely to be beneficial by (may choose more than one)

A. preventing chronic lung disease

B. reducing the incidence of pneumothorax

C. reducing mortality

D. more rapid improvement of RDS

E. preventing oliguria

33. On the second day of life, the patient in Questions 31 and 32 experiences bradycardia and hypotension with cyanosis and a metabolic acidosis. A CBC reveals a hematocrit of 28%. Likely diagnoses include (may choose more than one)

A. subcapsular hepatic hematoma

B. intraventricular hemorrhage

C. pneumomediastinum

D. hypoglycemia

E. hypocalcemia

34. A 4-day-old term breast-fed male appears icteric. The physical examination reveals mild pallor and significant jaundice with a palpable liver 2.5 cm below the right rib margin. His mother has a vague history of anemia and his older sister had prolonged neonatal jaundice. The next logical step to evaluate the patient includes all of the following EXCEPT

A. total and direct bilirubin levels

B. CBC with RBC morphology

C. reticulocyte count

D. Coombs test

E. hemoglobin electrophoresis

35. The serum total bilirubin of the patient in Question 34 is 20.0 mg/dL with a direct of 1.0 mg/dL. The hematocrit is 40%, the reticulocyte count is 5, and the smear reveals poikilocytosis and anisocytosis. The Coombs test result is negative. The next step in the management of the child's condition is

A. start phenobarbital

B. perform an exchange transfusion

C. start phototherapy

D. stop breast-feeding

E. check for galactosemia

36. After 3 days of phototherapy, the bilirubin level of the patient in Question 35 declines below 10 mg/dL. One day off phototherapy, the level of bilirubin remains less than 10 mg/dL. The patient is discharged home and grows well while breast-feeding. At 1 month of age, he returns with significant pallor, tachycardia, and a new heart murmur. The most likely problem at this time is

A. late-onset neonatal sepsis

B. ductal dependent congenital heart disease

C. hemolysis

D. myocarditis

E. supraventricular tachycardia

37. Jaundice appearing on day 1 of life suggests all of the above EXCEPT

A. TORCH infection

B. erythroblastosis fetalis

C. ABO incompatibility

D. sepsis

E. fetal-to-maternal transfusion

38. Direct-reacting hyperbilirubinemia on the 10th day of life suggest all of the following EXCEPT
    A. cystic fibrosis
    B. galactosemia
    C. neonatal hepatitis
    D. Byler syndrome
    E. Gilbert disease

39. Hyperbilirubinemia at 2 weeks of age suggests all of the following EXCEPT
    A. physiologic jaundice
    B. hypothyroidism
    C. pyloric stenosis
    D. biliary atresia
    E. breast milk jaundice

40. Late complications of Rhesus sensitization hyperbilirubinemia and its treatment include all of the following EXCEPT
    A. transient aregenerative anemia
    B. direct-reacting hyperbilirubinemia
    C. hypoglycemia
    D. graft-versus-host disease
    E. portal vein thrombosis

41. All of the following are associated with polycythemica EXCEPT
    A. hyperviscosity
    B. intrauterine growth retardation
    C. large-for-gestational-age infants
    D. twin-twin transfusion syndrome
    E. neonatal Graves disease

42. **Matching:** Hemorrhagic disease of the newborn
    1. Thrombocytopenia   A. Early onset
    2. Prolonged PT   B. Classic onset
    3. Maternal   C. Late onset
       phenytoin   D. None of the
    4. Breast-feeding   above
    5. Cholestasis   E. All of the
                                above

43. All of the following are problems of an infant of a diabetic mother (class B) EXCEPT
    A. hypoglycemia
    B. hypocalcemia

C. intrauterine growth retardation
D. hypomagnesemia
E. hyperbilirubinemia

44. Infants at risk for hyperinsulinemic hypoglycemia include all of the following EXCEPT
    A. infants with nesidioblastosis
    B. infants of diabetic mothers
    C. infants with galactosemia
    D. infants with leucine sensitivity with hyperammonemia
    E. infants with Beckwith syndrome

45. A 1500-g infant underwent extensive intestinal resection for severe necrotizing enterocolitis on the 10th day of life. The ileostomy began to function on the 15th day of life, and oral feedings were attempted on the 24th day of life. Each attempt to enterally feed the child was unsuccessful because excessive ileostomy fluid losses developed and the infant repeatedly became dehydrated. Total parenteral alimentation was initiated on the 14th day of life and continued throughout the next 2 months. In the second month of life, the child gradually manifested edema; an erythematous rash on the distal extremities, mouth, and perineal region; and alopecia. The serum alkaline phosphatase level was low, as was the serum albumin. The most appropriate therapy for this patient is to
    A. administer salt poor albumin
    B. increase the protein content in the hyperalimentation solution
    C. administer recombinant alkaline phosphatase
    D. administer zinc
    E. administer vitamin E

46. A 2100-g infant of a diabetic mother experiences seizures on the first day of life. Pregnancy was complicated by severe diabetic vasculopathy and placental insufficiency, with the development of late decelerations and the need for emergency caesarean section. The Apgar scores were 8 and 9 at 1 and 5 minutes, respectively. During the first 6 hours of

life, the child was well and tolerated formula feedings well. Jitteriness developed at 10 hours of age and progressed to tonic-clonic seizures at 18 hours of age. Laboratory studies revealed blood glucose of 80 mg/dL and calcium of 6.0 mg/dL. Thereafter, calcium gluconate (10%), 2 mL/kg, was given repeatedly without affecting the frequency of seizures. The most appropriate step to manage this infant's condition is to

A. administer glucose

B. administer pyridoxine

C. administer 1,35-dihydroxyvitamin D

D. administer magnesium sulfate

E. administer lorazepam

PART 12

Special Health Problems During Adolescence

Since antiquity (or even before), teenagers have held a special place in our hearts and our minds as physicians, as parents, and as former adolescents. Many diseases affect the physical and mental health of adolescents. Specific organ-related problems are often discussed in other parts of the *Nelson Textbook*. This part addresses adolescent epidemiology, depression, suicide, substance misuse, sleep and eating disorders, pregnancy, contraception, sexually transmitted diseases (STDs), menstrual problems, and disorders of the skin, breast, or bone.

Questions in this part are fairly straightforward and helpful in following and reinforcing the adolescent curriculum as discussed in the corresponding part and chapters in the *Nelson Textbook*.

1. Oral contraceptive agents are associated with all of the following risks EXCEPT
   A. thrombophlebitis
   B. carbohydrate intolerance
   C. high levels of high-density lipoproteins
   D. premature epiphyseal closure
   E. none of the above

2. False-positive VDRL test results would most likely occur in
   A. mononucleosis
   B. systemic lupus erythematosus
   C. endocarditis
   D. intravenous drug misuse
   E. tuberculosis
   F. all of the above

3. A foul-smelling vaginal discharge that emits a fishy odor with 10% potassium hydroxide and that demonstrates clue cells on the wet preparation is most likely due to
   A. gonorrhea
   B. *Chlamydia*
   C. chancroid
   D. *Gardnerella vaginalis*
   E. *Candida*

4. A 19-year-old man presents in an unresponsive state with miosis, slow respirations, and pulmonary edema. He has hypertrophic lesions over the dorsum of the left hand and the antecubital fossa. The most effective therapy is
   A. intravenous glucose
   B. flumazenil
   C. disulfiram
   D. naloxone (Narcan)
   E. intravenous calcium

5. Toluene (glue, solvents) misuse is associated with
   A. hallucinations
   B. tolerance
   C. pulmonary edema
   D. peripheral neuropathy
   E. rhabdomyolysis
   F. all of the above

6. Anabolic steroid use is associated with all of the following EXCEPT
   A. enhanced school performance
   B. testicular atrophy
   C. aggressive behavior
   D. cholestasis
   E. increased low-density lipoprotein levels

7. **Matching:** Eating disorders
   1. Increasing in   A. Anorexia
      frequency   nervosa

2. Primarily males

3. Most common disorder

4. "Feels fat" when emaciated

5. Amenorrhea

6. Binge eating with fear of not being able to stop

7. Bradycardia

8. Parotid swelling

9. Leukopenia

10. Hypothermia

11. Hyperthyroidism

12. Esophagitis

B. Bulimia
C. Both
D. Neither

8. A 15-year-old girl has experienced loss of 30 pounds during the past 6 months and has amenorrhea. She denies vomiting, diarrhea, and abdominal pain and claims to feel well. Physical examination reveals cachexia and a pulse of 40 per minute. Electrolyte determination reveals a serum potassium level of 3.0 and bicarbonate of 30. Hematocrit is 30, and erythrocyte sedimentation rate is 3 mm/hour. The most likely cause of this patient's condition is

A. inflammatory bowel disease

B. anorexia nervosa

C. bulimia nervosa

D. Addison disease

E. pituitary adenoma

9. Leading causes of hospitalization for adolescents include all of the following EXCEPT

A. pregnancy

B. mental health disorders

C. asthma

D. anemia

E. gastrointestinal disorders

F. injuries

10. Successful preventive measures to avoid morbidity and mortality from adolescent automobile accidents include all of the following EXCEPT

A. peer pressure TV commercials

B. graduated licensing systems

C. enforcement of drinking age laws

D. night-time driving restrictions

E. drivers' education classes

11. The American Academy of Pediatrics recommends annual health visits for adolescents for all of the following EXCEPT

A. learning problems

B. safety practices

C. scoliosis

D. breast examination

E. eating disorders

12. High-risk characteristics of adolescent sexuality include all of the following EXCEPT

A. young adolescents

B. late maturing boys

C. drug use

D. same-sex partner

E. coercive sex

13. An emancipated minor is one who is

A. able to understand health issues

B. lives with step parents

C. graduated high school

D. is a member of the U. S. military

E. travels overseas

14. Papanicolaou smears are indicated in

A. all young women over 16 years of age

B. a 14-year-old of a mother with cervical cancer

C. a 12-year-old exposed to diethylstilbestrol

D. all sexually active teenage females

E. none of the above

15. Depression in adolescents is characterized by all of the following EXCEPT

A. two to three times higher incidence in females

B. growth spurts

C. attention deficit disorder

D. substance abuse

E. death of a family member

16. A 17-year-old female manifests diminished interest in school, poor exercise participation, weight loss, and hypersomnia. The differential diagnosis includes all of the following EXCEPT

A. hypothyroidism

B. mononucleosis

C. exercise-induced asthma

D. chronic fatigue syndrome

E. depression

F. substance abuse

17. On further questioning of the patient in Question 16, you determine that she has inappropriate guilt, poor concentration, and low self-esteem. The most likely diagnosis is

A. pseudotumor cerebri

B. depression

C. lead poisoning

D. alcohol withdrawal

E. schizophrenia

18. Risk factors for adolescent suicide include all of the following EXCEPT

A. Native American race

B. chronic illness

C. access to guns

D. gender

E. gay and bisexual activity

19. Suicide ideation is

A. a significant risk factor for completed suicide in females

B. a significant risk for attempted suicide in young teens (12–14 years)

C. considered in about 25% of teens

D. less of a concern if there is no specific plan

E. does not require psychiatric consultation

20. **Matching:**

1. Defying adults

2. Harming animals

3. Legal label

4. Being arrested many times

5. Diagnosed by mental health practitioner

A. Juvenile delinquency

B. Oppositional defiant disorder

C. Conduct disorder

D. Neither *A, B,* nor *C*

E. All of the above

F. Both *B* and *C*

21. Diagnostic criteria for anorexia nervosa include all of the following EXCEPT

A. bradycardia and hypothermia

B. fear of becoming obese

C. feeling fat despite being emaciated

D. refusal to maintain body weight

E. absence of three consecutive menstrual cycles

22. Bulimia is characterized by the following EXCEPT

A. isocaloric nutrient malnutrition

B. self-induced vomiting and laxatives

C. fear of not being able to stop eating during a binge

D. at least two binge episodes per week for at least 3 months

E. binges lasting less than 2 hours

23. **Matching:** Drug use

1. Anticholinergic

2. Sympathomimetic

3. Opiate

4. Organic solvent

A. Propoxyphene

B. Jimson weed

C. Methamphetamine

D. Toluene

24. **Matching:** Drug misuse

1. Marijuana

2. Ecstasy

3. Angel dust

4. Acid

5. Ice

A. Methylenedioxyamphetamine

B. LSD

C. Methamphetamine

D. Weed

E. Phencyclidine

25. A 17-year-old white male presents with an exacerbation of acne and with aggressive behavior and poor school performance. Physical examination

reveals gynecomastia, testes that are smaller than expected for his sex maturity rating, and oily hair. The most likely diagnosis is

A. anabolic steroid abuse
B. adrenal hypertrophy
C. marijuana use
D. 17-hydroxylase deficiency
E. testicular feminization syndrome

26. A 16-year-old female has had headaches for 3 months, visual changes for 2 weeks, and now has galactorrhea. Her last normal menstrual period was 4 months ago. The most likely cause of her galactorrhea is

A. stress of having amenorrhea
B. elevated prolactin levels
C. elevated estrogen levels
D. migraines
E. adrenal insufficiency

27. All of the following may cause gynecomastia EXCEPT

A. Klinefelter syndrome
B. phenothiazines
C. anabolic steroids
D. heroin
E. albuterol

28. **Matching:** Menstrual cycle

1. Metrorrhagic
2. Menorrhagia
3. Hypermenor-rhea
4. Polymenorrhea
5. Menometror-rhagia

A. Excessive amount and increased du-ration of bleed-ing
B. Frequent, ir-regular, exces-sive, and pro-longed bleeding
C. Frequent regu-lar or irregular bleeding of less than 21-day intervals
D. Profuse men-strual flow of normal dura-tion

E. Intermenstrual irregular bleeding

29. A 16-year-old female has not had her first menstrual period. Her mother had her first period at the age of 12 years. The adolescent is short and has poor breast development. A vaginal smear shows no estrogen effect, and there is no withdrawal bleeding after administration of intramuscular progesterone. Her serum FSH level is high. The most likely diagnosis is

A. primary ovarian failure
B. FSH pituitary tumor
C. hypothyroidism
D. cervical stenosis
E. autoimmune endocrinopathy

30. A 14-year-old presents with vaginal bleeding that is more prolonged and profuse than her usual periods, which are irregular and first started 13 months ago. She has pallor and tachycardia. The next step in her evaluation is to

A. administer medroxyprogesterone (Provera)
B. administer conjugated estrogens (Premarin)
C. determine the hematocrit
D. determine the estrogen level
E. determine the platelet count

31. The most likely diagnosis of the patient in Question 30 is

A. ovarian tumor
B. fibroids
C. dysfunctional uterine bleeding
D. hemophilia
E. leukemia

32. The most appropriate therapy for the patient in Questions 30 and 31 is

A. Premarin
B. prednisone
C. 17-hydroxyprogesterone
D. ibuprofen
E. DDAVP

33. Serious complications of exogenous estrogens in oral contraceptive pills include all of the following EXCEPT

    A. thrombophlebitis

    B. myocardial infarction

    C. hepatic adenoma

    D. diabetes mellitus

    E. uterine rupture

34. A 19-year-old female tells you she had unprotected sex yesterday with her steady partner. She doesn't want to become pregnant. Your emergency treatment should be

    A. morgestrel (Ovral) 2 tablets once

    B. spermicide now and in 12 hours

    C. intravenous FSH and HCG

    D. Ovral 2 tablets now and in 12 hours

    E. Lo-Ovral 2 tablets now and in 12 hours

35. **Matching:** Genital ulcers
    1. Painless
    2. Purulent base
    3. Indurated
    4. Positive Tzanck smear
    5. Bubo formation
    6. Increased risk of HIV
    7. No risk to sexual partner

    A. Herpes simplex
    B. Syphilis
    C. Chancroid
    D. All of the above
    E. None of the above

36. The best contraceptive for a 16-year-old with a history of two pregnancies while on combination estrogen-progestin oral contraceptives and a steady sexual partner is

    A. an intrauterine device

    B. an all-progestin oral contraceptive

    C. condoms

    D. levo-norgestrel (Norplant)

    E. a cervical cap

PART 13

The Immunologic System and Disorders

Although acquired immunodeficiency syndrome (AIDS) is a common cause of childhood immunodeficiency, its differential diagnosis could include many of the diseases discussed in the chapters in this part of the *Nelson Textbook*. The chapters have been updated and include topics such as B-cell, T-cell, and combined B- and T-cell disorders in addition to diseases of the complement system and the leukocytes. Finally, the treatment of some of these disorders, bone marrow transplantation, is discussed in a separate and detailed chapter.

Questions in this part are related to the approach to children with recurrent infections and suspected immunodeficiency. The questions help distinguish the many different disorders according to the nature and extent of the infectious complications.

1. All of the following are associated with chronic granulomatous disease (CGD) EXCEPT
   A. autosomal recessive inheritance
   B. pyloric outlet obstruction
   C. *Aspergillus* pneumonia
   D. perianal abscess
   E. hypogammaglobulinemia

2. A 5-year-old boy presents with his third episode of painful cervical lymphadenitis. Each was treated with incision and drainage and grew *Staphylococcus aureus*. At the age of 2 years, he required surgical aspiration of a liver abscess. The most important laboratory test is
   A. PCR for ADA deficiency
   B. nitroblue tetrazolium test
   C. MAC-1 assay
   D. neutrophil count
   E. bone marrow aspiration

3. The most likely diagnosis in the patient described in Question 2 is
   A. Bruton agammaglobulinemia
   B. AIDS
   C. chronic granulomatous disease
   D. Kostmann disease
   E. cyclic neutropenia

4. Long-term effective therapy for the patient described in Question 2 is best accomplished with
   A. intravenous immunoglobulin
   B. interferon-γ
   C. interleukin-2
   D. bone marrow transplantation
   E. granulocyte transfusion

5. Neutropenia is noted in children in all of the following conditions EXCEPT
   A. Kostmann disease
   B. viral infection
   C. maternal preeclampsia
   D. Hunter syndrome
   E. Shwachman-Diamond syndrome
   F. glycogen storage disease type Ib
   G. neonatal alloimmune processes

6. **Matching:** Complement deficiency
   1. Lupus-like syndrome
   2. Recurrent neisserial infection
   3. Severe, recurrent pneumococcal infection

   A. C5, 6, 7, 8, 9
   B. C3
   C. C1q
   D. C1 inhibitor
   E. Properdin

4. Fatal meningococcal infection in males

5. Nonpitting edema

7. The complete DiGeorge syndrome is associated with all of the following EXCEPT

A. neonatal hypocalcemia

B. aortic atresia

C. graft-versus-host disease after blood transfusion

D. chromosomal deletion at 22q11.2

E. onset of infections after 12 months of age

F. micrognathia

8. **Matching:** Immunodeficiency

1. Fatal echovirus encephalitis
2. Splenomegaly
3. Chromosome 2q12
4. Mandibular hypoplasia
5. May be confused with AIDS
6. Most severe of congenital immuno-deficiencies
7. High frequency of autoimmune disorders
8. Rib cage anomalies
9. Lymphopenia plus severe neutropenia
10. Elevated IgE levels and eosinophilia

A. DiGeorge syndrome
B. Bruton syndrome
C. Common variable immuno-deficiency
D. Hyper IgM
E. CD8 lympho-cytopenia
F. Nezelof syndrome
G. Severe combined immunodefi-ciency (SCID)
H. Omenn syndrome
I. Reticular dysgenesis
J. Adenosine deaminase (ADA) deficiency

9. A 40-day-old, previously healthy, full-term female infant manifests fever, lethargy, and poor feeding for 12 hours. Physical examination reveals a lethargic child with vital signs of RR 70, HR 185, BP mean 25, T 39.50°C. The peripheral perfusion is poor, the chest reveals retractions, the abdomen is soft and reveals persistence of the umbilical cord, and the extremities are cool. Laboratory studies reveal a white blood cell count of 65,000 and a platelet count of 105,000. Family history reveals that a male sibling died suddenly at the age of 2 months, 10 years prior to the birth of this child. The most likely diagnosis is

A. chronic granulomatous disease

B. congenital leukemia

C. Kostmann syndrome

D. leukocyte adhesion deficiency

E. neutrophil myeloperoxidase deficiency

10. Evaluations of immune function should be initiated for otherwise healthy children with which of the following infections?

A. any serious documented bacterial infection (e.g., pneumonia)

B. any life-threatening bacterial infection (e.g., sepsis, meningitis)

C. four or more colds within 1 year

D. infections with unusual organisms (e.g., *Nocardia* spp.)

E. all of the above

11. The initial screening laboratory evaluation of a child with recurrent infections for possible immunodeficiency includes all of the following EXCEPT

A. complete blood count and differential

B. absolute lymphocyte count

C. immunoglobulins

D. platelet count

E. nitroblue tetrazolium test

12. Which of the following tests is an effective screening for T-cell function?

A. Absolute lymphocyte count

B. Flow cytometry for CD4 (helper) and CD8 (cytotoxic) T cells

C. Nitroblue tetrazolium test

D. *Candida* skin test

E. Mumps antibody test after mumps vaccination

13. A child is found to have a normal WBC count but serum concentrations of IgG, IgA, IgM, and IgE below the 95% lower limits for age. Which is the most likely diagnosis?
    A. Ataxia-telangiectasia
    B. X-linked lymphoproliferative syndrome
    C. DiGeorge syndrome
    D. Common variable immunodeficiency
    E. X-linked agammaglobulinemia

14. Which is the most common defined immunodeficiency disorder?
    A. Common variable immunodeficiency
    B. Selective IgA deficiency
    C. X-linked agammaglobulinemia
    D. X-linked lymphoproliferative syndrome
    E. Ataxia-telangectasia

15. The X-linked lymphoproliferative (XLP) syndrome is classically associated with overwhelming infection with which organism?
    A. Epstein-Barr virus
    B. Enteroviruses
    C. Catalase-positive organisms
    D. *Neisseria meningitidis*
    E. *Pneumocystis carinii*

16. Which is not true about DiGeorge syndrome?
    A. It occurs approximately equally in both males and females.
    B. Hypoplasia of the thymus and parathyroids is more common than aplasia.
    C. Children with partial DiGeorge have little trouble with infections.
    D. Absolute lymphocyte counts are usually markedly low.
    E. Concentrations of serum IgG, IgM, and IgA are usually normal.

17. Which of the following is not a prominent feature of Wiskott-Aldrich syndrome?
    A. Atopic dermatitis
    B. Thrombocytopenia

C. Recurrent infections with encapsulated bacteria
D. Leukopenia
E. X-linked recessive inheritance

18. In addition to recurrent staphylococcal abscesses and elevated serum IgE, the clinical manifestations of hyperimmunoglobulinemia E (hyper-IgE) syndrome frequently include which of the following?
    A. Recurrent pneumonia
    B. Pneumatoceles
    C. Recurrent fractures
    D. Hyperextensible joints
    E. All of the above

19. Which of the following is not true of monocytes and neutrophils?
    A. Monocytes, unlike neutrophils, have an unlimited capacity to divide.
    B. Monocytes remain longer in the circulation than do neutrophils.
    C. Monocytes in tissues (macrophages) can persist for months.
    D. Only neutrophils kill organisms by ingestion.

20. Which of the following is not typically associated with an eosinophilic response and eosinophilia?
    A. Allergic rhinitis
    B. Hypersensitivity drug reactions
    C. Trichinosis *(Trichinella spiralis)*
    D. Pinworms *(Enterobius vermicularis)*
    E. Wiskott-Aldrich syndrome

21. What is the phagocytic defect of chronic granulomatous disease?
    A. Defect of transendothelial migration
    B. Inability to ingest microorganisms
    C. Inability to activate the neutrophil respiratory burst
    D. Myeloperoxidase deficiency
    E. Excessive formation of H_2O_2

22. Delayed separation of the umbilical cord after birth suggests which type of immune dysfunction?
    A. B-cell defect

B. T-cell defect

C. Combined B- and T-cell defect

D. Phagocyte function defect

E. Complement component deficiency

23. A 4-month-old female presents with diarrhea and malabsorption, and on initial laboratory testing has a WBC count of 900/mm³. Which of the following is the most likely diagnosis?

A. Cystic fibrosis

B. Shwachman-Diamond syndrome

C. Cyclic neutropenia

D. Chronic granulomatous disease

E. Severe combined immunodeficiency

24. Which of the following is not associated with neutropenia?

A. Leukocyte adhesion deficiency

B. Shwachman-Diamond syndrome

C. Cartilage-hair hypoplasia

D. Chédiak-Higashi syndrome

E. Glycogen storage disease type Ib

25. Repeated meningococcal infections suggest what type of immune disorder?

A. B-cell defect

B. T-cell defect

C. Combined B- and T-cell defect

D. Phagocyte function defect

E. Complement component deficiency

26. Cyclic neutropenia is usually associated with all of the following EXCEPT

A. oral ulcerations

B. periodontal disease

C. cyclic reticulocytosis

D. septicemia

E. cellulitis

27. A 6-month-old presents with recurrent cellulitis and bacteremias due to *Staphylococcus aureus*. The white blood cell count is 2500 with 5% neutrophils, 10% eosinophils, 35% monocytes, and 50% lymphocytes. The platelet count is 650,000. A brother and a female cousin died at the age of 18 months and 2 years, respectively. The most likely diagnosis is

A. AIDS

B. severe combined immunodeficiency

C. Kostmann disease

D. cyclic neutropenia

E. chronic granulomatous disease

28. Long-term treatment of the disease described in Question 27 is best accomplished with

A. prophylactic antibiotics

B. intravenous immunoglobulin

C. interferon

D. G-CSF

E. bone marrow transplant

29. Reported complications of intravenous immunoglobulin therapy include all of the following EXCEPT

A. hepatitis C

B. anaphylaxis

C. fluid overload

D. AIDS

E. pain at site of injection

F. aseptic meningitis

PART 14

Allergic Disorders

It must be an "allergy"! This seems to be many patients' or parents' belief about many signs and symptoms. Alternatively, allergies may be mistakenly diagnosed as recurrent infections or other chronic disorders. Allergies may be relatively benign but annoying problems, such as allergic rhinitis; however, allergy-related immune problems, such as asthma or anaphylaxis, may create life-threatening crises. Furthermore, the prevalence of all allergies may be increasing, including the prevalence and possibly the severity of asthma. This part of the *Nelson Textbook* also discusses serum sickness, atopic dermatitis, urticaria, angioedema, insect and ocular allergies, and adverse food reactions. Finally, the treatments for these disorders are discussed in detail with current data.

Being able to answer the questions in this part will help readers identify and manage common, uncomplicated allergic problems in children.

1. The skin of patients with atopic dermatitis exhibits all of the following EXCEPT
   A. Wheal and flare reaction after intradermal injection of an allergen
   B. white dermographism
   C. abnormal rates of cooling
   D. blanching after intradermal histamine injection
   E. reduced threshold for skin infections

2. **Matching:**

   1. Begins on scalp   A. Eczema
   2. Weepy, crusty lesions   B. Seborrhea
   3. Responds more rapidly   C. Neither
      D. Both
   4. Greasy lesions
   5. Dry skin
   6. Pruritus
   7. Keratoconus
   8. Stomatitis
   9. Scales

3. A 12-year-old with repeated episodes of streptococcal pharyngitis experiences another episode of sore throat. The rapid strep test result is positive, and oral amoxicillin is started, with the first dose given in the office. One hour later, she experiences a funny feeling and a tingling sensation around her mouth. Next she becomes apprehensive, has difficulty swallowing, and develops a hoarse voice. On arrival at the emergency room, she has giant urticaria and the following vital signs: pulse 130, respiratory rate 32, blood pressure 70/30, and temperature 37.2°C. The most appropriate therapy is
   A. epinephrine
   B. prednisone
   C. diphenhydramine (Benadryl)
   D. cimetidine
   E. lactated Ringer's solution

4. The most likely diagnosis for the condition described in Question 3 is
   A. streptococcal toxic shock
   B. scarlet fever
   C. infectious mononucleosis
   D. anaphylaxis
   E. hay fever

5. Eosinophilia is observed in all of the following EXCEPT
   A. *Giardia* infection
   B. *Toxocara* infection
   C. drug hypersensitivity
   D. periarteritis nodosa
   E. allergy

6. All of the following may increase plasma levels of theophylline EXCEPT

A. cimetidine

B. erythromycin

C. influenza vaccine

D. smoking marijuana

E. ketoconazole

7. A 12-year-old presents with sneezing, clear rhinorrhea, and nasal itching. Physical examination reveals boggy, pale nasal edema with a clear discharge. The most likely diagnosis is

A. foreign body

B. vasomotor rhinitis

C. neutrophilic rhinitis

D. nasal mastocytosis

E. allergic rhinitis

8. Two weeks later, the patient described in Question 7 complains of headache, poor nasal airflow (mouth breathing), fever, and a change in the nature of the nasal discharge; it is now mucopurulent. The most likely diagnosis is

A. sinusitis

B. foreign body

C. rhinitis medicamentosa

D. choanal stenosis

E. ciliary dyskinesia

9. Immunotherapy provides symptomatic improvement in all of the following EXCEPT

A. ragweed allergy

B. local reaction to bee sting

C. tree pollen allergy

D. house dust mite allergy

E. anaphylaxis to a wasp sting

10. An 8-year-old boy experienced generalized urticaria immediately after a honeybee sting 2 months ago. He had no other symptoms except for a large local reaction at the site of the sting. Skin testing with honeybee venom has been strongly positive at a weak concentration. Appropriate recommendations include all of the following EXCEPT

A. immunotherapy

B. an epinephrine auto-injector (EpiPen) for administration if stung again

C. wearing shoes when outdoors

D. a Medic-Alert bracelet

E. wearing long pants

11. The mother of an 8-year-old boy with acute streptococcal tonsillitis calls to report that within 15 minutes after the first dose of penicillin V you prescribed, he is complaining of itching and has developed hives. You should recommend

A. oral Benadryl and call again if not improved within 30 minutes

B. immediate return to your office or the nearest emergency room

C. return to your office or the nearest emergency room if he becomes short of breath or loses consciousness

D. that they go to the laboratory for determination of serum tryptase level

E. substitution of erythromycin for penicillin

12. A 4-year-old boy with asthma has had mild wheezing only four times since you began treating him 6 months ago with theophylline (Slo-bid) Gyrocaps twice each day. He previously experienced coughing and wheezing at least three times each week. (A peak serum theophylline concentration 5 months ago was 16 µg/mL). For the past 4 days, he has again experienced mild coughing and wheezing responsive to inhaled albuterol. Two days ago, an emergency room physician began treatment with erythromycin/sulfisoxazole (Pediazole) for otitis media. This morning the youngster began vomiting. You should consider the likely cause of vomiting to be

A. provocation by coughing

B. infection

C. theophylline toxicity

D. albuterol toxicity

E. Pediazole intolerance

13. Which form of hypersensitivity reaction is characterized by antigen-antibody reactions on the cell membrane with activation of complement and destruction of the involved cell?

A. type I hypersensitivity

B. type II hypersensitivity

C. type III hypersensitivity

D. type IV hypersensitivity

E. type V hypersensitivity

14. Which factor is released from mast cells?

A. Eosinophil major basic protein

B. Platelet-activating factor

C. Histamine

D. Bradykinin

E. Serotonin

15. Which is not a sign of moderate to severe airway obstruction that might result from allergic response?

A. Dennie lines

B. Supraclavicular and intercostal retractions

C. Cyanosis

D. Pulsus paradoxus

E. Respiratory distress with minimal wheezing and a few rales

16. Which does the radioallergosorbent test (RAST) determine?

A. Bronchial reactivity to serotonin

B. Bronchial reactivity to specific toxins

C. Bronchial reactivity after inhalation bronchial challenge

D. Antigen-specific serum IgE concentrations

E. Allergic profile based on total eosinophils, total IgE, and skin testing

17. Which is not true concerning skin testing for allergic reactivity?

A. Antihistamines given prior to testing may inhibit the reaction.

B. Intradermal tests are more sensitive than puncture tests.

C. Positive skin test results by intradermal testing correlate better than puncture tests with clinical symptoms.

D. Positive skin test results do not necessarily indicate that the person will have clinical symptoms.

E. Larger reactions have greater clinical relevance.

18. Which is an advantage of skin testing compared with RAST to determine specific IgE?

A. Skin testing is not affected by administration of antihistamines.

B. Skin testing has greater sensitivity than RAST.

C. Skin testing is semiquantitative.

D. Skin testing is less expensive than RAST.

E. Skin testing is associated with less risk of allergic reaction.

19. Which is recommended as helpful in minimizing allergy to house dust mites?

A. Maximizing time spent in the house to a single room such as the bedroom

B. Washing bedding weekly in cold water

C. Installing new carpet

D. Keeping household humidity to less than 50%

E. All of the above are recommended.

20. Which anti-adrenergic activity of drugs is most desirable in treatment of allergic disorders?

A. α_1

B. α_2

C. $\beta_1 + \beta_2$

D. β_1

E. β_2

21. Which is true of antihistamines?

A. Classification of antihistamines from type I to type VI is based on increasing antihistamine activity.

B. Second-generation antihistamines are distinguished by greater effectiveness than first-generation antihistamines.

C. Antihistamines should not be administered in combination with decongestants.

D. Antihistamines are more effective in treating than preventing the action of histamine.

E. The choice of antihistamines should be based on associated adverse effects and cost.

22. Which is true of cromolyn?

A. It prevents antibody-mediated mast cell degranulation.

B. It prevents non–antibody-mediated mast cell degranulation.

C. It has no bronchodilator properties.

D. The incidence of adverse effects is low.

E. All of the above are true.

23. A 12-year-old child presents with watery rhinorrhea, paroxysmal sneezing, and nasal obstruction. The serum IgE level is normal, and skin test results are negative. A trial of antihistamine-decongestant therapy has not improved symptoms. Which is the recommended treatment?

A. Institute strict measures to avoid outdoor allergen exposure.

B. Begin seasonal use of sympathomimetic drugs.

C. Begin seasonal use of topical corticosteroids.

D. Amoxicillin for 10 days

E. Cefpodoxime for 10–14 days

24. A 10-year-old child has intermittent symptoms of mild asthma. Which treatment option is most appropriate?

A. Environmental control and patient education only; no medication is needed

B. Oral theophylline

C. Cromolyn

D. Inhaled β_2-agonist as needed for symptoms

E. Daily inhaled corticosteroid

25. The child in Question 24 has symptoms that worsen and are now persistent and of moderate severity. Which treatment option is most appropriate?

A. Oral theophylline

B. Inhaled β_2-agonist as needed for symptoms

C. Daily inhaled corticosteroid

D. Daily inhaled corticosteroid and a long-acting inhaled β_2-agonist

E. Daily inhaled corticosteroid, a long-acting inhaled β_2-agonist, and oral theophylline

26. Which is not a major criterion for diagnosis of atopic dermatitis in older children and adults?

A. Eczematous or lichenified dermatitis

B. Pruritus

C. Angioedema

D. Chronic or relapsing course

E. Family history of atopic disease

27. A 3-year-old is diagnosed with atopic dermatitis. Which environmental modification is recommended?

A. A bland diet, especially minimizing meats

B. Installation of wool carpeting instead of synthetic carpeting

C. Wear cotton garments

D. Use soaps and detergents that are especially effective in removing fatty substances

E. Avoid bath oils

28. Which is the most appropriate prognosis to relate to the parents of the 3-year-old in Question 27 with atopic dermatitis?

A. The child will be asymptomatic with standard local treatments.

B. Symptoms will gradually worsen during childhood, then gradually improve.

C. Symptoms will exhibit a remittent but progressively worsening course.

D. Symptoms will gradually improve over the next several years.

E. Symptoms will most likely resolve completely at puberty.

29. A 14-year-old presents with acute onset of urticaria that has gradually worsened over the past 10 days. Detailed history reveals no clues as to the possible etiology. The physical examination is normal except for urticaria. Which diagnostic option is recommended?

A. Systematic elimination diets to determine a possible ingestant cause

B. Allergy skin testing

C. Serum IgE and RAST

D. Skin biopsy

E. None of the above

30. Which treatment option is recommended for the patient in Question 29?

A. Oral prednisone

B. Wear cotton garments

C. A bland diet

D. Diphenhydramine

E. Loratadine

31. Which is not true concerning anaphylaxis?

A. Virtually any foreign substance can elicit an anaphylactic reaction.

B. Most anaphylactic reactions are due to drugs, foods, or Hymenoptera allergy.

C. Exercise alone can elicit an anaphylactic reaction.

D. Most anaphylactic reactions begin within 30 minutes of exposure.

E. The more rapid the symptoms appear after exposure, the more serious the reaction.

32. Which is the treatment of choice for anaphylaxis?

A. Diphenhydramine orally

B. Diphenhydramine by intravenous infusion

C. Aqueous epinephrine (1:1,000) by subcutaneous injection

D. Aqueous epinephrine (1:1,000) by intramuscular injection

E. Aqueous epinephrine (1:1,000) by intravenous infusion

33. A 16-year-old with history of anaphylaxis to Hymenoptera suffers a sting on an extremity. The first-aid kit that is available includes aqueous epinephrine, 1:1,000, and other necessary medical supplies. Which is *not* recommended for the management of this sting?

A. Infiltration of one half of the epinephrine dose subcutaneously around the site of the sting

B. Repeat doses of aqueous epinephrine at 15-minute intervals if necessary

C. A tourniquet placed above the site of the sting

D. Incision and suction of venom from the site of the sting

E. Transfer to an emergency room

34. A 2-year-old child who has just completed a course of cefaclor presents with low-grade fever, malaise, irritability, lymphadenopathy, and a generalized erythematous rash that is mildly pruritic. Which is the most likely diagnosis?

A. Partially treated meningitis

B. Infectious mononucleosis

C. Kawasaki disease

D. Type I hypersensitivity reaction

E. Type III hypersensitivity reaction

35. Which is not true concerning adverse drug reactions?

A. Topical administration is more likely to elicit sensitization than parenteral administration.

B. Parenteral administration is more likely to elicit sensitization than oral administration.

C. Frequent, intermittent administration is more likely to elicit sensitization than prolonged, continual administration.

D. The risk of sensitization is independent of dose.

E. Allergy to one antibiotic indicates an increased risk of allergy to an unrelated antibiotic.

36. Which is not a manifestation of insect allergy?

A. Rhinitis and conjunctivitis

B. Asthma

C. Wheal and flare

D. Anaphylaxis

E. Uveitis

37. Which is not true concerning allergic reactions to stinging insects?

A. The majority are due to Hymenoptera.

B. There is substantial cross-reactivity among vespid venoms.

C. Systemic reactions may occur after the first sting.

D. Most reactions are IgE-mediated.

E. Negative skin test and RAST results exclude the possibility of anaphylaxis.

38. A 15-year-old with a history of seasonal hay fever now also has itchy eyes, profuse tearing, and reddened and edematous conjunctivae. Which treatment option is effective for the ocular symptoms?

    A. Topical sympathomimetics (naphazoline or phenylephrine)
    B. Topical levocabastine (a selective H_1-receptor antagonist)
    C. Topical lodoxamide tromethamine (a mast cell stabilizer)
    D. Topical corticosteroids for severe cases
    E. All of these are effective.

39. Which is not true concerning allergic reactions to foods?

    A. Most adverse reactions to foods do not have an immunologic basis.
    B. Rashes and diarrhea after ingestion of fruit juices usually have an immunologic basis.
    C. Positive skin test results must be confirmed by food challenge.
    D. Persons with IgE-mediated food reactions consistently have positive skin test results.
    E. Negative skin test results reliably predict the absence of clinical symptoms.

PART 15

Rheumatic Diseases of Childhood

Rheumatic, autoimmune, connective tissue, and collagen vascular diseases are related terms of common disorders that are often difficult to manage, and rarely curable. The disorders are also difficult to distinguish from one another. This part teaches you to avoid the old statement, "When in doubt of a diagnosis with multiple organ involvement, say SLE." Indeed, this part has individual chapters on juvenile rheumatoid arthritis (JRA), the spondyloarthropathies, systemic lupus erythematosus (SLE), vasculitis syndromes (Henoch-Schönlein purpura, Kawasaki disease), dermatomyositis, scleroderma, mixed connective tissue disease, and many more.

Readers will not immediately become a rheumatologist wiz-kid, but they will find these questions educationally rewarding as they reiterate important concepts and points of diagnosis and management from the *Nelson Textbook*.

---

1. A 5-year-old boy develops severe abdominal pain of 3 days' duration. He is unable to eat and has occasional emesis. Physical examination reveals an anxious, acutely ill child with generalized abdominal tenderness, voluntary guarding of the anterior abdominal muscles, and normal findings on rectal examination. A surgical consultant believes the child has an acute abdomen, possibly appendicitis. Before the child is sent to the operating room, the urinalysis reveals 3 + hematuria and 1 + proteinuria. You should
   A. perform coagulation studies
   B. obtain a complete blood count
   C. perform renal ultrasonography
   D. proceed with the operation
   E. cancel the operation

2. On repeat physical examination, the patient described in Question 1 now has petechiae over the dorsal surfaces of the feet and hands and over the buttocks. His platelet count is 350,000. The most likely diagnosis is
   A. Kawasaki syndrome
   B. Henoch-Schönlein purpura
   C. Rocky Mountain spotted fever
   D. meningococcemia
   E. appendicitis with gram-negative sepsis

3. A 7-year-old white male presents with malaise, chest pain, high spiking fevers, and chills for 3 weeks. He has had no ill contacts, and he has missed school during the last week of the illness. Physical examination reveals an acutely ill child with a heart rate of 125, a temperature of 40.5°C, a fine but faint macular red-pink rash on the trunk and proximal extremities, lymphadenopathy, a liver 4 cm below the right costal margin, and a palpable spleen tip. Laboratory studies reveal a hemoglobin of 9.7 g/dL, a total white blood cell count of 26,000, and a platelet count of 650,000. The most important step in evaluating this patient would be to order
   A. an erythrocyte sedimentation rate (ESR)
   B. Lyme titers
   C. a chest radiograph
   D. an echocardiogram
   E. bone marrow aspiration

4. On further evaluation, the patient described in Question 3 has no evidence of pericardial tamponade or reduced cardiac function. His pulse normalizes when he defervesces. The approach to the management of this patient's pericardial effusion is to
   A. perform pericardiocentesis
   B. begin digitalization

C. improve preload with fluids

D. begin an oral nonsteroidal anti-inflammatory agent

E. begin methotrexate

5. The most likely diagnosis for the patient described in Question 3 is

A. systemic-onset juvenile rheumatoid arthritis

B. uremia

C. systemic lupus erythematosus

D. scleroderma

E. rheumatic fever

6. **Matching:**

1. High spiking fevers	A. Oligoarticular JRA
2. Predominantly affects knees and ankles	B. Polyarticular JRA
3. Affects large and small joints	C. Systemic-onset JRA
4. HLA-B27	D. Polyarticular rheumatoid factor positive
5. Most severe joint destruction	E. Spondyloarthropathy

7. A 9-year-old female notices that she has difficulty combing her hair and walking up stairs for approximately 1 month. Physical examination reveals a positive Gower sign and a faint maculopapular rash over the metacarpophalangeal joints. The most appropriate laboratory study to order is

A. erythrocyte sedimentation rate

B. serum creatinine phosphokinase

C. rheumatoid factor

D. motor nerve conduction study

E. antinuclear antibodies

8. The most likely diagnosis for the patient described in Question 7 is

A. muscular dystrophy

B. dermatomyositis

C. periarteritis nodosa

D. systemic lupus erythematosus

E. myotonic dystrophy

9. **Matching:**

1. Antibody to ribonuclear protein	A. Fasciitis
2. Tuberculosis	B. Relapsing panniculitis
3. Eosinophilia	C. Behçet syndrome
4. Painful red nodules on the thighs	D. Mixed connective tissue disease
5. Recurrent and chronic "croup"	E. Erythema nodosum
6. Uveitis	F. Relapsing polychondritis
7. Xerostomia	G. Sjögren syndrome

10. Erythema nodosum, an erythematous, nodular, often pretibial rash is associated with all of the following EXCEPT

A. inflammatory bowel disease

B. pseudotumor cerebri

C. sarcoidosis

D. *Yersinia*

E. group A *Streptococcus*

F. birth control pills

11. Positive ANA tests (titer $\geq$ 1:80) is associated with all of the following EXCEPT

A. systemic lupus erythematosus

B. juvenile rheumatoid arthritis

C. autoimmune hepatitis

D. dermatomyositis

E. salicylate intoxication

F. phenytoin

12. Low levels of complement may be associated with all of the following EXCEPT

A. nephrotic syndrome

B. vasculitis

C. nephritis

D. serum sickness

E. systemic lupus erythematosus

13. Pseudoporphyria is best described as a complication of

A. lupus

B. naproxen

C. dermatomyositis

D. prednisone

E. topical chloroquine

14. **Matching:** Drug therapy

1. Methotrexate	A. Blindness
2. Methylprednis-olone	B. Hypertension
3. Hydroxychloro-quine	C. Stevens-Johnson syn-drome
4. Sulfasalazine	D. Stomatitis
5. Intravenous immunoglobu-lins	E. Aseptic men-ingitis

15. **Matching:** JRA

1. Chronic uveitis	A. Polyarthritis
2. Erosive joint disease	B. Oligoarthritis
3. Cervical spine involvement	C. Systemic onset
4. Low back pain	D. All of the above
5. High spiking quotidian fever	E. None of the above
6. Erythematous diffuse macular rash	
7. Endocarditis	
8. Erythema migrans	

16. A 4-year-old white female has had joint swelling in multiple joints for over 6 months. She is slow to move in the morning and moves as if stiff for the first hours of the day. Thereafter she is a very active child. She has no rash and very little limitation of range of motion. Her ESR is 4. The most likely diagnosis is

A. hypermobility syndrome

B. dermatomyositis

C. SLE

D. JRA

E. Henoch-Schönlein purpura

17. The spondyloarthropathies are characterized by involvement of the axial skeleton and the presence of enthesitis (inflammation at the attachment of tendons to bone). These disorders include all of the following EXCEPT

A. polyarticular rheumatoid factor–negative JRA

B. psoriatic arthritis

C. inflammatory bowel disease arthritis

D. reactive arthritis secondary to diarrhea

E. reactive to arthritis due to genitourinary infection

18. Infectious agents associated with arthritis (nonpurulent) include all of the following EXCEPT

A. rubella vaccine

B. parvovirus

C. *Yersinia*

D. *Campylobacter*

E. respiratory syncytial virus

F. hepatitis B

19. All of the following are diagnostic criteria for the diagnosis of SLE EXCEPT

A. malar rash

B. arthritis

C. seizures

D. Raynaud phenomenon

E. thrombocytopenia

F. pericarditis

20. A 12-year-old white female presents with arthralgias of the knees and elbow and swollen hands of 6 months' duration. She has intermittent fever and has lost 15 pounds. Other than swollen joints, her physical examination is normal. Three years prior to this time, she was found to have thrombocytopenia and was diag-nosed with idiopathic thrombocytopenic purpura (ITP). In addition, one summer she had severe sunburn, and 2 years ago she had mouth sores. Today she has a he-matocrit of 25% and a positive Coombs test result; in addition, the urinalysis re-veals multiple red blood cells. The most likely diagnosis is

A. JRA

B. ITP

C. Evans syndrome

D. periarteritis

E. SLE

21. Laboratory data in the patient in Question 20 reveals a positive antibody to double-stranded DNA, a positive antinuclear antibody (ANA), and undetectable complement levels. The best approach to treatment is
    A. intravenous immune globulin (IVIG)
    B. plasmapheresis
    C. cyclosporine
    D. prednisone
    E. ibuprofen

22. After all symptoms have resolved in the patient in Questions 20 and 21, the serum complement levels remain very low. The family history is also positive for an aunt with lupus. The most likely reason for the low complement at this time is
    A. immune complex formation
    B. subclinical nephritis
    C. congenital complement deficiency
    D. prednisone therapy
    E. familial angioedema

23. A 12-year-old female has had difficulty in getting out of chairs and combing her hair for 3 months. Physical examination reveals tenderness over the quadricep muscles and 4/5 strength. In addition, there is a faint erythematous rash over both upper eyelids. The next step in the diagnosis is
    A. serum ANA
    B. serum creatine phosphokinase (CPK)
    C. complement
    D. muscle biopsy
    E. nerve conduction study

24. The patient in Question 23 begins to have difficulty swallowing solids and starts to drool. The most likely problem is
    A. palatopharyngeal muscle weakness
    B. bulbar neuropathy
    C. anterior horn cell disease
    D. botulism
    E. trichinosis

25. The most likely diagnosis of the patient in Questions 23 and 24 is

    A. polio
    B. JRA
    C. dermatomyositis
    D. scleroderma
    E. viral myositis

26. All of the following are true about Kawasaki disease EXCEPT
    A. it occurs in outbreaks
    B. it is a vasculitis
    C. exposure to an affected patient greatly increases the risk of the disease
    D. Asian children have the highest risk
    E. 80% of patients are less than 5 years old
    F. it is the leading cause of acquired heart disease in children in the United States

27. Possible complications of Kawasaki disease include all of the following EXCEPT
    A. arthritis
    B. splenic rupture
    C. aseptic meningitis
    D. urethritis
    E. hydrops of the gall bladder

28. The most common cause of death from Kawasaki disease in the early phase of disease is
    A. myocardial infarction
    B. rupture of an aneurysm
    C. stroke
    D. myocarditis
    E. pericarditis

29. The differential diagnosis of Kawasaki disease includes all of the following EXCEPT
    A. dermatomyositis
    B. toxic shock syndrome
    C. scarlet fever
    D. Stevens-Johnson syndrome
    E. measles
    F. Rocky Mountain spotted fever

30. A 4-year-old white female has a low grade fever, intermittent crampy

abdominal pain with emesis, and swollen knees of 3 days' duration. There is a petechial rash of the lower extremity. The most likely diagnosis is
A. meningococcemia
B. idiopathic thrombocytopenia purpura
C. Henoch-Schönlein purpura
D. SLE
E. Rocky Mountain spotted fever

31. All of the following are complications of Henoch-Schönlein purpura EXCEPT
A. seizures
B. coronary aneurysms
C. pancreatitis
D. pulmonary hemorrhage
E. neuropathy

32. Serious persistent renal disease occurs in what percent of children with HSP?
A. <0.1%
B. <10%
C. 2% of males
D. None
E. 5% of females

33. **Matching:**
1. Relapsing polychondritis
2. Sweet syndrome
3. Hypertrophic osteoarthropathy
4. Plant thorn synovitis
5. Diabetes mellitus

A. Neutrophilic perivascular infiltrates
B. Clubbing
C. Monoarticular chronic arthritis
D. Thick and tight soft tissue of hands
E. External ear involvement

34. A 12-year-old black female has had a 2-year history of chronic sinusitis. Today she has an episode of hemoptysis and respiratory distress. Her urinalysis reveals hematuria. The most helpful laboratory test is
A. Sm antibody
B. antiPR3 ANCA
C. angiotensin converting enzyme level

D. ANA speckled
E. ESR

35. The most likely diagnosis for the patient in Question 34 is
A. SLE
B. Goodpasture disease
C. Wegener granulomatosis
D. sarcoidosis
E. tuberculosis

36. The most appropriate therapy is (may choose more than one)
A. cyclosporine
B. Imfliximab
C. prednisone
D. cyclophosphamide
E. vincristine

37. An 18-year-old male has a swollen right wrist and left ankle with bilateral pain over both Achilles tendons. Two weeks before this, he received an antibiotic for a urethral discharge; his girlfriend was also treated. Physical examination reveals tenderness over both Achilles tendons, swollen painful joints (right wrist, left ankle), and limited forward bending at the waist. The most likely course of treatment would be
A. ceftriaxone
B. doxycycline
C. prednisone
D. nonsteroidal anti-inflammatory agents
E. intravenous immunoglobulin

38. Which of the following are associated with poor prognosis of juvenile rheumatoid arthritis?
A. Female sex
B. Older age
C. Involvement of the joints of the hands and wrists
D. Seropositive for rheumatoid factor
E. All of the above

39. Which organism is associated with reactive arthritis?
A. *Shigella*
B. *Chlamydia trachomatis*

C. *Yersinia enterocolitica*

D. *Campylobacter jejuni*

E. All of the above

40. Which of the following is the preferred initial choice of therapy for most rheumatic diseases?
    A. Nonsteroidal anti-inflammatory drugs
    B. Cyclophosphamide
    C. Methotrexate
    D. Sulfasalazine
    E. Azathioprine

41. Which is a component of the diagnostic criteria for systemic lupus erythematosus?
    A. Leukocytosis (>15,000/mm³)
    B. Seizures
    C. Subcutaneous nodules
    D. False-positive heterophil test
    E. Erosive arthritis involving two or more peripheral joints

42. A 4-year-old Middle-Eastern boy presents with a history of brief acute episodes of fever and abdominal pain. The most likely diagnosis is
    A. Beçhet syndrome
    B. Sjögren syndrome
    C. juvenile dermatomyositis
    D. familial Mediterranean fever
    E. amyloidosis

43. **Matching:** Physical findings of rheumatic or vasculitic diseases
    1. Gottron papules
    2. Malar rash
    3. Raynaud phenomenon
    4. Enlarged salivary glands
    5. Coronary artery aneurysms
    6. Palpable petechiae

    A. Sjögren syndrome
    B. Scleroderma
    C. Henoch-Schönlein purpura
    D. Kawasaki disease
    E. Systemic lupus erythematosus
    F. Juvenile dermatomyositis

PART 16

Infectious Diseases

Talk about a "play within a play"—this mega part is a book within a book. The part is divided into 15 sections with a total of more than 200 chapters and subchapters. The sections include an overview in addition to clinical syndromes caused by various infectious agents (fever, sepsis, meningitis, pneumonia, gastroenteritis, and others); there are sections on bacterial, viral, mycotic, rickettsial, and parasitic infections as well as one on prevention. Because infections are common pediatric problems at all ages of development, many new and authoritative contributors have extensively updated this part of the *Nelson Textbook*. Cross-references are provided to pertinent organ-specific infections produced by a particular pathogen and discussed in these sections.

Readers should enjoy working on the questions in this part of the book. You will not become an immediate infectious disease consultant, but you should be more knowledgeable about the common and occasionally the uncommon infectious diseases of children. By the way—beware of the uncommon. If one of the physician contributors can encounter malaria and typhoid fever in Wisconsin, almost anything may appear in your own clinic, emergency room, hospital ward, or intensive care unit.

---

1. You are asked to investigate an outbreak among children with profuse watery diarrhea in a daycare center. Likely etiology agents that you should consider include all of the following EXCEPT
   A. *Cryptosporidium*
   B. *Giardia*
   C. Rotavirus
   D. *Ascaris lumbricoides*

2. A 7-month-old child presents in late October with 3 days of fever to 103°F, a mildly injected pharynx, mild cervical adenopathy, and diarrhea. On the fourth day of the illness, the fever ceases and a measles-like rash appears. The most likely diagnosis is
   A. measles
   B. rubella
   C. drug reaction to antipyretics
   D. HHV-6 infection
   E. enteroviral infection

3. After diagnosis of pertussis in a toddler, erythromycin should be given to the patient and to which family members?
   A. Only those with a cough
   B. Only those younger than 7 years old

   C. Only those who are incompletely immunized
   D. Only those with compromised immunity
   E. All regardless of age, symptoms, or immunization status

4. A 3-year-old boy presents with a 7-day history of fever, cervical adenopathy, foul breath, and painful oral lesions on his tongue, gums, and lips. For the past 3 days, he has had a red, painful swollen area about the nail of his right thumb with an area of fluid by the nail bed, unresponsive to warm soaks and a first-generation cephalosporin. The most likely etiology is
   A. *Staphylococcus aureus*
   B. mucocutaneous candidiasis
   C. coxsackievirus
   D. adenovirus
   E. herpes simplex virus

5. A 13-month-old previously healthy child presents on New Year's Eve with a 1-day history of fever, lethargy, and left-side focal motor seizure activity. The cerebrospinal fluid (CSF) reveals 170 lymphocytes/mm³, 400 red blood cells/mm³, protein of 150 mg/dL, and

normal glucose level. MRI scan reveals right temporal abnormalities. The single most appropriate therapy to begin empirically while awaiting definitive diagnosis would be

A. ceftriaxone

B. nafcillin, cefotaxime, and metronidazole

C. acyclovir

D. amphotericin B

E. isoniazid, rifampin, pyrazinamide, and streptomycin

6. A full-term newborn male whose mother had reactive Venereal Disease Research Laboratory (VDRL) and microhemagglutination assay—*Treponema pallidum* (MHA-TP) results at the time of delivery was evaluated. He was anemic and had thrombocytopenia and mild hepatomegaly. He also had a desquamative skin rash consistent with congenital syphilis. His CSF was clear, with 5 white blood cells (WBCs), 0 RBCs, protein of 80 mg/dL, and glucose of 49 mg/dL; the CSF VDRL result was nonreactive. Based on this examination, which of the following is true?

A. The patient has symptomatic congenital syphilis but not neurosyphilis and can therefore be treated with benzathine penicillin.

B. The patient may be treated with a combination of ampicillin and gentamicin for 7–10 days.

C. Neurosyphilis cannot be ruled out in this infant; therefore, he should be treated as though he had neurosyphilis.

D. All cases of neurosyphilis would have CSF pleocytosis and a reactive CSF VDRL result.

7. *Nocardia* infection is an acute, subacute, or chronic suppurative infection that primarily causes pulmonary disease in immunocompromised patients. The hallmark of *Nocardia* infection is

A. a tendency to remissions and exacerbations

B. involvement of bone

C. a self-limited disease with scar formation

D. association in the pelvis with intrauterine device (IUD) placement

E. an association with sickle cell disease

8. A 16-year-old female presents with signs and symptoms of appendicitis. Her past medical history is significant only for sexual activity and placement of an IUD 1 year previously. She undergoes an appendectomy, in which her appendix is found to be normal. One month postoperatively, she has local pain and has an irregular, hard mass in her ileocecal area. The most likely diagnosis is

A. *Yersinia* pseudoappendicitis

B. lymphoma

C. inflammatory bowel disease

D. pelvic actinomycosis

E. amebiasis

9. A 15-year-old female wishes to play soccer in school and needs medical clearance. On physical examination, her liver edge is palpable and seems minimally enlarged. Ultrasonography of the liver shows one cyst approximately 3 cm in diameter. Her menstruation is normal. Results of serologic test results for *Echinococcus* and hepatitis are negative, and liver enzyme values are normal. She has lived her whole life in Salt Lake City, Utah, and has never traveled abroad. Which factor is most important in allowing her to play this sport?

A. Her travel history

B. Negative echinococcal serology

C. Negative hepatitis serology

D. Normal liver enzymes

E. Normal menstrual periods

10. The prognosis with cholera is poor if

A. illness is complicated by hypokalemia

B. acidosis develops

C. acute tubular necrosis develops

D. tachycardia and tachypnea develop

E. hypoglycemia and seizures occur

11. A 2-week illness characterized by gradually increasing fever that eventually reaches 104°F and is associated with headache, malaise, cough, and abdominal pain in a child who has recently returned from a visit to a developing country most likely is
    A. cholera
    B. diphtheria
    C. shigellosis
    D. typhoid fever
    E. tetanus

12. Antimotility agents have a role in therapy of acute diarrhea in infants and toddlers with gastroenteritis due to
    A. *Shigella*
    B. *Salmonella*
    C. enterohemorrhagic *E. coli*
    D. *Campylobacter*
    E. none of the above

13. Oral rehydration is the treatment of choice for all children with gastroenteritis EXCEPT those with
    A. high fever
    B. ileus and coma
    C. *Shigella dysenteriae*
    D. poor skin turgor, sunken fontanel, dry mouth, and decreased urine output

14. A 1-year-old child experiences ascending paralysis with peripheral neuropathy (cranial nerves are normal); the CSF is normal except for an elevated protein level. The likely infectious agent precipitating this syndrome is
    A. *Corynebacterium diphtheriae*
    B. *Clostridium botulinum*
    C. *S. dysenteriae* serotype 1
    D. *Campylobacter jejuni*
    E. *Clostridium tetani*

15. A 20-month-old develops hemolytic anemia, anuria, azotemia, and thrombocytopenia after a bout of febrile bloody diarrhea. What is the most likely cause of this illness?
    A. *C. jejuni*

B. *S. typhi*
C. Enterohemorrhagic *E. coli*
D. *Aeromonas*
E. non-typhi *Salmonella*

16. A 10-month-old child presents with a temperature of 105°F, watery diarrhea, and a generalized seizure. The most likely cause of this syndrome is
    A. *Salmonella* gastroenteritis
    B. *Aeromonas* gastroenteritis
    C. *Shigella* gastroenteritis
    D. Rotavirus gastroenteritis
    E. drug ingestion

17. Hemorrhagic cystitis, conjunctivitis, pneumonia, and diarrhea all have been linked to which of the following?
    A. Respiratory syncytial virus
    B. Adenovirus
    C. Rhinovirus
    D. Herpes simplex virus
    E. Parainfluenza virus

18. Toxoplasmosis causes all of the following patterns of disease EXCEPT
    A. congenital infection in neonates manifested by chorioretinitis, cerebral calcifications, and hydrocephalus due to first-trimester infection
    B. congenital infection in neonates who appear normal at birth but become blind in adolescence because they have retinal (macular) lesions that recrudesce at that time
    C. brain abscess that results in confusion, seizures, and paralysis in a patient with acquired immunodeficiency syndrome (AIDS)
    D. asymptomatic acute infection in a pregnant woman that places her unborn child at significant risk for congenital toxoplasmosis
    E. myocarditis in a previously healthy young adult
    F. pectoral lymphadenopathy that is mistaken for breast cancer in a middle-aged woman
    G. congenital malformations, such as

cleft palate, or patent ductus arteriosus

19. Patients who should receive prophylaxis for *P. carinii* pneumonia are those afflicted with
    A. X-linked agammaglobulinemia
    B. severe combined immunodeficiency disorder
    C. chronic granulomatous disease
    D. sickle cell disease
    E. congenital neutropenia

20. A 4-year-old male is brought to your office because of a circular reddish rash under his armpit. The child has been afebrile and has had no other systemic symptoms. The rash is not pruritic. The child's parents state that they have recently returned from a vacation in Massachusetts on Cape Cod and that a small tick had been removed from the same area where the rash is now. The only abnormality on the examination is the circular, flat, erythematous rash that is about 6 cm in diameter and is not tender. The appropriate next step in treating this patient is to
    A. order a test for serum antibodies against *Borrelia burgdorferi* to confirm that the child has Lyme disease
    B. begin treatment with doxycycline
    C. begin treatment with amoxicillin
    D. begin treatment with ceftriaxone
    E. perform a lumbar puncture to be certain that the child's central nervous system (CNS) is not involved

21. A 6-year-old child is brought to your office because a tiny tick was found and removed from his forearm. The parents are unsure how long the tick had been attached, although they thought that it probably had not been there for more than 1 day. They live in an area in which Lyme disease is common. The next step in the proper treatment of this patient should be to
    A. send the tick to be tested for infection with *B. burgdorferi*
    B. reassure the parents that the risk of

infection is small and have them observe the area around the bite for the development of a rash
    C. begin prophylactic treatment with amoxicillin
    D. order a serologic test for antibodies against *B. burgdorferi* in the child
    E. wait 1 month and then order a serologic test for antibodies against *B. burgdorferi* in the child

22. Nodular lymphangitis in a child bitten by a cat is most likely caused by
    A. *Mycobacterium marinum*
    B. *Sporothrix schenckii*
    C. *Pasteurella multocida*
    D. *Nocardia brasiliensis*
    E. *Aeromonas hydrophilia*

23. All of the following are requirements for the diagnosis of allergic bronchopulmonary aspergillosis EXCEPT
    A. asthma
    B. cutaneous reactivity to *Aspergillus fumigatus* antigens
    C. elevated serum IgE level
    D. peripheral eosinophilia
    E. hyperexpansion and hilar adenopathy

24. *T. gondii* is acquired by all of the following means EXCEPT
    A. ingestion of oocysts excreted by cats
    B. ingestion of oocysts excreted by dogs
    C. ingestion of cysts in undercooked meat
    D. transplacental transmission from an acutely infected mother to her fetus in utero
    E. organ transplantation of an infected to a previously uninfected recipient

25. The Fitz-Hugh–Curtis syndrome is characterized by
    A. right upper quadrant pain caused by gonococcal perihepatitis
    B. polyarticular arthritis and rash of disseminated gonococcal infection
    C. lower quadrant pain caused by gonococcal endometritis
    D. gonococcal meningitis

E. monoarticular arthritis and urethral exudate caused by *N. gonorrhoeae*

26. The drug that is recommended as initial therapy for nondisseminated gonococcal disease in children and adults is

   A. penicillin
   B. tetracycline
   C. ceftriaxone
   D. cefazolin
   E. erythromycin

27. Because cerebral malaria can be fatal in as little as 24 hours, in any child having suggestive symptoms and/or history of recent tropical travel, what confirmatory procedure should immediately be invoked?

   A. Serologic testing for specific antibodies
   B. CT scan of the brain
   C. Urinalysis for hematuria
   D. Temperature readings at 6-hour intervals to ascertain fever intermittency
   E. Microscopic examination of blood films

28. A child who returned 2 weeks ago from equatorial Africa is admitted in a coma, with high fever and a palpable spleen. The liver is not enlarged. Laboratory studies reveal hypoglycemia, but the CSF is essentially normal. An immediate working diagnosis would be

   A. pancreatic neoplasm
   B. pneumococcal meningitis
   C. falciparum malaria
   D. visceral leishmaniasis
   E. dengue hemorrhagic fever

29. A 15-year-old male presents to your office with complaint of fever, malaise, headache, cough, and shortness of breath. A chest radiograph reveals left upper and lower lobe infiltrates. His WBC count is elevated. He states that he recently received a pet cockatiel that became ill and died. What is the most likely diagnosis?

   A. *Mycoplasma* pneumonia

B. Pneumococcal pneumonia
C. Psittacosis
D. Q fever
E. Legionnaires' disease

30. What is the most appropriate step in the diagnosis of the case described in Question 29?

   A. Blood culture
   B. Routine throat culture
   C. Sera sampling for chlamydial complement fixation (CF) test
   D. Sputum or throat culture for *Chlamydia*
   E. Viral culture

31. The most common clinical manifestation of atypical cat-scratch disease is

   A. seizures and coma
   B. systemic disease
   C. erythema nodosum
   D. oculoglandular syndrome of Parinaud
   E. neuroretinitis

32. All of the following are true of cat-scratch disease EXCEPT that

   A. lymph nodes are tender in 80% of patients
   B. lymph nodes vary in size from 1 to 12 cm
   C. fever (≥38.1°C) occurs in 90% of patients
   D. malaise and fatigue occur in 30% of patients
   E. splenomegaly occurs in 9% of patients

33. Which is the characteristic incubation period for development of cutaneous papules from *Bartonella henselae* after a cat bite or scratch?

   A. <24 hours
   B. 2–4 days (range: 1–7 days)
   C. 7–12 days (range: 3–30 days)
   D. 6–8 months (range: 4–12 months)

34. Which of the following routes of transmission has been associated with several large outbreaks of human listeriosis?

   A. Aerosol transmission

B. Person-to-person spread

C. Zoonotic transmission

D. Drinking contaminated water

E. Food-borne transmission

35. Which of the following diagnostic tests is LEAST useful in establishing a diagnosis of mesenteric adenitis due to *Yersinia pseudotuberculosis*?

A. Stool culture

B. Mesenteric lymph node histology

C. Abdominal ultrasonography

D. Mesenteric lymph node culture

E. Endoscopy

36. Which of the following blood products has been shown to be of greatest risk in transfusion-associated disease due to *Y. enterocolitica*?

A. Albumin

B. Fresh frozen plasma

C. Platelet concentrates

D. Intravenous immune globulin

E. Packed RBCs after 2-week storage

37. All of the following have been shown to be routes of transmission for tularemia EXCEPT

A. the bite of an infected tick

B. the bite of a mosquito

C. aerosol transmission

D. drinking contaminated water

E. person-to-person transmission

38. On examining a full-term newborn, the physician noted mild hepatomegaly. The remainder of the physical findings was normal, including head circumference and retinas. A urine culture grew cytomegalovirus (CMV). Results of head ultrasonography were normal. Subsequent testing disclosed no metabolic disorders. What deficit is most likely to occur in the next year?

A. Visual loss

B. Hearing loss

C. Cirrhosis

D. Patent ductus arteriosus

E. Immunoglobulin deficiency

39. During springtime, an infectious disease spread through a small community in the United States. The main signs and symptoms were fever, mild rash, and arthralgia. One pregnant woman in late gestation contracted the illness but recovered without difficulty. However, 1 month later she was delivered of a stillborn infant. The pathology report listed the diagnosis "hydrops fetalis." What is the most likely infectious disease?

A. Congenital rubella virus

B. Congenital CMV

C. Congenital parvovirus

D. Congenital herpes simplex virus (HSV)

E. Congenital HIV

40. An HIV-seropositive female comes to her physician for advice because she is pregnant. She has never been on any antiviral medication because she had remained healthy without symptoms of AIDS. However, she wonders whether antiviral treatment might diminish the likelihood of fetal HIV infection. Which one of the following statements is correct?

A. Treatment of the pregnant woman will produce maternal thrombocytopenia.

B. Treatment will result in viral resistance in all infected infants.

C. Treatment will decrease the likelihood of fetal infection but adversely affect the woman, so it should be avoided.

D. Treatment will decrease the likelihood of fetal infection by greater than 50%.

E. Treatment will adversely affect the fetus and should be avoided.

41. A 5-year-old urban male was admitted to the hospital because of low-grade fever, flaccid paralysis of both legs, sensory changes, and absent ankle deep tendon reflexes. The child had received only two immunizations with OPV at the age of 2 and 6 months. His diagnosis is most probably

A. acute paralytic poliomyelitis due to wild poliovirus

B. paralysis due to nonpolio enteroviruses

C. vaccine-associated poliomyelitis

D. Guillain-Barré syndrome

E. tick-bite paralysis

42. **Matching:** Match each syndrome with the appropriate parasite exposure history.

1. Cercarial dermatitis
2. Eosinophilic meningitis
3. Jaundice, biliary stricture, and cholangio-carcinoma
4. Iron deficiency anemia and protein malnutrition
5. Fever, jaundice, eosinophilia, and multiple hypodense lesions on imaging of the liver

A. Consumption of uncooked snails infested with *Angiostrongylus*

B. Prolonged residence in Southeast Asia, consumption of raw fish

C. Walking barefoot in hookworm-endemic areas

D. Wading in freshwater streams infested with *Schistosoma mansoni*

E. Consumption of wild watercress sandwiches in areas endemic for *Fasciola hepatica*

43. The 12-year-old son of diplomat parents presents with crampy abdominal pain, fever, migratory arthralgias, and hepatosplenomegaly. During the past 5 years, his family has lived in the Philippines, Kampuchea, Senegal, and Mali. Ultrasound examination of his abdomen shows periportal fibrosis consistent with schistosomiasis. His kidneys and bladder are normal. Which of the following schistosome species is UNLIKELY to be the cause of his illness?

A. *Schistosoma mansoni*

B. *Schistosoma japonicum*

C. *Schistosoma intercalatum*

D. *Schistosoma haematobium*

E. *Schistosoma mekongi*

44. Which of the following therapeutic options is the optimal method to manage symptomatic nontuberculous mycobacterial lymphadenitis?

A. Complete surgical excision

B. Isoniazid and rifampin for 6 months

C. Await suppuration and then incise and drain

D. Perform partial biopsy, begin antituberculous therapy

E. Oral clarithromycin until the swelling resolves

45. Which of the following vaccines should NOT be given to children with severe combined immunodeficiency syndrome?

A. diphtheria, tetanus, pertussis (DTP) vaccine

B. Measles virus vaccine

C. Salk poliovirus vaccine

D. Hepatitis B virus vaccine

E. Pneumococcal vaccine

46. A 6-month-old breast-fed infant presents with a 24-hour history of diarrhea but no emesis. On examination, the child is afebrile, has normal vital signs, but has slightly sunken eyes and fontanel. She continues to nurse fairly well. The most appropriate therapy is

A. slow intravenous rehydration and nothing by mouth

B. clear liquid diet for 24 hours, followed by dilute formula or breast milk for several days until stools reduce in frequency

C. rapid infusion of intravenous saline

D. oral electrolyte solution given by mouth to make up a 5–10% volume deficit over 6 hours and continuation of breast-feeding

E. begin tincture of opium or loperamide (Imodium)

47. The most useful information in

diagnosing the cause of fever of undetermined origin (FUO) comes from

A. history and physical examination
B. laboratory test results
C. diagnostic scanning
D. provocative tests
E. radiographs

48. In regions where penicillin-resistant pneumococci are prevalent, patients who are strongly suspected of having bacterial meningitis should receive which of the following antimicrobial agents added to ceftriaxone or cefotaxime for empirical antimicrobial therapy?

A. Clindamycin
B. Azithromycin
C. Vancomycin
D. Streptomycin
E. Any of the above

49. Febrile children with sickle cell anemia are at an increased risk for having overwhelming sepsis. Some of these children can be given intramuscular ceftriaxone and treated as outpatients. Which of the following should lead to hospitalization?

A. Temperature greater than 40°C
B. WBC count less than 5,000 cells/μL
C. WBC count greater than 30,000 cells/μL
D. Apparent respiratory distress
E. All of the above

50. Pyelonephritis is a frequent cause of fever in young infants. All of the following infants have an increased risk of urinary tract infections EXCEPT

A. uncircumcised male infants
B. those with urinary tract anomalies
C. young girls
D. those with Mediterranean ancestors
E. those with vesicoureteral reflux

51. A 5-year-old black male has had fever, headache, abdominal pain, and muscle aches for the preceding 3–4 days. His temperature is 103.4°F, heart rate is 130, and respirations are 40 per minute. He appears acutely ill and dehydrated. He has no rash. No history of tick bite is obtained, and the child had recently been camping in rural Wisconsin. Laboratory findings include WBC count of 2,300/mm³, 24% segmented neutrophils, 65% bands, 8% lymphocytes, and platelet count 57,000/mm³. Elevations in serum AST (465 IU/L; normal, 0–40 IU/L) were also present. A peripheral blood smear reveals small blue clusters of bacteria-like bodies in an aggregate within the cytoplasm of 1% of circulating mononuclear WBCs. What is the most appropriate diagnosis?

A. Staphylococcal septicemia
B. Ehrlichiosis
C. Meningococcemia
D. Hemolytic uremic syndrome
E. Rocky Mountain spotted fever

52. Which is the most common cause of osteomyelitis?

A. *Staphylococcus aureus*
B. Group A *Streptococcus*
C. Group B *Streptococcus*
D. *Pseudomonas aeruginosa*
E. *Salmonella*

53. Which is true concerning infections in immunocompromised persons?

A. Fever is an insensitive sign of infection.
B. Normal skin flora can cause life-threatening infection.
C. Absolute neutrophil counts of <5000 cells/mm³ are predictive of infection.
D. The risk of serious infection is highest in the first 48 hours of neutropenia.
E. Multiple infections are uncommon.

54. Strains of *Staphylococcus aureus* can produce which of the following toxins?

A. Exfoliatin A and B
B. Enterotoxins A–E
C. Toxic shock syndrome toxin-1 (TSST-1)
D. All of the above

55. A 16-year-old female has abrupt onset

of high fever, vomiting, and diarrhea, with a diffuse sunburn-like rash, hyperemia of the pharyngeal and conjunctival membranes, oliguria, and postural hypotension. The most likely diagnosis is

A. hemolytic-uremic syndrome

B. Kawasaki disease

C. Rocky Mountain spotted fever

D. toxic shock syndrome

E. Henoch-Schönlein purpura

56. Production of an exopolysaccharide protective biofilm (slime) is an attribute of which organism?

A. *Staphylococcus aureus*

B. Coagulase-negative staphylococci

C. Group A *Streptococcus*

D. *Haemophilus influenzae*

E. *Moraxella catarrhalis*

57. The drug of choice for empirical treatment of indwelling line and prosthesis infections caused by coagulase-negative staphylococci is

A. nafcillin

B. cephalexin

C. ceftriaxone

D. clindamycin

E. vancomycin

58. Scarlet fever is caused by

A. *Staphylococcus aureus* strains that produce exfoliatins

B. *Staphylococcus aureus* that produce enterotoxins

C. group A *Streptococcus* that produce pyrogenic exotoxins

D. human herpesvirus type 6

E. parovirus B19

59. Which of the following is not a finding of scarlet fever?

A. Pastia lines

B. Desquamation

C. White strawberry tongue

D. Red strawberry tongue

E. Preauricular lymphadenopathy

60. Which is not true about cat-scratch disease?

A. The causative organism is *Bartonella henselae*

B. The diagnosis can only be confirmed by culture of the organism

C. Treatment affords minimal, if any, benefit

D. Recovery usually occurs slowly over many months

E. The prognosis is generally excellent

61. The preferred treatment of infant botulism is

A. penicillin G

B. clindamycin

C. hydration and cathartics

D. botulism immune globulin (BIG)

E. supportive treatment only, including intensive care if necessary

62. A 14-year-old child develops a nontender, solitary nodule that slowly enlarged over several weeks and that began at the site of an abrasion that occurred while cleaning his fish aquarium. Which is the most likely infecting organism?

A. *Sporothrix schenckii*

B. *Mycobacterium avium* complex

C. *Mycobacterium marinum*

D. *Mycobacterium leprae*

E. *Chlamydia trachomatis* (LGV biovar)

63. The preferred treatment of Lyme disease in a child 13 years of age is

A. doxycycline

B. amoxicillin

C. ceftriaxone

D. erythromycin

E. trimethoprim-sulfamethoxazole

64. The recommended treatment of *Mycoplasma pneumoniae* illness is

A. amoxicillin or ampicillin

B. ceftriaxone, cefotaxime, or cefotetan

C. erythromycin, clarithromycin, or azithromycin

D. gentamicin or kanamycin

E. trimethoprim-sulfamethoxazole

65. Which of the following is true concerning measles?
    A. There is no animal reservoir.
    B. There is no vector.
    C. There is no transmissible latent virus.
    D. There is only one serotype.
    E. All of the above

66. Which is true concerning measles and vitamin A?
    A. There is no confirmed relationship of vitamin A to measles.
    B. Measles causes vitamin A deficiency.
    C. Treatment with vitamin A reduces measles severity for children in developing countries.
    D. Subacute sclerosing panencephalitis (SSPE) is more likely in children with underlying vitamin A deficiency.
    E. Treatment with vitamin A reduces the incidence of SSPE.

67. Which is not a common manifestation of congenital rubella syndrome?
    A. Snuffles
    B. Intrauterine growth retardation
    C. Cataracts
    D. Structural cardiac defects
    E. Sensorineural hearing loss

68. Which contacts should receive erythromycin after diagnosis of pertussis in a child?
    A. Unimmunized children younger than 4 years in the same household
    B. All unimmunized children in the same household
    C. Symptomatic children and adults in the same household
    D. Unimmunized children in the same household and in the same daycare, and symptomatic adults in the same household
    E. All children and adults in the same household or daycare regardless of immunization history or symptoms

69. The only absolute contraindication to subsequent administrations of acellular pertussis vaccine is

A. collapse or shock-like state within 2 days of pertussis vaccination
B. persistent, inconsolable crying lasting ≥3 hours within 2 days of pertussis vaccination
C. an anaphylactic reaction to a previous dose of whole-cell pertussis vaccine
D. convulsions with or without fever within 3 days of pertussis vaccination
E. history of sudden infant death syndrome (SIDS) in the family

70. Diphtheria and tetanus toxoids and acellular pertussis vaccine (DTaP) should be administered at which ages?
    A. 2 and 4 months and 1–6 years
    B. 2, 4, 6, and 12 months, and 10–12 years
    C. 2, 4, 6, and 15–18 months, and 4–6 years
    D. 2, 4, 6, and 15–18 months, 4–6 years, and every 5 years thereafter
    E. 2, 4, 6, and 15–18 months, 4–6 years, and every 10 years thereafter

71. Enteroviruses include all of the following viruses EXCEPT
    A. coxsackieviruses
    B. echoviruses
    C. polioviruses
    D. polyomaviruses
    E. hepatitis A virus

72. What percentages of poliovirus infections are inapparent?
    A. 5–10%
    B. 20–25%
    C. 50%
    D. 75–80%
    E. 90–95%

73. Which feature of paralytic polio distinguishes it from Guillain-Barré syndrome?
    A. Pleocytosis is uncommon in paralytic polio.
    B. Paralysis is usually asymmetric in paralytic polio.
    C. The paralysis of polio is usually spastic.

D. Sensory changes are common in paralytic polio.

E. Paralytic polio only occurs in unimmunized persons.

74. Which is not true of the risk of vaccine-associated paralytic poliomyelitis (VAPP)?

A. The risk is associated *only* with OPV and not IPV.

B. The risk is higher after second and third doses than after the first dose.

C. The risk is higher for immunocompromised persons.

D. The risk is present for household contacts as well as vaccinees.

E. The risk for VAPP in the United States has exceeded the risk for wild-type polio since 1979.

75. Which is not a manifestation of enterovirus infection?

A. Aseptic meningitis

B. Herpangina

C. Hand, foot, and mouth disease

D. Aphthous stomatitis

E. Vomiting and diarrhea

76. Which is not a manifestation of parvovirus B19 infection?

A. Facial rash ("slapped-cheek" appearance)

B. Lacy, reticulated rash over the trunk and proximal extremities

C. Arthritis

D. Temporary reversal of the CD4:CD8 ratio

E. Reticulocytopenia

77. Which is not true of herpes simplex virus (HSV) infections in neonates?

A. Most cases are caused by HSV type 2.

B. Women with primary HSV genital tract infection are more likely to transmit infection to their offspring than women with recurrent HSV infection.

C. Most mothers of newborns with perinatal HSV have a history of genital HSV.

D. Most mothers of newborns with

perinatal HSV are asymptomatic at delivery.

E. Most cases are transmitted at delivery and are not true congenital infections.

78. Which is recommended for a woman with active genital HSV infection during labor?

A. Culture of the newborn with treatment based on culture results

B. Culture of the newborn and empirical acyclovir

C. Intravenous acyclovir treatment of the mother

D. Cesarean section within 4 hours of rupture of membranes

E. Intravenous acyclovir treatment of the mother and cesarean section within 4 hours of rupture of membranes

79. Which is true concerning antiviral treatment of varicella-zoster virus infections?

A. It has a high risk of drug toxicity

B. It significantly modifies the course of chickenpox in immunocompetent persons

C. It significantly modifies the course of zoster

D. It is associated with a greater risk of recurrences

80. Which serologic titers are most consistent with acute primary Epstein-Barr virus infection?

A. IgM-VCA negative; IgG-VCA negative; EA 1:40; EBNA negative

B. IgM-VCA negative; IgG-VCA 1:160; EA 1:40; EBNA negative

C. IgM-VCA 1:16; IgG-VCA 1:160; EA 1:40; EBNA negative

D. IgM-VCA 1:16; IgG-VCA 1:160; EA 1:40; EBNA 1:8

E. IgM-VCA 1:16; IgG-VCA 1:160; EA negative; EBNA 1:8

81. Which tumor is not associated with Epstein-Barr virus?

A. Burkitt lymphoma

B. Lymphoproliferative disease in immunocompromised persons

C. Leiomyosarcoma

D. Nasopharyngeal carcinoma

E. Kaposi sarcoma

82. Which is not a cause of an infectious mononucleosis-like syndrome?

A. Cytomegalovirus

B. Epstein-Barr virus

C. Parvovirus B19

D. Human immunodeficiency virus (HIV)

E. *Toxoplasma gondii*

83. Which is not true concerning congenital cytomegalovirus infection?

A. It is the most common congenital infection.

B. Approximately 5% of infected newborns have severe disease.

C. Approximately 60% of infected newborns have mild disease.

D. The diagnosis is best confirmed by neonatal urine culture.

E. Treatment with ganciclovir is investigational.

84. The peak age group of HHV-6 infection is

A. in newborns, acquired as a congenital infection

B. 0–3 years

C. 5–15 years

D. Over 13 years

E. Over 16 years as a sexually transmitted infection

85. The recommended treatment of HHV-6 infection complicated by seizures is

A. acyclovir

B. ganciclovir

C. famciclovir

D. foscarnet

E. symptomatic treatment only

86. Match the disease with the causative organism:

1. Lyme disease

2. Cat-scratch disease

3. Relapsing fever

4. Syphilis

5. Yaws

6. Weil syndrome

7. Chancroid

8. Lymphogranuloma venereum

9. Hand, foot, and mouth syndrome

10. Fifth disease

11. Roseola

A. *Haemophilus ducreyi*

B. *Treponema pallidum*

C. Human herpesvirus type 6

D. Coxsackievirus

E. *Chlamydia trachomatis*

F. *Treponema pertenue*

G. *Borrelia burgdorferi*

H. Leptospira

I. *Borrelia recurrentis*

J. Parvovirus B19

K. *Bartonella henselae*

87. Which is not a complication of influenza?

A. Pneumonia

B. Otitis media

C. Reye syndrome

D. Hemolytic-uremic syndrome

E. Acute myositis

88. Indications for influenza vaccine for persons at least 6 months of age include all of the following EXCEPT

A. Immunosuppression caused by medications

B. Residence in a chronic care facility

C. Family member who is at risk of complications of influenza

D. Family history of SIDS

E. Women in the second or third trimester of pregnancy

89. A 4-year-old child has an acute illness of coryza, barky cough, hoarseness, and anorexia. There are no fever or lower respiratory tract findings. The most likely etiology is

A. influenza virus

B. parainfluenza virus

C. respiratory syncytial virus

D. calicivirus

E. adenovirus

90. A 7-month-old infant has rhinorrhea, cough, audible wheezes, and chest retractions. There is a low-grade fever and irritability. The most likely etiology is
    A. influenza virus
    B. parainfluenza virus
    C. respiratory syncytial virus
    D. adenovirus
    E. *Chlamydia trachomatis*

91. A 2-month-old infant has conjunctivitis, tachypnea, and mild cough. There is no fever. Rales are present bilaterally. The most likely etiology is
    A. influenza virus
    B. parainfluenza virus
    C. respiratory syncytial virus
    D. adenovirus
    E. *Chlamydia trachomatis*

92. Manifestations of *Chlamydia trachomatis* pneumonia include all of the following EXCEPT
    A. fever
    B. conjunctivitis
    C. cough
    D. tachypnea
    E. eosinophilia

93. Which is the recommended treatment of *Chlamydia trachomatis* conjunctivitis or pneumonia?
    A. erythromycin eye drops for 7 days
    B. erythromycin eye drops and erythromycin orally for 7 days
    C. erythromycin orally for 2 weeks
    D. trimethoprim-sulfamethoxazole for 7 days
    E. ceftriaxone as a single intramuscular dose

94. Following your request for an x-ray of a 2-year-old child, the radiologist calls you to report finding a steeple sign. The most likely etiology is
    A. influenza virus
    B. parainfluenza virus
    C. respiratory syncytial virus
    D. adenovirus
    E. *Chlamydia trachomatis*

95. Indications for RSV prophylaxis with palivizumab or RSV-IVIG include all of the following EXCEPT
    A. children < 2 years of age with congenital cyanotic heart disease
    B. Children < 2 years of age with bronchopulmonary dysplasia who require oxygen
    C. Infants ≤ 12 months of age who were born at ≤ 28 weeks' gestation
    D. Infants ≤ 6 months of age who were born at ≤ 32 weeks' gestation
    E. All of the above should receive palivizumab

96. Which of the following is frequently caused by adenoviruses?
    A. Pharyngitis
    B. Pertussis-like syndrome
    C. Conjunctivitis
    D. Acute diarrhea
    E. All of the above

97. Which is the cell receptor for most rhinoviruses?
    A. ICAM-1
    B. CD23
    C. Tumor necrosis factor (TNF)
    D. IL-10
    E. IFN-γ

98. Which is not associated with gastroenteritis?
    A. Rotavirus
    B. Polyomavirus
    C. Astrovirus
    D. Adenovirus
    E. Calicivirus

99. Which is not associated with papillomaviruses?
    A. Common skin warts
    B. Laryngeal papillomatosis
    C. Condylomata acuminata
    D. Cervical cancer
    E. All of the above are associated with papillomaviruses

100. Which is true about treatment for papillomaviruses?
    A. Warts, especially hand warts, often resolve spontaneously
    B. Effective treatments are painful
    C. Effective treatments are physician-applied
    D. Most cervical warts should be treated by a generalist
    E. Treatment of cervical warts greatly decreases the risk of cervical cancer

101. Which is true about eastern equine encephalitis?
    A. It is the most common of the arboviral encephalitides.
    B. The area of highest incidence is the northeastern United States.
    C. Asymptomatic infections are uncommon.
    D. Death or residual neurologic deficits are common.
    E. Zanamivir is an effective treatment but is not usually required.

102. Which is not a typical symptom of dengue fever?
    A. Headache
    B. A transient macular rash for the first 1–2 days of fever
    C. A maculopapular rash after defervescence
    D. Mild interstitial pneumonia
    E. Arthralgias

103. Which is not a feature of dengue hemorrhagic fever?
    A. Hematocrit decreased by ≤ 20%
    B. Pleural effusion (by chest radiograph)
    C. Hypoalbuminemia
    D. Thrombocytopenia (≤100,000/mm³)
    E. Arthralgias

104. Which is a risk factor for hantavirus pulmonary syndrome caused by Sin nombre virus?
    A. Tick bites
    B. Mosquito bites
    C. Exposure to infected rodents
    D. Swimming in stagnant or brackish water
    E. Contaminated food

105. A child suffers a provoked bite from a stray dog that was captured by animal control and appears healthy. Which is the appropriate action?
    A. Confine and observe the dog for 10 days for signs suggestive of rabies.
    B. Submit the dog's head for examination for rabies.
    C. Begin rabies vaccination.
    D. Administer human rabies immune globulin (HRIG) and begin rabies vaccination.
    E. No postexposure prophylaxis is necessary because it was a provoked attack.

106. Which describes the recommended use of HRIG for postexposure rabies prophylaxis in the United States?
    A. One half of the HRIG dose at the exposure site, the remainder at another intramuscular site, always with rabies vaccine
    B. As much of the HRIG dose as possible at the exposure site, the remainder at another intramuscular site, always with rabies vaccine
    C. One half of the HRIG dose at the exposure site, the remainder at another intramuscular site, with rabies vaccine for high-risk bites
    D. As much of the HRIG dose as possible at the exposure site, the remainder at another intramuscular site, with rabies vaccine for high-risk bites
    E. Rabies immune globulin is no longer recommended in the United States

107. Which animals should be regarded as rabid in the United States?
    A. Rabbits and hares
    B. Feral mice and rats
    C. Squirrels and chipmunks
    D. Bats
    E. Woodchucks and beavers

108. Which is not a feature of prion proteins?
    A. They are glycoproteins.
    B. They are susceptible to chemical and physical treatments.
    C. They are transmissible.
    D. Their primary structure is encoded by the host.
    E. Prions from different species are very similar in structure.

109. Which is not true of the spongiform encephalopathies?
    A. Creutzfeldt-Jakob disease (CJD) is the most common human spongiform encephalopathy.
    B. Kuru occurs primarily in young persons.
    C. Some forms show autosomal dominant inheritance.
    D. There is no effective treatment.
    E. Most patients die within 1 year.

110. Which is not true of HIV gp120?
    A. It shows little heterogeneity among HIV strains.
    B. It is a transmembrane glycoprotein.
    C. It is highly immunogenic.
    D. It is a major component of the viral envelope.
    E. It binds with the CD4 cell receptor.

111. Which mechanism is responsible for vertical transmission of HIV infection?
    A. Intrauterine fetal infection
    B. Intrapartum (peripartum) transmission
    C. Breast-feeding
    D. All of the above

112. Which is not diagnostic of HIV infection in an 8-month-old child?
    A. Positive test result for p24 antigen
    B. Positive HIV culture
    C. Positive HIV Western immunoblot
    D. Positive test result for HIV DNA
    E. Positive test result for HIV RNA

113. Which is not true concerning HIV infection?
    A. HIV suppression is best achieved by regularly rotating antiretroviral regimens.
    B. Therapy can reduce HIV burden to undetectable levels.
    C. Viral burden predicts disease progression.
    D. CD4 cell counts reflect the risk of opportunistic infections.
    E. Adherence to therapy is crucial.

114. Which is not true concerning treatment of HIV infection?
    A. Multiple-drug regimens are superior to single-drug therapy.
    B. Protease inhibitors prevent uncoating of infectious virions.
    C. Nucleoside and non-nucleoside reverse transcriptase inhibitors act at different sites of reverse transcription.
    D. Drug-drug interactions are common with protease inhibitors.
    E. Antiretroviral treatment is most successful in treatment-naive patients.

115. Which infants born to HIV-infected mothers should receive prophylaxis for *Pneumocystis carinii*?
    A. Infants with a positive HIV culture, DNA or RNA PCR, or p24 antigen
    B. Infants with an AIDS-defining diagnosis
    C. Infants after a first episode of *P. carinii* pneumonia
    D. Infants with a CD4 cell count of < 750 cells/mm³ or CD4 percentage < 15%
    E. All infants 6 weeks of age until HIV infection is excluded

116. Which is not a component of the recommended prophylactic regimen to prevent vertical HIV transmission?
    A. Zidovudine orally to the mother after the first trimester
    B. Zidovudine intravenously to the mother during delivery
    C. Zidovudine orally to the newborn for the first 6 weeks of life
    D. All of the above are recommended.

117. Which is not recommended as part of

the care for an asymptomatic 2-year-old HIV-infected child with a CD4 cell count of 45 cells/mm^3?

A. Trimethoprim-sulfamethoxazole prophylaxis for *Pneumocystis carinii*

B. Clarithromycin prophylaxis for *Mycobacterium avium* complex

C. Monthly IVIG prophylaxis for bacterial infections

D. Tuberculin skin testing

E. All of the above are recommended.

118. Which is not true of infections with human T-cell lymphotrophic virus type I (HTLV-I)?

A. It is the cause of adult T-cell leukemia/lymphoma.

B. Breast-feeding is safe.

C. It is transmitted by sexual contact.

D. All donated blood in the United States is tested for anti-HTLV antibodies.

E. All of the above are true.

119. An 8-year-old child presents with acute onset of meningitis and encephalitis in late summer after swimming in a stagnant pond. Which etiology should be suspected?

A. *Pseudomonas*

B. Herpes simplex virus

C. *Mucor*

D. *Naegleria*

E. Malaria

120. A 4-year-old child presents with acute onset of colicky abdominal pain, blood-stained diarrhea, and tenesmus. There is no fever. Trophozoites are seen in the stool. The family has recently returned from a trip to Mexico. Which etiology should be suspected?

A. *Giardia lamblia*

B. *Entamoeba dispar*

C. *Entamoeba histolytica*

D. *Naegleria*

E. *Cryptosporidium*

121. Which is not true concerning the treatment of *Entamoeba histolytica* amebiasis?

A. Asymptomatic cyst excreters usually do not need to be treated.

B. Iodoquinol is recommended for asymptomatic persons.

C. Metronidazole is recommended for invasive intestinal amebiasis.

D. Metronidazole is recommended for hepatic amebiasis.

E. Metronidazole therapy should always be followed by iodoquinol.

122. Which is not a recognized source of *Giardia lamblia*?

A. Swimming pools

B. Mountain streams

C. Children in child-care centers

D. Food

E. All of the above are sources of *Giardia lamblia*.

123. Which is not true concerning the treatment of *Giardia lamblia* infections?

A. Asymptomatic cyst excreters usually do not need to be treated.

B. Children with acute diarrhea require treatment.

C. Children with chronic diarrhea require treatment.

D. Metronidazole is the treatment of choice.

E. Metronidazole therapy should always be followed by iodoquinol.

124. Which is not a spore-forming intestinal protozoa?

A. *Giardia lamblia*

B. *Cryptosporidium*

C. *Isospora*

D. *Cyclospora*

E. Microsporidia

125. Which is not true concerning *Cryptosporidium parvum* infections?

A. Infection is common in children.

B. It causes a bloody colitis.

C. Diarrhea may persist for several weeks.

D. Treatment is not recommended for immunocompetent persons.

E. Paromomycin is recommended for

treatment of immunocompromised persons.

126. A sexually active adolescent presents with copious malodorous yellow vaginal discharge with vulvovaginal irritation. Which is the most likely etiology?
    A. *Candida albicans*
    B. *Trichomonas vaginalis*
    C. *Giardia lamblia*
    D. *Haemophilus ducreyi*
    E. *Enterobius vermicularis*

127. Match the disease with the causative organism:
    1. Kala-azar
    2. African sleeping sickness
    3. Chagas disease
    4. Malaria
    5. Hookworms
    6. Cutaneous larva migrans
    7. Visceral larva migrans
    8. Pinworms
    9. Whipworms
    10. Cysticercosis
    11. Hydatid disease

    A. *Ancylostoma braziliense*
    B. *Trypanosoma cruzi*
    C. *Trichuris trichiura*
    D. *Ancylostoma duodenale* and *Necator americanus*
    E. *Leishmania*
    F. *Plasmodium*
    G. *Toxocara canis*
    H. *Echinococcus*
    I. *Trypanosoma brucei*
    J. *Enterobius vermicularis*
    K. *Taenia solium*

128. Which *Plasmodium* species causes the most severe form of malaria and has the highest fatality rate?
    A. *P. falciparum*
    B. *P. malariae*
    C. *P. ovale*
    D. *P. vivax*
    E. All malaria species are similar in severity.

129. Which is the most useful method for diagnosis of malaria?
    A. Serologic testing for IgM antibodies
    B. Serologic testing for IgG antibodies
    C. Rapid antigen testing
    D. Thick and thin blood smears
    E. Polymerase chain reaction (PCR) testing

130. Which is not true concerning *Pneumocystis carinii* infections?
    A. Most persons are infected before 4 years of age.
    B. Most primary infections are usually associated with only low-grade fever and nonspecific symptoms.
    C. Cell-mediated immunity is more important than humoral immunity.
    D. Severe *P. carinii* pneumonia occurs almost exclusively in immunocompromised persons.
    E. All of the above are true.

131. Which is the recommended treatment of pinworms *(Enterobius vermicularis)*?
    A. Ketoconazole, in a single dose
    B. Albendazole or mebendazole, in a single dose
    C. Albendazole or mebendazole, in two doses 2 weeks apart
    D. Trimethoprim-sulfamethoxazole, in a single dose
    E. Trimethoprim-sulfamethoxazole, in two doses 2 weeks apart

132. A child presents with several days of increasing myalgias, especially while chewing and with breathing, and fever. There is a history of eating undercooked meat. Laboratory testing shows 8% eosinophilia. Which is the most likely etiology?
    A. *Trichuris trichiura*
    B. *Trichinella spiralis*
    C. *Strongyloides stercoralis*
    D. *Toxocara canis*
    E. *Ascaris lumbricoides*

133. Which is the most useful test for diagnosis of neurocysticercosis?
    A. Serologic testing
    B. Stool examination
    C. Rapid antigen testing
    D. Computed tomography (CT)

E. Polymerase chain reaction (PCR) testing

134. Match the type of vaccine preparation with the organism:
  1. Inactivated whole infectious agent
  2. Toxoid
  3. Polysaccharide
  4. Conjugated polysaccharide
  5. Recombinant protein
  6. Purified protein(s)
  7. Live attenuated infectious agent

  A. Meningococcus
  B. Hepatitis B
  C. *Haemophilus influenzae* type b
  D. Tetanus
  E. Acellular pertussis vaccine
  F. Hepatitis A
  G. Varicella

135. Vaccines against the same infectious agent but produced by different manufacturers are considered interchangeable with the exception of
  A. *Haemophilus influenzae* type b vaccines
  B. hepatitis A vaccines
  C. hepatitis B vaccines
  D. acellular pertussis vaccines
  E. Lyme disease vaccines

136. Which information about vaccination is not required to be documented in the patient's medical record?
  A. Date of administration
  B. Site of administration
  C. Manufacturer
  D. Lot number
  E. Name of the person administering the vaccine

137. Which infection is not readily transmissible among children attending child daycare?
  A. Cytomegalovirus
  B. Rhinoviruses
  C. Human immunodeficiency virus (HIV)
  D. *Giardia lamblia*
  E. Otitis media

138. Match the rickettsial disease with the causative organism:
  1. Rocky Mountain spotted fever
  2. Rickettsialpox
  3. Murine typhus
  4. Epidemic typhus and Brill-Zinsser disease
  5. Scrub typhus
  6. Human monocytic ehrlichiosis
  7. Human granulocytic ehrlichiosis

  A. *Rickettsia akari*
  B. *Rickettsia prowazekii*
  C. *Rickettsia typhi/ Rickettsia felis*
  D. *Ehrlichia phagocytophilia* group
  E. *Rickettsia rickettsii*
  F. *Ehrlichia chaffeensis*
  G. *Orientia tsutsugamushi*

139. Which is not suggestive of Rocky Mountain spotted fever?
  A. History of tick exposure
  B. Presentation during the spring through fall
  C. Headache and myalgias
  D. Nausea and vomiting
  E. Rash on the palms and soles

140. Which is not a laboratory finding suggestive of Rocky Mountain spotted fever?
  A. Normal to slightly low leukocyte count
  B. Shift to the left
  C. Reticulocytopenia
  D. Thrombocytopenia
  E. Low serum sodium

141. Which is the recommended treatment of Rocky Mountain spotted fever in a child less than 8 years of age?
  A. Ceftriaxone
  B. Chloramphenicol
  C. Doxycycline
  D. Clindamycin
  E. Quinidine

142. Which is the recommended treatment of human ehrlichiosis?
  A. Ceftriaxone

B. Chloramphenicol

C. Doxycycline

D. Clindamycin

E. Quinidine

143. Which is the most likely to cause of fungal pneumonia in immunocompetent persons living in the Ohio and Mississippi River valleys?

A. *Aspergillus*

B. *Cryptococcus neoformans*

C. *Histoplasma capsulatum*

D. *Blastomyces dermatitidis*

E. *Coccidioides immitis*

144. An adolescent with a history of spelunking presents with 2 weeks of weight loss, fatigue, dyspnea, and fever. Which is most likely?

A. *Aspergillus*

B. *Cryptococcus neoformans*

C. *Histoplasma capsulatum*

D. *Blastomyces dermatitidis*

E. *Coccidioides immitis*

145. Which is the most likely cause of fungal pneumonia in immunocompetent persons living in arid areas of California, Arizona, and southwestern Texas?

A. *Aspergillus*

B. *Cryptococcus neoformans*

C. *Histoplasma capsulatum*

D. *Blastomyces dermatitidis*

E. *Coccidioides immitis*

146. Which of the following is not a sign that is consistent with the diagnosis of mild diarrhea and dehydration?

A. Normal respiratory rate

B. Slightly decreased urine output

C. Sunken eyes

D. Weight loss of 3–5%

E. Capillary refill time of 1–2 seconds

147. Which of the following is appropriate for oral rehydration of a child with mild-moderate dehydration?

A. Coca-Cola left for 1 hour to allow the carbonation to dissipate

B. WHO solution

C. Weak tea with a teaspoon of sugar

D. Apple juice

E. Rice water

148. Which of the following most strongly suggests a bacterial etiology in a child with diarrhea?

A. Stool rate of one stool per hour

B. Temperature of $\leq 38.5°C$

C. Liquid stool that soaks into the diaper

D. Microscopic finding of leukocytes in the stool

E. Absence of blood and mucus in the stool

149. Antibiotic treatment speeds the recovery from diarrhea caused by

A. *Salmonella enteritidis*

B. *Shigella*

C. rotavirus

D. *Staphylococcus aureus*

E. all of the above

150. Which is the recommended treatment for neonatal listeriosis?

A. Ceftriaxone

B. Ampicillin with or without an aminoglycoside

C. Cefotaxime with or without an aminoglycoside

D. Erythromycin

E. Vancomycin

151. Which serogroup is not included in the quadrivalent meningococcus vaccine?

A. A

B. B

C. C

D. W135

E. Y

152. Which organism is *not* a well-recognized cause of occult bacteremia of infants and children?

A. *Streptococcus pneumoniae*

B. *Neisseria meningitidis*

C. *Haemophilus influenzae* type b

D. *Moraxella catarrhalis*

E. *Salmonella* spp.

153. Which is associated with a poorer prognosis for persons presenting with meningococcal disease?
    A. Presence of petechiae for < 12 hours
    B. Meningitis
    C. Thrombocytosis
    D. Leukoytosis
    E. Low circulating levels of tumor necrosis factor

154. In addition to genital tract infections, which is not a well-recognized form of *Neisseria gonorrhoeae* infection?
    A. Asymptomatic infection
    B. Lymphadenitis
    C. Conjunctivitis
    D. Suppurative arthritis
    E. Disseminated disease with bacteremia

155. Which contacts should receive rifampin chemoprophylaxis following diagnosis of invasive *Neisseria meningitidis* in a child?
    A. Unimmunized or partially immunized children less than 4 years of age in the same household
    B. All unimmunized or partially immunized children in the same household
    C. All children and adults in the same household if there is an unimmunized or partially immunized child less than 48 months of age
    D. Unimmunized or partially immunized children in the same household and in the same daycare
    E. All children and adults in the same household or daycare regardless of immunization history

156. Which contacts should receive rifampin chemoprophylaxis after diagnosis of invasive *Haemophilus influenzae* type b in a child?
    A. Unimmunized or partially immunized children less than 4 years of age in the same household
    C. All children and adults in the same household if there is an unimmunized or partially immunized child less than 48 months of age

    D. Unimmunized or partially immunized children in the same household and in the same daycare
    E. All children and adults in the same household or daycare regardless of immunization history

157. An adolescent living in rural New Mexico with domestic cats that roam freely presents with sudden onset of fever, chills, and extraordinarily painful lymphadenopathy and appears toxic. Which is the most likely etiology?
    A. *Bartonella henselae*
    B. *Francisella tularensis*
    C. *Yersinia pestis*
    D. *Rickettsia rickettsii*
    E. Hantavirus pulmonary syndrome

158. Which organism causes acute respiratory symptoms in persons with cystic fibrosis?
    A. *Aeromonas*
    B. *Plesiomonas*
    C. *Pseudomonas aeruginosa* (nonmucoid strains)
    D. *Stenotrophomonas maltophilia*
    E. *Burkholderia cepacia*

159. Which is not a means of transmission of *Francisella tularensis*?
    A. Tick bite
    B. Contact with infected animals
    C. Consumption of contaminated foods
    D. Inhalation
    E. Person-to-person spread

160. Which is the recommended treatment for tularemia?
    A. Gentamicin or streptomycin
    B. Ceftriaxone or cefotaxime
    C. Trimethoprim-sulfamethoxazole
    D. Chloramphenicol
    E. Vancomycin

161. Which is the most useful test for prompt diagnosis of *Legionella* pneumonia?
    A. Culture of respiratory secretions
    B. Direct detection in respiratory secretions

C. Detection of antigen in urine

D. Serologic testing for IgM antibodies

E. Serologic testing for IgG antibodies

162. Which is the recommended treatment for *Legionella*?

A. Gentamicin or streptomycin

B. Ceftriaxone or cefotaxime

C. Trimethoprim-sulfamethoxazole

D. Erythromycin

E. Vancomycin

163. Which is the most common cause of systemic and focal infections in the newborn?

A. *Staphylococcus aureus*

B. Group A *Streptococcus*

C. Group B *Streptococcus*

D. *Escherichia coli*

E. Herpes simplex virus

164. Which is not true concerning perinatal group B *Streptococcus* neonatal infections?

A. Approximately 20–40% of pregnant women are colonized.

B. Colonization rates are increased in women over 40 years of age, whites, and in higher socioeconomic groups.

C. Pregnant women who are colonized are usually asymptomatic.

D. Approximately 40–70% of infants born to colonized women become colonized.

E. Approximately 0.5–2% of colonized infants become infected.

165. According to the consensus of American Academy of Pediatrics (AAP) and CDC recommendations using the approach based only on risk factors, which is not a risk factor for which intrapartum prophylaxis should be given for group B *Streptococcus* infections?

A. Previous infant with invasive group B *Streptococcus* disease

B. Maternal group B *Streptococcus* bacteriuria during pregnancy

C. Delivery at < 37 weeks' gestation

D. Maternal age > 35 years

E. Intrapartum temperature ≥ 38°C (100.4°F)

166. Which is the recommended regimen for selective intrapartum prophylaxis for group B *Streptococcus*?

A. Penicillin G 5,000,000 units intravenously to the mother at the onset of labor

B. Penicillin G 5,000,000 units intravenously to the mother at the onset of labor, followed by 2,500,000 million units intravenously every 4 hours until delivery

C. Penicillin G 5,000,000 units intravenously to the mother at the onset of labor, followed by continuous infusion of 500,000 units per hour until delivery

D. Crystalline penicillin G 50,000 units intramuscularly to the newborn

E. Procaine penicillin G 150,000 units intramuscularly to the newborn

167. A 9-year-old child is found to have a positive PPD test result on routine screening. There are no symptoms. Laboratory tests, including chest x-ray, are normal. Which of the following is the best interpretation of this finding?

A. *Mycobacterium tuberculosis* infection

B. *Mycobacterium tuberculosis* disease

C. *Mycobacterium tuberculosis* or atypical *Mycobacterium* infection

D. *Mycobacterium tuberculosis* or atypical *Mycobacterium* disease

E. Recent exposure to *Mycobacterium tuberculosis* but neither infection nor disease

168. What is the risk of the child in Question 167 developing clinical and radiographic evidence of tuberculosis if untreated?

A. <1%

B. 5–10%

C. 50%

D. 90–95%

E. Almost 100%

169. Which is the most common form of

transmission of *Mycobacterium tuberculosis*?

A. Inhalation of organisms originating from soil or other environmental sources

B. Ingestion of organisms originating from soil or other environmental sources

C. Person-to-person spread by direct contact with infected discharge or contaminated fomite

D. Person-to-person spread by infected airborne droplet

E. All of the above

170. Which is true concerning the 5-unit PPD skin test for tuberculosis?

A. It is administered by subcutaneous injection.

B. The reaction is measured 24–48 hours after administration.

C. Persons with tuberculosis meningitis often do not react to PPD skin test.

D. Corticosteroid therapy may increase the amount of reaction.

E. Reaction is measured by the amount of erythema and induration.

171. A 3-year-old child, in whose mother tuberculosis was just diagnosed, has a positive PPD skin test result. A chest x-ray shows a localized, nonspecific infiltrate in the peripheral segments of the right lower lobe. Which is the most appropriate course to confirm the diagnosis of tuberculosis disease in this child?

A. Culture of sputum

B. Culture of pulmonary secretions obtained by bronchoscopy

C. Culture of gastric contents obtained by gastric aspiration

D. Percutaneous lung and pleural biopsies for culture and histopathology

E. Segmental lobectomy for culture and histopathology

172. Which is true concerning drug resistance of *Mycobacterium tuberculosis*?

A. Naturally resistant organisms occur at a frequency of about 10^{-2} to 10^{-3}.

B. Drug resistance is transferable between organisms.

C. Drug resistance to each drug is independent of resistance to other drugs.

D. Isoniazid, rifampin, and pyrazinamide are bacteriostatic.

E. None of the above

173. Which is not true concerning isoniazid?

A. It penetrates all body tissues and fluids.

B. It can be given orally or intramuscularly.

C. Rapid acetylation is associated with lower rates of peripheral neuritis and hepatotoxicity.

D. Peripheral neuritis is rare in children.

E. Hepatotoxicity is rare in children.

174. Which is the recommended treatment of active pulmonary tuberculosis in children?

A. Isoniazid for 9 months

B. Isoniazid and rifampin for 6 months

C. Isoniazid, rifampin, and pyrazinamide for 6–9 months

D. Isoniazid and rifampin for 6 months, with pyrazinamide during the first 2 months

E. Isoniazid and rifampin for 6 months, with ethambutol during the first 2 months

175. A mother of a newborn is found to have an abnormal-appearing admission chest x-ray and acid-fast bacilli on sputum smear. The mother has no other symptoms and is ready to be discharged from the hospital and is willing to comply with her recommended treatment. Which is the recommended management strategy for the newborn?

A. Treat the mother and isolate her from the newborn until the mother has been treated for 2 weeks.

B. Treat the mother and isolate her from the newborn until the mother has three consecutive negative sputum smears and cultures.

C. Treat the mother; no isolation is necessary.

D. Treat the mother and treat the infant with isoniazid and rifampin for 6 months, with pyrazinamide during the first 2 months; no isolation is necessary.

E. Treat the mother and treat the infant with isoniazid until the mother is sputum culture–negative for 3 months; no isolation is necessary.

176. Which best describes the pathogenesis of *Clostridium difficile*–associated diarrhea?

A. Invasion of the small bowel wall by *C. difficile*

B. Invasion of the large bowel wall by *C. difficile*

C. Production of toxins A, B, or C

D. Enteroaggregative strains of *C. difficile*

E. Unknown

177. Which is not a risk factor for *Clostridium difficile*–associated diarrhea?

A. Antibiotics that affect normal gut flora but not *C. difficile*

B. Chemotherapy

C. Bowel surgery

D. Oral ingestion of *Lactobacillus* (e.g., yogurt)

E. Bowel stasis

178. A previously healthy 6-month-old who just completed antibiotic treatment for acute otitis media and now is healthy and asymptomatic undergoes a stool culture to check for antibiotic-associated diarrhea. The stool culture grows *C. difficile*. Which is the preferred antibiotic treatment?

A. Clindamycin orally

B. Vancomycin orally

C. Vancomycin intravenously

D. Metronidazole orally

E. No antibiotic treatment should be given

179. Which is not a clue of anaerobic infection?

A. Sterile pus

B. Polymorphic organisms on Gram stain

C. Sweet-smelling odor

D. Gas formation in tissues

E. Tissue necrosis

180. Which form of leprosy is characterized by a single, large lesion that slowly enlarges, heavy cellular infiltration in the dermis, destruction of the cutaneous nerve fibers, a vigorous and specific cell-mediated immune response, and granulomas composed of epithelioid cells and lymphocytes but few or absent bacilli?

A. Lepromatous leprosy

B. Borderline lepromatous leprosy

C. Borderline leprosy

D. Borderline tuberculoid leprosy

E. Tuberculoid leprosy

181. Which is the most frequent disease associated with atypical mycobacteria in children?

A. Cellulitis

B. Lymphadenitis

C. Skeletal infections

D. Pneumonia

E. Urinary tract infections

182. Which is the recommended treatment for cervical lymphadenitis caused by atypical mycobacteria?

A. Isoniazid and rifampin for 6 months

B. Isoniazid and rifampin for 6 months, with pyrazinamide during the first 2 months

C. Clarithromycin and rifampin for 6 months

D. Complete surgical excision followed by clarithromycin and rifabutin for 6 months

E. Complete surgical excision alone

183. Which serologic pattern is most consistent with successful treatment of primary syphilis in an adolescent 2 years previously?

A. RPR 1:8, VDRL 1:16

B. Negative VDRL, negative MHA-TP

C. VDRL 1:8, negative MHA-TP

D. Negative VDRL, positive MHA-TP

E. VDRL 1:8, positive MHA-TP

184. A sexually active adolescent who has never been treated for syphilis is found to have a negative VDRL and a positive MHA-TP. What is the most likely explanation?

A. Primary syphilis

B. Secondary syphilis

C. Latent syphilis

D. Lyme disease

E. False-negative VDRL

185. A sexually active adolescent who lives in a rural area with contact with farm animals presented 1 week ago with an acute febrile illness with headache, emesis, and myalgias that resolved briefly. He now returns with hematuria, proteinuria, hepatomegaly, and icterus. Which diagnosis is most likely?

A. Relapsing fever

B. Leptospirosis

C. Infection mononucleosis

D. Hantavirus pulmonary syndrome

E. Acute HIV infection

186. Which is the most common result of primary *Toxoplasma gondii* infection in children?

A. Cellulitis

B. Lymphadenitis

C. Meningitis

D. Pneumonia

E. No specific symptoms

187. A 2-week-old neonate experiences high fever, severe respiratory distress, and hepatomegaly. The chest x-ray shows a fine, nodular infiltrate throughout both lungs, and congenital tuberculosis is suspected. Which is not an expected finding?

A. Positive PPD skin test result

B. Positive PPD skin test results in family members

C. Acid-fast organisms on gastric aspirate

D. Meningitis

E. Hepatitis

188. Which is not a risk factor for the congenital syphilis of a newborn to a mother treated for syphilis during pregnancy?

A. Treatment of the mother with erythromycin

B. Treatment of the mother with doxycycline

C. Change in maternal VDRL from 1:32 at treatment to 1:16 at delivery

D. Treatment of the mother more than 30 days before delivery

E. All of the above are risk factors.

189. Periostitis of the long bones is characteristic of which congenital infection(s)?

A. Cytomegalovirus and rubella

B. *Toxoplasma gondii*

C. Syphilis

D. Herpes simplex virus

E. Parvovirus B19

190. Which is not true concerning congenital toxoplasmosis?

A. Fetal infection is more common if maternal infection is acquired in late pregnancy.

B. Severe disease is more common if maternal infection is acquired in early pregnancy.

C. Almost all persons with untreated congenital infection eventually experience symptoms or signs of infection.

D. Chorioretinitis is common at birth but infrequently develops afterward.

E. Central nervous system involvement is common.

191. Which congenital infection is associated with cats?

A. Cytomegalovirus

B. Rubella

C. *Toxoplasma gondii*

D. Syphilis

E. Parvovirus B19

192. Which is not true concerning the clinical manifestations of hepatitis A?
    A. The incubation period is about 4 weeks.
    B. Hepatitis A infection can be differentiated from other forms of viral hepatitis on the basis of clinical manifestations.
    C. Children are more likely to experience asymptomatic infection than adults.
    D. Hepatitis A can have a relapsing course for several months.
    E. Hepatitis A is not associated with chronic liver disease.

193. Which is associated with an increased risk of hepatitis A infection?
    A. Attendance at daycare centers
    B. Household contacts of children in daycare
    C. Men who have sex with men
    D. Contaminated food and water
    E. All of the above

194. A 1-year-old attends a daycare facility where an outbreak of hepatitis A infection has been identified in the past week. Which is the recommended prevention strategy for this child?
    A. Hepatitis A vaccine once
    B. Hepatitis A vaccine now and in 6–12 months
    C. IVIG 200 mg/kg once
    D. IG 0.02 mL/kg once
    E. IG 0.02 mL/kg once and hepatitis A vaccine once

PART 17

The Digestive System

We are now moving to organ system–based parts of the *Nelson Textbook* and this accompanying review book. Gastrointestinal diseases are quite common if we consider all of the children whom we have seen with vomiting, abdominal pain, diarrhea, or constipation. Parents and society are preoccupied with what goes into and comes out of the mouth and what exits the bottom. Fortunately, we have many diagnostic approaches that enable us to test, image, or directly visualize the entire gastrointestinal system.

The questions should help build on the educational foundation of the *Nelson Textbook*. Questions cover the full spectrum of gastrointestinal and hepatic disorders from the oral to the peritoneal cavity and from the esophagus to the rectum, including the hepatobiliary pancreatic structures.

1. The recommended procedure for a physician to follow for an avulsed central incisor in an 8-year-old child is to
   A. call the dentist for an appointment
   B. keep the tooth moist until dental care is available
   C. reimplant the tooth to resemble the one on the other side
   D. place the tooth in apple juice

2. Although the toxic dose of fluoride is many times greater than the dose needed to cause mild fluorosis (mottling), the dose associated with mottling in young infants is how many times the dose from fluoridated water?
   A. 2–5 times
   B. 10–20 times
   C. 100–200 times
   D. 1000 times

3. Complications of appendicitis include
   A. wound infection
   B. intra-abdominal abscess
   C. infertility
   D. liver abscess
   E. all of the above

4. Abdominal pain, weight loss, anemia, and a chronic or recurrent course in an adolescent female suggest
   A. Henoch-Schönlein purpura
   B. inflammatory bowel disease
   C. pregnancy
   D. pelvic inflammatory disease
   E. irritable bowel disease

5. **Matching:** Gastrointestinal tumors
   1. Familial polyposis
   2. Gardner syndrome
   3. Lip and gum pigmentation
   4. Diarrhea, achlorhydria
   5. Facial flushing
   6. Hypertension

   A. VIPoma
   B. Carcinoid
   C. Pheochromocytoma
   D. Osteomas
   E. Annual colonoscopy
   F. Peutz-Jeghers syndrome

6. A 16-year-old female with a past history of hypothyroidism, which developed at age 10, now manifests fever, anorexia, amenorrhea, and jaundice of 4 months' duration. Her direct bilirubin level is 6 mg/dL, and her total bilirubin value is 11 mg/dL. Results of the tests for hepatitis A, B, and C are negative, and her serum IgG level is 16.5 g/L. The most likely diagnosis is
   A. mononucleosis
   B. chronic active hepatitis
   C. α_1-antitrypsin deficiency
   D. cystic fibrosis
   E. Wilson disease

7. An 18-year-old male complains of right upper respiratory quadrant pain and fever for 2 weeks. Physical examination reveals hepatomegaly, no icterus, and right lower quadrant fullness. Four weeks before admission, he returned from Mexico, where he received an over-the-counter medication for an illness characterized by abdominal pain, nausea, and emesis. The most likely diagnosis is

   A. giardiasis
   B. hepatitis
   C. hepatic abscess
   D. cholangitis
   E. Crohn disease

8. A 10-year-old female who had biliary atresia treated with the Kasai procedure in infancy now manifests increasing clumsiness, reduced deep tendon reflexes, and ataxia. The most likely diagnosis is

   A. hepatic encephalopathy
   B. vitamin A deficiency
   C. encephalitis
   D. vitamin E deficiency
   E. kernicterus

9. **Matching:** Jaundice

   1. Hemolysis
   2. Breast milk jaundice
   3. Viral hepatitis
   4. Sepsis
   5. Hypothyroidism
   6. Pyloric stenosis
   7. Cystic fibrosis
   8. Biliary atresia
   9. Crigler-Najjar syndrome
   10. Zellweger syndrome
   11. Galactosemia
   12. Gilbert disease

   A. Indirect hyperbiliru-binemia
   B. Mixed (cholestatic) jaundice
   C. Either

10. A 15-year-old female is placed in a total body cast after repair of scoliosis. The cast is to be in place for 2 months. Two weeks after cast placement, she experiences abdominal pain, emesis, and nausea. The most likely diagnosis is

    A. peptic ulcer disease
    B. pancreatitis
    C. pyelonephritis
    D. appendicitis
    E. sepsis

11. **Matching:** Malabsorption

    1. Acanthocytes
    2. Pellagra-like rash
    3. IgA-endomysial antibody
    4. Attends daycare
    5. Chronic sinopulmonary disease
    6. Responds to oral zinc sulfate
    7. Neutropenia

    A. Cystic fibrosis
    B. *Giardia*
    C. Celiac disease
    D. Hartnup disease
    E. Abetalipopro-teinemia
    F. Acrodermatitis enteropathica
    G. Shwachman-Diamond syndrome

12. An 11-year-old Tanner stage 2 female experiences intermittent periumbilical abdominal pain 2 days before emergently visiting her pediatrician. Six hours later, she is nauseated and has one or two episodes of emesis. She also has had two soft bowel movements without blood or relief of symptoms. She walks cautiously into your office and lies still on your examining table. When you begin your examination, she is apprehensive and watches every move of your examining hand. You notice guarding and tenderness throughout her abdomen; the most tender area is the right lower quadrant. The most likely diagnosis is

    A. pelvic inflammatory disease
    B. ruptured ectopic pregnancy
    C. Crohn disease
    D. appendicitis
    E. mesenteric adenitis

13. A 2-year-old female was well until 12 hours ago, when lethargy, vomiting, and intermittent crying episodes began during which she appears to be in pain. During these painful episodes, she draws her legs up to her abdomen. In the office, she

passes a maroon-colored stool and has a slightly tender but full abdomen. The most likely diagnosis is

A. pyloric stenosis

B. appendicitis

C. urinary tract infection

D. intussusception

E. peptic ulcer disease

14. A 6-week-old male born to para 1, gravida 1, 44-year-old woman presents with a week of recurrent nonbilious emesis and dehydration. The serum levels of sodium are 138, potassium 2.9, and bicarbonate 34. The most likely diagnosis is

A. duodenal stenosis

B. annular pancreas

C. adrenogenital syndrome

D. galactosemia

E. pyloric stenosis

15. The proper instructions to the family of a child with an avulsed permanent tooth include all of the following EXCEPT

A. rinse the tooth

B. insert the clean tooth in the tooth socket

C. scrub the root of the tooth

D. place the tooth in cold cow's milk

E. avoid having the child swallow the tooth

16. False-positive elevations of serum amylase levels may be found in all of the following EXCEPT

A. viral pneumonia

B. renal failure

C. mumps

D. appendicitis

E. anorexia nervosa

17. All of the following conditions are associated with a higher incidence of inguinal hernia EXCEPT

A. cystic fibrosis

B. a family history of inguinal hernia

C. adrenogenital syndrome

D. testicular feminization syndrome

18. An asymptomatic 2-year-old swallowed a hearing aid battery 4 hours previously. A radiograph at 11:00 p.m. located it in the upper third of the esophagus. The most appropriate next step is to

A. observe the patient to see if it will pass through the esophagus during the next 24 hours

B. schedule esophagoscopy the next morning to remove the battery

C. observe the patient in expectation that it will pass into the stomach during the next 6 hours

D. Attempt to retrieve the battery using a Foley catheter and fluoroscopy

E. Schedule immediate esophagoscopy to retrieve the battery

19. A 5-year-old female with cirrhosis and portal hypertension experiences increasing abdominal distension. Shifting dullness and a puddle sign are noted on physical examination. Paracentesis reveals cloudy fluid. Culture of the ascitic fluid is most likely to reveal

A. *Pseudomonas*

B. *Candida albicans*

C. Pneumococci

D. *Serratia*

E. *H. influenzae*

20. The most common indication for pediatric liver transplantation is

A. neonatal hepatitis

B. biliary atresia

C. metabolic liver disease

D. fulminant hepatic failure

21. The expected 5-year survival rate after a pediatric liver transplantation is

A. 25%

B. 50%

C. 75%

D. 90%

22. The following immunizations should be given on schedule prior to liver transplantation because immunosuppression may prevent administration

A. measles-mumps-rubella

B. oral polio

C. varicella

D. all of the above

23. Which common complication after liver transplantation can later lead to lymphoma?

A. Epstein-Barr infection

B. Cytomegalovirus infection

C. Hepatitis C infection

D. Chronic rejection

24. Nondigestive causes of vomiting include all of the following EXCEPT

A. atrial septal defect

B. migraine

C. pregnancy

D. labyrinthitis

E. adrenal insufficiency

F. urinary tract infection

25. Dysphagia is best described as

A. pain on swallowing

B. emesis without nausea

C. drooling due to obstruction

D. difficulty swallowing

E. reflux dyspepsia

26. All of the following are true about cyclic vomiting EXCEPT

A. the onset is between 3 and 5 years

B. episodes last 2–3 days

C. there are four or more emesis episodes per hour

D. it is a migraine equivalent

E. it is associated with nystagmus

27. **Matching:** Diarrhea

1. Secretory
2. Osmotic
3. Increased motility
4. Decreased motility
5. Decreased surface area
6. Invasiveness

A. Laxative abuse

B. Irritable bowel disease

C. Celiac disease

D. Cholera

E. Blind loop

F. Amebiases

28. Potential causes of constipation include all of the following EXCEPT

A. hypothyroidism

B. hypokalemia

C. lead

D. ibuprofen

E. narcotics

29. Cross-bite malocclusion exists when

A. maxillary molars are slightly forward to the mandibular molar

B. maxillary molars are perfectly in line with the mandibular molar

C. the maxillary tooth is missing

D. the mandibular tooth is missing

E. the mandibular tooth erupts earlier than the maxillary tooth

30. Palatopharyngeal incompetence is characterized by all of the following EXCEPT

A. hypernasal speech

B. presence of a submucosal cleft

C. difficulty in pronouncing *p, b, d, t, h, v, f, s*

D. improvement after adenoidectomy

E. difficulty whistling

31. After blunt facial trauma, a 12-year-old appears to have a missing incisor. There is no evidence of the tooth at the scene, and the child does not remember swallowing the tooth. The next step in evaluating the child is

A. plan for a bridge

B. abdominal x-ray to search for the avulsed tooth

C. dental x-ray to look for intrusion

D. ceramic tooth

E. penicillin to prevent facial cellulitis

32. A 10-year-old presents with dysphagia, regurgitation of undigested food, and failure to thrive. Chest radiograph reveals bronchiectasis. The most likely diagnosis is

A. cystic fibrosis

B. chalasia

C. achalasia

D. foreign body

E. cleft epiglottis

33. Gastroesophageal reflux in children may be associated with all of the following EXCEPT
    A. Sandifer syndrome
    B. esophagitis
    C. aspiration pneumonia
    D. pylorospasm
    E. occult blood loss

34. A 3-year-old manifests the sudden onset of drooling and coughing. He is anxious and refuses to eat. His voice is normal, and his lung examination results also are normal. The most likely diagnosis is
    A. laryngospasm
    B. croup
    C. epiglottitis
    D. esophageal foreign body
    E. gastroesophageal reflux

35. A 4-week-old first-born male with vomiting is suspected of having pyloric stenosis. At the time you examine the patient, the physical examination results are normal. The best way to demonstrate the abnormal physical findings is
    A. keep the patient NPO
    B. give intravenous glucagon
    C. give intravenous gastric
    D. feed the infant
    E. examine the infant under anesthesia

36. Acquired causes of gastric outlet obstruction include all of the following EXCEPT
    A. cystic fibrosis
    B. epidermolysis bullosa
    C. prostaglandin E infusions
    D. eosinophilic gastritis
    E. Crohn disease

37. A 5-year-old has a history of chronic recurrent abdominal pain and emesis. A diagnosis of cyclic vomiting was made at 3 years of age. Therapy with antimigraine medications was unsuccessful. During each episode, the serum ammonia, pH, glucose, and bicarbonate were normal. He now manifests bile-stained emesis, a tender distended abdomen, and bright-

red blood per rectum. The most likely diagnosis is
    A. stress ulcers
    B. intussusception
    C. malrotation
    D. superior mesenteric artery syndrome
    E. meconium ileus equivalent

38. A 2-year-old presents with painless rectal bleeding of 2 days' onset. Physical examination, including a rectal examination, yields negative results. The most appropriate test to perform at this time is
    A. barium enema
    B. colonoscopy
    C. upper GI study
    D. tagged RBC scan
    E. Meckel scan

39. The next therapeutic step for the patient in Question 38 is
    A. H_2-blocking agents
    B. transfuse 1 unit of packed red blood cells
    C. surgical resection of the diverticulum
    D. gastrotomy
    E. endoscopic ablation of the diverticulum

40. A premature infant was demonstrated to have intestinal malrotation. After surgical repair, she experienced repeated episodes of emesis and abdominal distention. The differential diagnosis should include all of the following EXCEPT
    A. adhesions
    B. electrolyte disturbance
    C. intestinal pseudo-obstruction
    D. acquired lactase deficiency
    E. cystic fibrosis

41. The patient in Question 40 is carefully evaluated. All electrolytes are normal, a plain abdominal x-ray (KUB) reveals multiple air fluid levels, but the barium small bowel follow-through is negative for an anatomic site of obstruction. The most likely etiology of the patient's distention and vomiting is

A. hypothyroidism

B. congenital microvillus inclusion disease

C. pancreatitis

D. intestinal pseudo-obstruction

E. hypermagnesemia

42. All of the following are true about Hirschsprung disease EXCEPT

    A. it is uncommon in preterm infants

    B. males are affected more than females

    C. it is associated with VATER syndrome

    D. it is associated with trisomy 21

    E. breast-fed infants may appear less ill than formula-fed infants

43. An 8-month-old manifests fussiness and emesis and refuses to eat. At presentation to the hospital on the second day of admission, he is difficult to arouse. Vital signs are normal, there is abdominal distention, and the rectal examination reveals occult blood in the stool. The most likely diagnosis is

    A. food poisoning

    B. intussusception

    C. colic

    D. adrenal hyperplasia

    E. infant botulism

44. The best approach to the treatment of the patient in Question 43 is

    A. cisapride

    B. hydrostatic reduction enema

    C. immediate surgery

    D. H₂-blocking agents

    E. prednisone

45. A 1-day-old neonate of 35 weeks of gestational age presents with drooling and respiratory distress. A nasogastric tube is placed, oxygen is given, and a chest x-ray obtained. After reviewing the chest x-ray, Figure 17–1, the most likely diagnosis is

    A. meconium aspiration pneumonia

    B. tracheoesophageal fistula

    C. tetralogy of Fallot

    D. foreign body

    E. VATER syndrome

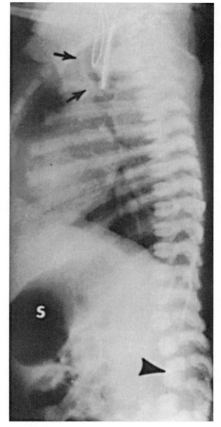

Figure 17–1

46. A 9-year-old white male presents with a 3-month history of epigastric abdominal pain that is intermittent, aching, and lasts for 10–15 minutes. Pain is also present at night. Stool examination for occult blood is positive. The most likely diagnosis is

    A. pancreatitis

    B. urinary tract infection

    C. left lower lobe pneumonia

    D. peptic ulcer disease

    E. giardiasis

47. The hematocrit of the patient in Question 46 is 29%, and the vital signs are stable. The next appropriate test is

    A. upper gastrointestinal endoscopy

    B. ESR

    C. angiography

    D. Meckel scan

    E. barium enema

48. The most appropriate medical treatment of the patient in Questions 46 and 47 is
    A. cimetidine and clarithromycin
    B. omeprazole and metronidazole
    C. sucralfate and bismuth subsalicylate
    D. omeprazole, clarithromycin, and metronidazole
    E. metronidazole and bismuth subsalicylate

49. All are true about Crohn disease and ulcerative colitis (IBD) EXCEPT
    A. the risk of IBD is higher if a family member is affected by IBD
    B. Crohn disease carries a higher risk of malignancy than does ulcerative colitis
    C. the two diseases may be present in the same family
    D. there is an association between IBD and glycogen storage disease type 1b
    E. cigarettes protect against ulcerative colitis

50. **Matching:**
    1. Hypoalbuminemia
    2. FUO
    3. Tenesmus
    4. Sclerosing cholangitis
    5. Growth failure
    6. Strictures
    7. Cardiac involvement
    8. Perianal disease
    9. Oral ulceration
    10. Exacerbations

    A. More common in ulcerative colitis
    B. More common in Crohn disease
    C. Both *A* and *B*
    D. Neither *A* nor *B*

51. An 18-month-old white male manifests failure to thrive, poor appetite, abdominal distention, diarrhea, and irritability. He had been well until 9 months of age. Thereafter, he was weaned from breast milk to regular foods. His growth curve is noted in Figure 17–2. The most likely diagnosis is
    A. giardiasis
    B. celiac disease
    C. cystic fibrosis
    D. pancreatitis
    E. mitochondrial myopathy

52. The disease in Question 51 is also noted with higher prevalence in patients with all of the following EXCEPT
    A. IgA deficiency
    B. Down syndrome
    C. juvenile rheumatoid arthritis
    D. diabetes mellitus
    E. systemic lupus erythematosus

53. The best diagnostic serum test for the disease in Question 51 is
    A. ANA
    B. IgA endomysial antibody
    C. IgA antigluten antibody
    D. IgA antigliadin antibody
    E. antineutrophil cytoplasmic antibody

54. **Matching:** Malabsorptive syndromes
    1. Intestinal lymphangiectasia
    2. Microvillus inclusion disease
    3. Autoimmune enteropathy
    4. Tufting enteropathy
    5. Tropical sprue
    6. Enterokinase deficiency

    A. Membranous glomerulonephritis
    B. Elevated stool α-fetoprotein
    C. Cell-cell matrix disorder
    D. Autosomal recessive
    E. Normal lipase, low tryptic activity in duodenal fluid
    F. Responds to antibiotics

55. Complications of appendicitis include all of the following EXCEPT
    A. male sterility
    B. hepatic abscess
    C. peritonitis
    D. intestinal obstruction
    E. ARDS

56. **Matching:** Cholestasis
    1. Alagille syndrome
    2. Byler disease
    3. Aagenaes syndrome
    4. Zellweger syndrome
    5. Δ⁴-3-oxosteroid 5 β reductase
    6. Biliary atresia

    A. Amish families
    B. Peroxisomal disorder
    C. Tetralogy of Fallot
    D. Lymphedema
    E. Kasai operation
    F. Resembles tyrosinemia

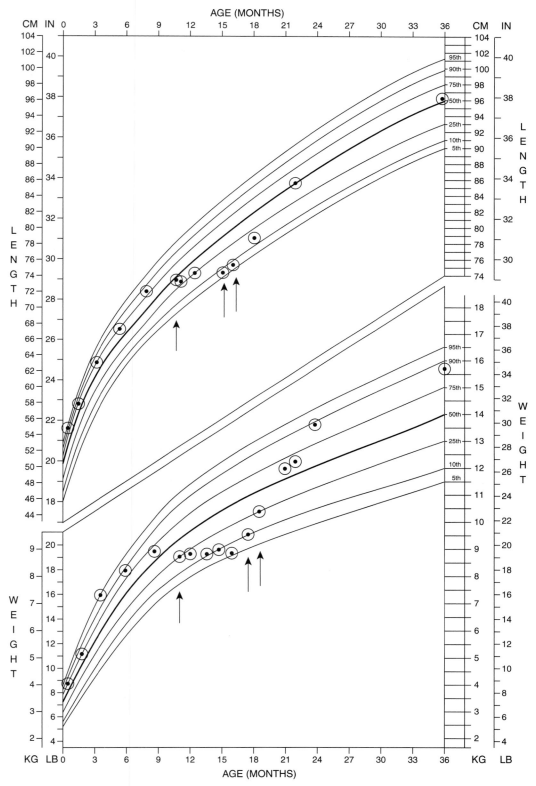

Figure 17-2

57. Wilson disease is associated with all of the following EXCEPT
    A. cardiomyopathy
    B. hepatomegaly
    C. ascites and portal hypertension
    D. dystonia and tremor
    E. hemolysis
    F. Fanconi syndrome

58. A 12-year-old black female presents with malaise, fatigue, anorexia, and jaundice. The differential diagnosis should include all of the following EXCEPT
    A. mononucleosis
    B. chronic active hepatitis
    C. hepatitis B
    D. chronic fatigue syndrome
    E. Wilson disease

59. Laboratory studies for the patient in Question 58 reveal serum aminotransferases of 900 IU/L, a total bilirubin of 8 and a direct of 4, serum IgG of 16 g/L, a positive ANA, and a positive anti-liver kidney microsomal antibody titer. The most likely diagnosis is
    A. α_1-antitrypsin deficiency
    B. chronic active hepatitis
    C. ulcerative colitis
    D. hepatitis A
    E. serum sickness

60. The best approach to therapy of the patient in Questions 58 and 59 is
    A. vitamin A
    B. ribavirin
    C. interferon
    D. IVIG
    E. prednisone

61. The most common cause of facial swelling without facial tenderness or erythema in the maxillary area of a 12-year-old is
    A. localized trauma
    B. an abscessed tooth
    C. a bee sting
    D. *Haemophilus influenzae* type b
    E. angioedema

62. The most reliable physical finding in appendicitis is
    A. the psoas sign
    B. abdominal distension
    C. direct tenderness
    D. abnormal bowel sounds
    E. rebound tenderness

63. An 18-month-old is discovered with his mouth over a storage bottle containing a strong alkali. The parents remove the bottle, and the boy seems well. Some fluid is missing from the bottle, but no external signs are found on the child's clothing and the child has no burns on his face or his lips. The most appropriate advice to give the parents, who are on their way to the hospital, is
    A. administer ipecac
    B. administer milk
    C. administer toast
    D. administer acetaminophen

64. After the child described in Question 63 arrives in the emergency room, results of his physical examination, including an examination of his posterior pharynx, are found to be unremarkable. The most appropriate approach now is to
    A. administer prednisone to decrease stricture formation
    B. administer penicillin to prevent infection
    C. administer an acidic fluid to neutralize the alkali
    D. perform endoscopy to assess the severity of the ingestion
    E. place a nasogastric tube to feed the child

65. **Matching:** Constipation
    1. Onset at birth
    2. Enterocolitis
    3. Stool in ampulla
    4. Encopresis
    5. Poor weight gain

    A. Hirschsprung disease
    B. Functional constipation

66. A 2-year-old child is evaluated 18 months after an unsuccessful portoenterostomy (Kasai) procedure to treat extrahepatic

biliary atresia. He is jaundiced and has signs of cirrhosis and portal hypertension. In addition, he is not walking well, has an ataxic gait, and shows no deep tendon reflexes. He has received inadequate medical care and no nutritional supplementation. The most likely explanation of his neuromuscular disorder is

A. vitamin A deficiency

B. vitamin B_{12} deficiency

C. vitamin D deficiency

D. biotin deficiency

E. vitamin E deficiency

67. A 10-year-old male is admitted to the hospital for his third episode of pancreatitis. The test most likely to lead to a diagnosis of the cause of these episodes is

A. serum amylase determination

B. abdominal CT scan with intravenous

C. abdominal ultrasonography

D. endoscopic retrograde cholangiopancreatography (ERCP)

E. a sweat test

68. The differential diagnosis of an inguinal hernia in an infant includes

A. inguinal adenitis

B. retractile testis

C. hydrocele of the cord

D. isolated hydrocele

E. all of the above

69. The anorectal defect most frequently encountered in male patients is

A. perineal fistula

B. rectourethral fistula

C. rectum-bladder neck fistula

D. rectal atresia

E. imperforate anus without a fistula

PART 18

The Respiratory System

Respiratory problems are leading causes of morbidity and death among children throughout the world. Respiratory physiology has been a challenging topic for most medical students and practitioners. This part of the *Nelson Textbook* does an excellent job of integrating the physiology, anatomy, and pathology with the clinical disease entities. This part moves through an initial section on pulmonary development and function to more specific anatomically based sections on the upper and lower respiratory tracts, diseases of the pleura, and neuromuscular or skeletal diseases that affect pulmonary function.

Questions in this area should help readers review their knowledge in clinical pulmonology and otorhinolaryngology. In addition, readers will be in a better position to recognize and manage acute and chronic respiratory illnesses.

---

1. A 3.5-kg full-term infant is born after an uncomplicated delivery with Apgar scores of 9 and 9 at 1 and 5 minutes. The infant cries vigorously after birth but then goes into a quiet state. Within 10 minutes, the infant experiences cyanosis and respiratory arrest. During resuscitation, the nurse is unable to pass a nasogastric tube. The most likely diagnosis is
   A. tracheoesophageal fistula
   B. pneumothorax
   C. persistent fetal circulation
   D. choanal atresia
   E. laryngotracheomalacia

2. **Matching:** Upper airway infection
   1. Parainfluenza virus   A. Croup
   2. *Staphylococcus aureus*   B. Epiglottitis
   3. Steeple sign   C. Bacterial
   4. Thumb sign   tracheitis
   5. Ragged tracheal air column
   6. *Haemophilus influenzae* type b
   7. Requires urgent endotracheal intubation
   8. Corticosteroids of benefit
   9. Barking cough
   10. Drooling

3. A 1-year-old presents with an acute onset of cough, choking, and respiratory distress. Physical evaluation reveals a respiratory rate of 45 and wheezing. There is no family history of asthma, and no one at home is ill. The older sister states that they were both playing house and that they both had eaten sunflower seeds. The most likely diagnosis is
   A. anaphylaxis
   B. bronchiolitis
   C. cystic fibrosis
   D. foreign body aspiration
   E. angioedema

4. An 18-year-old female presents with an acute onset of chest pain, tachypnea, and cyanosis 1 week after the birth of her first child. Her chest radiograph is nondiagnostic, but her Pao_2 is 60 mm Hg on 40% oxygen. The most likely diagnosis is
   A. pre-eclampsia
   B. *Legionella* pneumonia
   C. a fractured rib
   D. a pulmonary embolism
   E. hysterical hyperventilation

5. All of the following are gastrointestinal manifestations of cystic fibrosis EXCEPT
   A. intussusception
   B. appendicitis
   C. colonic mucosal thickening

D. gastric outlet obstruction

E. inguinal hernias

6. A 13-year-old male presents with fever, sore throat, difficulty swallowing, and a garbled "hot potato" voice. He was well until 7 days before admission, when he had a mild sore throat that did not remit and then rapidly worsened 1 day before admission. The most likely diagnosis is

A. foreign body

B. rheumatic fever

C. retropharyngeal abscess

D. peritonsillar abscess

E. diphtheria

7. Which of the following is the most likely diagnosis in an otherwise normal adolescent with the sudden onset of respiratory distress, cyanosis, retractions, and markedly decreased breath sounds over his left lung?

A. Empyema

B. Chylothorax

C. Pneumothorax

D. *Staphylococcal* pneumonia

E. Aspiration of a foreign body

8. Which of the following is appropriate in the treatment of bronchial foreign body?

A. Flexible fiberoptic bronchoscopy

B. Rigid open tube bronchoscopy

C. Bronchodilators and postural drainage

D. Fogarty catheter

E. Foley catheter

9. **Matching:** Restrictive lung disease

1. Respiratory rate   A. Decreased
2. Inspiration time   B. Increased
3. Expiration time   C. Normal
4. Retractions   D. Present
5. Amplitude of breaths   E. Absent

10. **Matching:** Extrathoracic obstruction

1. Respiratory rate   A. Decreased
2. Inspiratory time   B. Increased
3. Expiratory time   C. Normal
4. Retractions   D. Present
5. Inspiration studies   E. Absent

11. **Matching:** Intrathoracic obstruction

1. Respiratory rate   A. Decreased
2. Inspiratory time   B. Increased
3. Expiratory time   C. Normal
4. Retractions   D. Present
5. Expiratory wheeze   E. Absent

12. All of the following are true about congenital central hypoventilation syndrome (Ondine curse) EXCEPT

A. there is an association with Hirschsprung disease

B. some cases are familial

C. most patients present as adolescents

D. patients hypoventilate during sleep

E. blood gases are normal when the patient is awake at the onset of the illness

13. The best way to identify the anatomy of a child with choanal atresia is

A. ultrasonography

B. rhinoscopy

C. rhinogram

D. MRI

E. CT scan

14. A 3-year-old presents to your office with a 3-week history of unilateral nasal discharge. The discharge is malodorous and lately has been blood tinged. The most likely diagnosis is

A. tertiary syphilis

B. unilateral choanal atresia

C. chronic rhinovirus infection

D. foreign body

E. Wegener granulomatosis

15. The appropriate treatment of the 3-year-old in Question 14 is

A. amoxicillin

B. Cerumenex

C. hydrogen peroxide

D. local anesthesia followed by suction

E. catheter snare removal

16. A 12-year-old male presents with recurrent left-sided unilateral epistaxis that has been present for 6 months.

Possible causes include all of the following EXCEPT

A. juvenile nasopharyngeal angiofibroma
B. von Willebrand disease
C. idiopathic thrombocytopenia purpura
D. hereditary hemorrhagic telangiectasia
E. Henoch-Schönlein purpura

17. The patient in Question 16 is noted to have a mass in the same nostril in which the epistaxis is noted. The most likely diagnosis is
A. encephalocele
B. neuroepithelioma
C. juvenile nasopharyngeal angiofibroma
D. Hodgkin disease
E. Ewing sarcoma

18. The most common cause of a nasal polyp in children is
A. aspirin allergy
B. juvenile nasopharyngeal angiofibroma
C. Peutz-Jeghers syndrome
D. renal failure
E. cystic fibrosis

19. Common causes of the common cold include all of the following EXCEPT
A. respiratory syncytial virus
B. reovirus
C. coronavirus
D. parainfluenza virus
E. rhinovirus

20. All of the following have been found to be effective for treating the common cold in young children EXCEPT
A. zinc
B. vitamin C
C. chicken soup
D. antihistamines
E. Sudafed
F. none of the above

21. All of the following are true about streptococcal pharyngitis EXCEPT
A. reculturing is not necessary if signs have abated
B. once-a-day amoxicillin is ineffective therapy

C. the carrier state is not a risk for rheumatic fever
D. the patient is no longer infective 24 hours after penicillin
E. treatment within 10 days of onset prevents rheumatic fever

22. The most common nasopharyngeal tumor in children is
A. neuroendothelioma
B. Askin tumor
C. Ewing sarcoma
D. nasopharyngeal carcinoma
E. rhabdomyosarcoma

23. Predisposing risk factors for obstructive sleep apnea and hypoventilation include all of the following EXCEPT
A. obesity
B. trisomy 21
C. sickle cell anemia
D. cleft palate
E. Hashimoto disease

24. Common manifestations of obstructive sleep apnea in children include all of the following EXCEPT
A. restlessness during sleep
B. snoring
C. mouth breathing
D. daytime hypersomnolence
E. respiratory pauses during sleep

25. A 1-month-old male has had noisy breathing since birth. He is worse when supine. The physical examination reveals retractions, mild thoracic deformity, and inspiratory stridor. The most likely diagnosis is
A. diaphragmatic hernia
B. tracheoesophageal fistula
C. laryngomalacia
D. choanal atresia
E. vocal cord paralysis

26. The differential diagnosis for the patient in Question 25 includes all of the following EXCEPT
A. laryngeal papillomatosis
B. laryngeal hemangioma

C. laryngeal web

D. Pierre Robin syndrome

E. choanal atresia

27. **Matching:** Sequestration

   1. Surgical resection needed
   2. Hemoptysis
   3. Heart failure
   4. Infection
   5. Lower lobe
   6. Left lung

   A. Intralobular
   B. Extralobular
   C. Both
   D. Neither

28. A 3-year-old presents with stridor and a barking cough. There is mild respiratory distress, tachypnea, respiratory stridor, and a temperature of 99°F. The most likely diagnosis is

   A. laryngotracheobronchitis

   B. epiglottitis

   C. bacterial tracheitis

   D. retropharyngeal abscess

   E. peritonsillar abscess

29. The most likely pathogen responsible for the signs of the patient in Question 28 is

   A. *H. influenzae* type b

   B. *S. aureus*

   C. RSV

   D. parainfluenza virus

   E. enterovirus

30. The approach to the management of the patient in Questions 28 and 29 is

   A. racemic epinephrine and systemic steroids

   B. aerosolized steroids and albuterol

   C. oxacillin and intubation

   D. racemic epinephrine and oxacillin

   E. systemic steroids and intubation

31. The patient in Questions 28–30 improves slightly but 3 days later manifests increasing respiratory distress, cyanosis, cough, and high spiking fevers to 105°F. The most likely diagnosis is

   A. epiglottitis

   B. supraglottitis

   C. retropharyngeal abscess

D. laryngeal papillomatosis

E. bacterial tracheitis

32. The pathogens responsible for the acute deterioration in the patient in Question 31 include all of the following EXCEPT

   A. *H influenzae* type b

   B. *H influenzae* untypable

   C. *M. catarrhalis*

   D. *S. aureus*

   E. all are responsible

33. A 3-year-old has a sudden onset of cough and respiratory distress while playing with siblings in the playroom. There is wheezing over the left lung. The chest x-ray is shown in Figure 18–1. The most likely diagnosis is

   A. tuberculosis

   B. asthma

   C. aspergillosis

   D. foreign body aspiration

   E. anaphylaxis

34. The treatment of choice for the patient in Question 33 is

   A. steroids

   B. albuterol

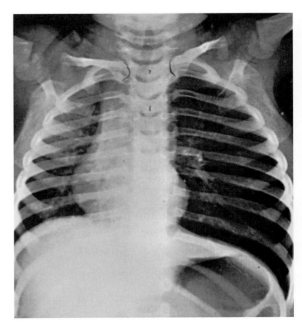

Figure 18-1

C. flexible fiberoptic bronchoscopy

D. rigid bronchoscopy

E. postural drainage

35. A 12-year-old is found unconscious in his family's tool shed. He is tachypneic, coughing, and cyanotic and he has rales in both lung fields. His breath smells like gasoline. The best approach to this patient is to

A. give ipecac

B. perform gastric lavage

C. begin antibiotics

D. begin steroids

E. begin oxygen

36. All of the following are true about desquamative interstitial pneumonitis EXCEPT

A. association with adenovirus infection

B. cyanosis and dyspnea

C. clubbing and fever

D. some familial cases

E. immune complex formation

F. slow onset

37. Possible causes of secondary pulmonary hemorrhage/hemosiderosis include all of the following EXCEPT

A. mitral valve stenosis

B. pulmonary arteriovenous malformation

C. hemolytic uremic syndrome

D. Henoch-Schönlein purpura

E. aortic valve insufficiency

38. A 10-year-old male with a history of asthma presents with respiratory distress and decreased breath sounds over his entire right lung. His chest x-ray is shown in Figure 18–2. This x-ray demonstrates

A. left-sided pneumothorax

B. right-sided pneumothorax

C. right-sided atelectasis

D. right-sided pleural effusion

E. acute chest syndrome

39. Hiccups (singultus) that are chronic and disruptive may be associated with all of the following EXCEPT

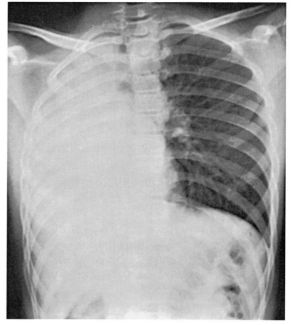

Figure 18-2

A. posterior fossa tumors

B. insects lodged in the ear canal

C. pleural effusion

D. chocolate (theobromine)

E. pericarditis

40. Indicators for serious lower respiratory tract disease in children with chronic pulmonary symptoms include all of the following EXCEPT

A. clubbing

B. cough that disappears with sleep

C. cyanosis

D. failure to thrive

E. chronic purulent sputum

41. **Matching:** Cough

1. Disappears with sleep
2. With vigorous exercise
3. Nocturnal
4. Severe on wakening
5. Paroxysmal

A. Asthma
B. Sinusitis
C. Habit
D. Cystic fibrosis

42. All of the following are true about cystic fibrosis EXCEPT

A. incidence of 1 per 3,500 black and 1 per 17,000 white infants

B. autosomal recessive inheritance

C. more than 700 gene mutations

D. F508 as the dominant mutation

E. WI282X mutation in 60% of Ashkenazi Jews

F. severity of lung disease is not predictable by the gene mutation

43. The most common manifestation of preliminary involvement in children with cystic fibrosis is
A. cyanosis
B. clubbing
C. cough
D. wheezing
E. nasal polyps

44. Intestinal manifestations of cystic fibrosis include all of the following EXCEPT
A. intussusception
B. esophagitis
C. rectal prolapse
D. appendicitis
E. increased susceptibility to viral enteritis
F. malabsorption
G. biliary cirrhosis
H. pancreatitis

45. **Matching:** Treatment complications of cystic fibrosis

1. Intestinal obstruction   A. Chloramphenicol
    B. Aminoglycoside

2. Optic atrophy
3. Hearing loss
4. Hyperuricemia
5. Enamel hypoplasia
6. Hyperglycemia

C. Tetracycline
D. High-dose pancreatic enzymes
E. Steroids

46. A 3-year-old has had recurrent episodes of cough, pneumonia, and sinusitis. Repeated sweat chloride levels are normal, and the F508 mutation is not present. In the last year, the child has had repeated episodes of otitis media. The chest x-ray reveals dextrocardia. The next diagnostic test should be
A. quantitative immunoglobulins
B. IgG subclass determination
C. CBC
D. nasal scraping for electron microscopy
E. HIV serology

47. Empyema is associated with all of the following pathogens EXCEPT
A. *Staphylococcus aureus*
B. *Haemophilus influenzae* type b
C. group A *Streptococcus*
D. *Pneumococcus*
E. *Mycoplasma*

PART 19

The Cardiovascular System

What clinician hasn't been perplexed by a heart murmur in a newborn infant or an athlete during a pre-participation sports examination? The ability to differentiate pathologic lesions from benign murmurs is occasionally difficult and may require consultation or ancillary testing. This extensively updated part is usefully divided into eight sections: evaluation, the transitional circulation, congenital heart disease (left-to-right shunts, obstructive lesions, cyanotic congenital heart disease), cardiac arrhythmias, acquired heart disease, myocardial diseases, therapy, and diseases of the peripheral vascular system including hypertension. The chapters on heart and heart-lung transplantation are exciting and state of the art.

In developing questions, we could not provide you with auscultatory findings. Nonetheless, the questions in this part of the *Nelson Review* will help add to your sound foundation of knowledge in pediatric cardiology.

---

1. A 1-day-old is noted to be cyanotic. Physical examination reveals a grade 2–3/6 systolic murmur and a single loud second heart sound. The chest radiograph reveals a normal-sized heart and decreased pulmonary vascular markings. The electrocardiogram (ECG) reveals left ventricular dominance. The next step in the management of this neonate is to administer
   A. sodium bicarbonate
   B. morphine
   C. prostaglandin E_1
   D. digoxin
   E. positive-pressure ventilation

2. The most likely diagnosis in the patient described in Question 1 is
   A. persistent pulmonary hypertension
   B. transposition of the great arteries
   C. truncus arteriosus
   D. pulmonary atresia
   E. total anomalous venous return

3. An 18-month-old is noted to assume a squatting position frequently during playtime at the daycare center. The mother also notices occasional episodes of perioral cyanosis during some of these squatting periods. The day of admission, the child becomes restless, hyperpneic, and deeply cyanotic. Within 10 minutes, the child becomes unresponsive. The most likely underlying lesion is
   A. cardiomyopathy
   B. anomalous coronary artery
   C. tetralogy of Fallot
   D. constipation
   E. breath-holding spell

4. Therapy of a "blue" or "tet" spell could include all of the following EXCEPT
   A. epinephrine
   B. knee-chest position
   C. oxygen
   D. morphine
   E. sodium bicarbonate
   F. phenylephrine

5. A 2-day-old experiences cyanosis, hypotension, and metabolic acidosis. On examination, the infant is lethargic, tachycardic, and gray-blue, with hepatomegaly, a grade 2–3/6 systolic murmur, and poor radial and femoral pulses. A chest radiograph reveals cardiomegaly, and an ECG demonstrates right ventricular dominance with markedly reduced R waves in V_5 and V_6. The most likely diagnosis is
   A. myocarditis
   B. hypoplastic left heart syndrome
   C. anomalous coronary arteries

D. total anomalous venous return

E. tetralogy of Fallot

6. A 3-day-old presents with fussiness and poor feeding. On examination, the heart rate is noted to be 250. The ECG reveals a rate of 250, a QRS of 0.07 seconds, and no visible P waves. The most likely diagnosis is

A. ventricular tachycardia

B. supraventricular tachycardia with aberrant conduction

C. supraventricular tachycardia

D. heart block

E. none of the above

7. The first approach to the therapy of the dysrhythmia described in Question 6 is

A. fluid challenge

B. iced saline bag placed over the face

C. carotid massage

D. propranolol

E. verapamil

8. **Matching:** Congenital heart disease—syndromes

1. Endocardial Cushing defect   A. DiGeorge syndrome

2. Bicuspid aortic valve   B. Congenital rubella

3. Conotruncal anomalies   C. Trisomy 21

4. Complex multiple cyanotic lesions   D. Turner syndrome

   E. Asplenia syndrome

5. PDA

6. Dextrocardia   F. Williams syndrome

7. Supravalvular aortic stenosis   G. Kartagener syndrome

9. **Matching:** Systemic illnesses and heart disease

1. Pericarditis   A. Lyme disease

2. Heart block (acquired)   B. Homocystinuria

3. Coronary thrombosis   C. Juvenile rheumatoid arthritis

4. Aortic insufficiency   D. Hypothyroidism

5. Cardiac rhabdomyoma   E. Marfan syndrome

6. Bradycardia   F. Tuberous sclerosis

7. Short PR interval   G. Carnitine deficiency

8. Cardiomyopathy   H. Pompe disease

9. Congenital heart block   I. Maternal systemic lupus erythematosus

10. A previously well 3½-month-old presents with poor feeding, diaphoresis during feeding, and poor growth. Vital signs reveal respirations of 70, pulse of 175, and blood pressure of 90/65 mm Hg in the upper and lower extremities. The cardiac examination reveals a palpable parasternal lift and a systolic thrill. A grade 4 holosystolic murmur and a mid-diastolic rumble are noted. The chest radiograph reveals cardiomegaly. The most likely diagnosis is

A. cardiomyopathy

B. myocarditis

C. VSD

D. coarctation of the aorta

E. transposition of the great arteries

11. The initial treatment of choice for a symptomatic patient with isolated pulmonic stenosis is

A. closed surgical blade valvotomy

B. open surgical valvotomy

C. balloon catheter valvuloplasty

D. Blalock-Taussig shunt

E. valve replacement

12. Pulsus paradoxus is associated with

A. pericarditis

B. endocarditis

C. rheumatic fever

D. myocarditis

E. postperfusion syndrome

13. The radiographic finding of notching of the ribs is associated with

A. pulmonary hypertension

B. anomalous pulmonary venous return above the diaphragm

C. coarctation of the aorta

D. systemic hypertension

E. aortic insufficiency

14. **Matching:** Syndromes and congenital heart disease
    1. Hypoplasia of right lung, anomalous pulmonary venous return
       A. Noonan
       B. Polysplenia
       C. Fetal alcohol
       D. Scimitar
    2. Biliary atresia
    3. Pulmonary stenosis
    4. VSD

15. **Matching:** Systemic diseases
    1. Fenfluramine
       A. Heart block
    2. Kearns-Sayre syndrome
       B. Aortic stenosis
    3. Hemochro-matosis
       C. Rhabdomyoma
       D. Cardiomyopathy
    4. Tuberous sclerosis

16. All of the following are true about an ostium secundum defect (atrial septal defect) EXCEPT
    A. females outnumber males
    B. symptoms usually begin in infancy
    C. wide and fixed splitting of the second heart sound is present
    D. right ventricular volume overload is present
    E. cardiac catheterization is unnecessary for diagnosis

17. An atrioventricular septal defect is different from an ostium secundum ASD because the AV septal defect
    A. does not manifest heart failure
    B. does not create volume overload
    C. has the same ECG findings
    D. produces an early tendency for pulmonary hypertension
    E. creates an atrial level shunt

18. A 5-month-old previously well infant is found to have a loud holosystolic murmur (4/6) at the left sternal border. The first and second heart sounds are normal; there is no tachycardia, rumble, or gallop; and hepatomegaly is not noted. The child feeds well and has grown adequately. You suspect
    A. a restrictive VSD
    B. anomalous left coronary artery
    C. a VSD with a 4:1 shunt
    D. tetralogy of Fallot
    E. single ventricle

19. All of the following are true about a small VSD EXCEPT
    A. spontaneous closure is more common in muscular vs. membranous defects
    B. closure usually occurs in the first 2 years of life
    C. there is no risk of endocarditis
    D. pulmonary pressures are normal
    E. surgical repair is not recommended

20. A 6-month-old presents with tachycardia, tachypnea, and poor feeding for 3 months. Physical examination reveals a continuous machinery murmur and a wide pulse pressure with a prominent apical impulse. The most likely diagnosis is
    A. pulmonic stenosis
    B. aortic stenosis
    C. ventricular septal defect
    D. patent ductus arteriosus
    E. anomalous coronary artery

21. The differential diagnosis of the lesion in Question 20 includes all of the following EXCEPT
    A. truncus arteriosus
    B. aorticopulmonary window
    C. sinus of Valsalva aneurysm rupture
    D. aortic valve insufficiency
    E. critical aortic stenosis from a bicuspid valve

22. The treatment of the patient in Questions 20 and 21 is best performed by which methods (may choose more than one)?
    A. Intravenous indomethacin
    B. Surgical closure
    C. Catheter coil closure
    D. Digoxin until the PDA closes spontaneously
    E. Angiotensin converting enzyme inhibitor

23. A neonate manifests cyanosis and hepatomegaly. There is a grade 4/6 systolic ejection murmur without an audible ejection click. The ECG reveals tall, spiked P waves and right ventricular hypertrophy. The best method to evaluate this patient is to perform a
    A. chest x-ray
    B. vector cardiogram
    C. immediate cardiac catheterization
    D. MRI
    E. Echocardiogram

24. The most likely diagnosis in the patient in Question 23 is
    A. patent ductus arteriosus
    B. critical aortic stenosis
    C. critical pulmonic stenosis
    D. tetralogy of Fallot
    E. truncus arteriosus

25. The treatment of choice for the lesion of the neonate in Questions 23 and 24 is
    A. digoxin
    B. propranolol (Inderal)
    C. surgical shunt
    D. balloon valvuloplasty
    E. valve replacement

26. A 12-year-old male tries out for a middle school hockey team. He has a history of a heart murmur as an infant, but the doctor thought it would go away. During the tryout, he experiences severe dyspnea and becomes light headed. At your office, he has a normal rhythm, pulse, and blood pressure and is no longer dizzy. There is a grade 4/6 systole ejection murmur that radiates to the neck. There is also an ejection click. An ECG reveals left ventricular hypertrophy. The next approach to his management includes
    A. chest x-ray
    B. exercise test
    C. digitalization
    D. echocardiography
    E. tilt table testing

27. The patient in Question 26 most probably has
    A. pulmonic stenosis
    B. mild aortic stenosis

C. severe aortic stenosis
    D. patent ductus arteriosus
    E. Williams syndrome

28. Complications of aortic stenosis include all of the following EXCEPT
    A. sudden death with exercise
    B. endocarditis
    C. exercise intolerance
    D. syncope
    E. rheumatic fever

29. Treatment of the patient in Question 27 is best accomplished with
    A. immediate valve replacement
    B. a shunt
    C. digoxin
    D. propranolol
    E. balloon valvuloplasty

30. A 4-day-old previously healthy term infant presents in heart failure. There is a gallop, a grade 3/6 systole murmur, hepatomegaly, and cardiomegaly on chest x-ray. The blood pressure is 95/70. All of the following will be helpful in evaluating the patient EXCEPT
    A. arterial blood gas
    B. blood pressure in the upper and lower extremities
    C. complete blood count
    D. determination of splenomegaly
    E. chest x-ray

31. The blood pressure in the right arm is 95/70, and in the lower extremity it is 45/25. The most likely diagnosis is
    A. patent ductus arteriosus
    B. truncus arteriosus
    C. asplenia
    D. DiGeorge syndrome
    E. coarctation of the aorta

32. Complications after successful coarctation repair include all of the following EXCEPT
    A. postoperative hypertension
    B. delayed chronic "essential" hypertension
    C. postoperative mesenteric arteries

D. pheochromocytoma

E. restenosis

33. An 8-year-old from the former Soviet Union is brought to your office because of a heart murmur and dusty blue skin. He has marked clubbing of his fingers and toes, and his hematocrit is 70%. He has a grade 4/6 holosystolic murmur. His chest x-ray reveals a normal pulmonary blood flow as well as a right-sided aortic arch (see Figure 19–1). What is the likely diagnosis?

A. Total anomalous venous return

B. Tetralogy of Fallot

C. Eisenmenger syndrome

D. Transposition of the great vessels

E. Single ventricle

34. The reason that the hematocrit is so high is

A. chronic hypoxia

B. it was taken in a low cardiac output state

C. it was a peripheral finger stick

D. polycythemia improves flow through VSD

E. hyperviscosity aids flow to the pulmonary artery

35. The patient in Question 33 experiences a headache and is unable to move the left side of his body. The most likely cause is

A. embolic stroke

B. cerebral thrombosis

C. cerebral abscess

D. migraine

E. moyamoya disease

36. A 2-month-old male presents with tachycardia, dyspnea, tachypnea, and a gallop rhythm with no heart murmur. He was perfectly well until 1 day prior to the episode. The physical examination reveals a heart rate of 235, a temperature of 37.8°C, and a normal blood pressure with warm, well-perfused extremities. The most likely diagnosis is

A. sepsis

B. supraventricular tachycardia

C. ingestion

D. ventricular tachycardia

E. sinus rhythm

37. Ice applied to the face has been ineffective in the patient in Question 36. The treatment of choice is

A. adenosine

B. verapamil

C. digoxin

D. lidocaine

38. Prior to the patient in Questions 36 and 37 being given medication, he becomes hypotensive, mottled, and cold. His heart rate is 240. The next therapeutic step should be

A. digoxin

B. verapamil

C. lidocaine

D. defibrillation

E. synchronized DC cardioversion

39. Sudden death in an athlete immediately after forceful blunt trauma to the chest is most likely

A. commotio cordis

B. myocardial infarction

C. lacerated coronary artery

D. ruptured cardiac tendineae

E. hemorrhagic pericarditis

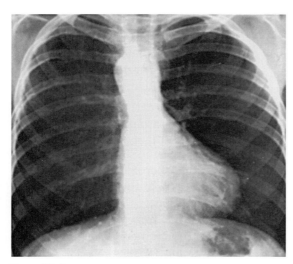

Figure 19-1

40. Patients at risk for bacterial endocarditis include those with all of the following EXCEPT
    A. repaired simple atrial septic defect
    B. aortic stenosis
    C. rheumatic fever heart disease
    D. palliative vascular shunts
    E. previous endocarditis

41. Manifestations of endocarditis include all of the following EXCEPT
    A. Gottron nodules
    B. hematuria
    C. petechiae
    D. splenomegaly
    E. Roth spots
    F. stroke

42. An 8-year-old female presents with chest pain of 1-day's duration. Five days prior to the pain, she had fever, chills, and myalgias. Physical examination reveals an uncomfortable, anxious, afebrile patient with tachycardia, no murmur, and distant heart sounds. The chest x-ray is shown in Figure 19–2. There is a paradoxical pulse of 22 mm Hg. The most likely diagnosis is
    A. myocarditis
    B. cardiomyopathy

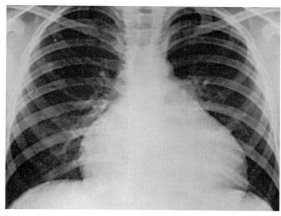

Figure 19-2

    C. Kawasaki disease
    D. pericarditis
    E. sepsis

43. The differential diagnosis of the patient in Question 42 includes all of the following EXCEPT
    A. rheumatic fever
    B. SLE
    C. juvenile rheumatoid arthritis
    D. postmeningococcal immune complexes
    E. chronic atrial fibrillation

PART 20

Diseases of the Blood

This part covers all aspects of hematology, from the many common and uncommon anemias to polycythemia, pancytopenias, transfusion therapy, coagulopathies and thrombosis, the spleen, and the lymphatics. The individual chapters are well written and can help reinforce the multiple genetic and structural relationships of hemoglobin in the different thalassemias. The growing areas of thrombotic and bleeding disorders are also well covered. A clinical approach to all of these disorders is emphasized; the history and physical examination and some simple inexpensive laboratory studies become paramount tools for hematologists and general pediatricians.

The questions help confirm your understanding of the coagulation pathways; microcytic, macrocytic, and normocytic anemias; and other common and important pediatric hematology topics.

1. A 5-year-old white female has multiple bruises on her lower extremities and oral-mucosal bleeding of 3 days' duration. Two weeks before these signs, she had a mild respiratory tract infection. Physical examination reveals multiple ecchymoses and petechiae; no lymphadenopathy or hepatosplenomegaly is noted. The next diagnostic step is
   A. a complete blood count
   B. a prothrombin time
   C. a bleeding time
   D. a partial thromboplastin time
   E. an antinuclear antibody titer

2. The most likely diagnosis for the condition described in Question 1 is
   A. leukemia
   B. neuroblastoma
   C. aplastic anemia
   D. idiopathic thrombocytopenia purpura
   E. systemic lupus erythematosus

3. A 10-month-old white male presents with a 1-day history of persistent bleeding after cutting his lip slightly. The family history is unremarkable, and the patient is receiving no medications. Laboratory data reveal a hemoglobin value of 11 g/dL, platelets of 350,000, a prothrombin time of 11.8 seconds, and a partial thromboplastin time (PTT) of 100 seconds, which is corrected by mixing of normal plasma. The most likely diagnosis is
   A. von Willebrand disease
   B. hemophilia A
   C. Hageman factor deficiency
   D. scurvy
   E. anti-cardiolipin antibody syndrome

4. Appropriate long-term management of the disease described in Question 3 includes all of the following EXCEPT
   A. avoiding aspirin
   B. hepatitis B vaccination
   C. home replacement factor VIII therapy
   D. splenectomy
   E. desmopressin for mild hemorrhage

5. Ten years later, the patient described in Questions 3 and 4 experiences recurrent hemarthroses that become refractory to standard doses of factor VIII. The most likely cause of this is
   A. worsening hemophilia
   B. factor VIII antibodies
   C. development of AIDS
   D. development of hepatitis
   E. aspirin therapy

6. A 5-day-old full-term male presents with intense cyanosis, tachypnea, and tachycardia. Physical examination reveals cyanosis of the skin and mucous

membranes; the lungs, heart, pulses, and general examination show no abnormalities. Arterial blood gas determination reveals a Pao₂ of 95 while the patient is breathing room air and an oxygen saturation of 40%. The most likely diagnosis is

A. transposition of the arteries
B. pulmonary atresia
C. pulmonary hypoplasia
D. methemoglobinemia
E. Heinz body anemia

7. **Matching:** Hemolytic anemia

1. Dactylitis	A.	Hereditary spherocytosis
2. Decay-accelerating factor deficiency	B.	Autoimmune hemolytic anemia
3. Oxidant stressors	C.	Hereditary pyropoikilocytosis
4. Spectrin deficiency	D.	Sickle cell anemia
5. Microcytosis	E.	Paroxysmal nocturnal hemoglobinuria
6. Coombs positive	F.	Glucose-6-phosphate dehydrogenase (G-6-PD) deficiency
7. Thermal sensitivity	G.	Hemoglobin E

8. **Matching:** Anemia

1. Thalassemia	A.	Microcytic
2. Aplastic anemia	B.	Normocytic
3. Copper deficiency	C.	Macrocytic
4. Enzymopathy		
5. Orotic aciduria		
6. Iron deficiency		
7. Hypothyroidism		
8. Leukemia		

9. **Matching:** Red blood cell aplasia

1. Onset before age 4 months	A.	Diamond-Blackfan syndrome
2. X-linked recessive	B.	Transient erythroblastopenia of childhood
3. Rarely needs multiple transfusions	C.	Both
4. Elevated hemoglobin F	D.	Neither
5. Normal MCV		

10. An 18-month-old Caucasian male is brought to your office for a routine health maintenance visit. The mother reveals that the child always appears hungry; in fact, he drinks a quart of whole milk a day and also eats dirt. Intake of solid foods is sporadic, but the mother states that she thought all 18-month-olds were "picky eaters." Physical examination reveals mild pallor of the conjunctivae. He has no hepatosplenomegaly, and the rest of the examination findings are normal. Based on the information, which of the following would be the most likely to determine the diagnosis?

A. Complete blood count, including blood smear
B. Reticulocyte count
C. Lead screen
D. Ophthalmologic consultation
E. Testing stools for occult blood

11. A blood smear taken from the patient described in Question 10 shows microcytic hypochromic anemia. Iron supplementation therapy is started. When will the reticulocyte response be at maximum?

A. 1–2 days
B. 5–7 days
C. 14–21 days
D. 3–4 weeks
E. About 6 weeks

12. In the patient described in Questions 10 and 11, when the hemoglobin and hematocrit return to normal, which should be done?

A. Stop iron supplementation
B. Continue iron for 1–2 weeks
C. Continue iron for 4–8 weeks
D. Continue iron for 4–7 days

13. If the patient described in Questions 10–12 does not experience improvement in his anemia, which of the following should be explored (choose as many as are appropriate)?

A. Gastrointestinal blood loss
B. Thalassemia

C. Sickle cell anemia

D. Urinary tract infection

E. Milk protein allergy-reduced colitis

14. **Matching:** For each of the following disorders, select the appropriate platelet presentation.

    1. Henoch-Schönlein purpura
    2. Aspirin toxicity
    3. ITP
    4. Wiscott-Aldrich
    5. Kawasaki disease
    6. Disseminated intravascular coagulation (DIC)
    7. TTP
    8. Kasabach-Merritt syndrome

    A. Platelets decreased in number
    B. Platelet count normal
    C. Platelets increased

15. A 10-year-old undergoes total splenectomy because of trauma. The best statement about the risk of postsplenectomy infection is that

    A. the risk is increased in older children

    B. the most common organisms are staphylococci

    C. post-traumatic splenosis reliably protects patients

    D. postsplenectomy vaccinations reliably protect patients

    E. the risk is increased and may be lifelong

16. A previously normal African-American army recruit was assigned to Southeast Asia and given malarial prophylaxis. He experienced pallor, fatigue, and dark urine. His hemoglobin level decreased from 14.8 to 9 g/dL. The most likely diagnosis is

    A. hereditary spherocytosis

    B. sickle cell disease

    C. hepatitis

    D. G-6-PD deficiency

    E. Immune hemolytic anemia

17. The diagnosis of the condition described in Question 16 can be confirmed by

    A. hemoglobin electrophoresis

    B. enzyme assay

    C. sucrose hemolysis test

    D. osmotic fragility

    E. Coombs test

18. The best treatment for the patient described in Questions 16 and 17 includes

    A. immediate transfusion

    B. discontinuing current malarial prophylaxis

    C. iron therapy

    D. oxygen

    E. prednisone

19. A previously normal 10-year-old male experiences pallor, fatigue, and a fall in hemoglobin level from 13 to 8 g/dL without evidence of bleeding. His spleen is slightly enlarged. The reticulocyte count is 10%, and his WBC and platelet counts are normal. Many spherocytes are observed on the blood film. The most likely diagnosis is

    A. hereditary spherocytosis

    B. G-6-PD deficiency

    C. pyruvate kinase (PK) deficiency

    D. occult bleeding

    E. acquired immune hemolytic anemia

20. The definitive diagnostic test for the condition described in Question 19 is

    A. an enzyme assay

    B. a stool Hemoccult test

    C. chest radiography

    D. direct and indirect Coombs tests

    E. an osmotic fragility test

21. For the patient described in Questions 19 and 20, initial treatment at the time of diagnosis may include (may choose more than one)

    A. splenectomy

    B. intravenous gamma-globulin

    C. ferrous sulfate

D. glucocorticoids

E. transfusion

22. A 2-month-old child is found to have sickle cell anemia (hemoglobin SS) from a cord blood screening study. Appropriate measures for the treatment of this infant should include which of the following?

A. Prophylactic oral penicillin G to be given twice daily

B. Prophylactic transfusion of packed RBCs to be given at 4- to 6-week intervals

C. Monthly deferoxamine injections to prevent iron overload

D. Splenectomy

E. None of the above

23. The prothrombin time, which is a test of the extrinsic tissue coagulation pathway, is abnormally prolonged in

A. hemophilia A

B. von Willebrand disease

C. congenital factor XIII deficiency

D. congenital factor VII deficiency

E. congenital factor XI deficiency

24. The bleeding time is a test for

A. fibrinogen

B. antithrombin III activity

C. platelet function

D. factor VIII coagulant activity

E. lupus-type anticoagulant

25. A 3.2-kg, 40-week's-gestational age male is born by spontaneous vaginal delivery to a 20-year-old white female. Past maternal medical problems reveal a history of easy bruising that required splenectomy at 18 years of age. Current coagulation studies of the mother include a prothrombin time of 12 seconds, a partial thromboplastin time of 25 seconds, fibrinogen of 300 mg/dL, and a platelet count of 175,000. At 3 hours of age, the infant is noted to have multiple petechiae and a platelet count of 15,000. The most likely diagnosis is

A. neonatal alloimmune thrombocytopenia

B. congenital von Willebrand disease

C. maternal idiopathic thrombocytopenic purpura

D. congenital leukemia

E. congenital syphilis

26. Elevated serum transferrin receptor levels signify

A. iron deficiency

B. ferritinemia

C. acute phase responses

D. erythrocyte marrow hypoproliferation

E. hemorrhage

27. All of the following are true about congenital hypoplastic anemia EXCEPT

A. dominant inheritance

B. recessive inheritance

C. high erythropoietin levels

D. a defect in erythroid precursors

E. a defect in the erythropoietin receptor gene

28. Iron deficiency anemia is associated with all of the following EXCEPT

A. milk protein allergy

B. obesity

C. plumbism

D. hookworm

E. pulmonary hemosiderosis

29. All of the following are true about Fanconi anemia EXCEPT

A. autosomal recessive inheritance

B. stable chromosomes

C. median survival of 30 years

D. increased risk of leukemia

E. aplastic anemia in $> 95\%$ of cases

30. Indications for platelet transfusions in infants less than 4 months of age include all of the following platelet counts and clinical situations EXCEPT

A. $<100 \times 10^9/L$ and bleeding

B. $<50 \times 10^9/L$ and invasive procedure

C. $<20 \times 10^9/L$ and stable

D. $<50 \times 10^9/L$ and immune mediated

E. $<100 \times 10^9/L$ and unstable

31. All of the following are true about the reptilase time EXCEPT
    A. it is not sensitive to heparin
    B. it is prolonged by reduced fibrinogen
    C. it is prolonged by dysfunctional fibrinogen
    D. it is prolonged by fibrin split products
    E. it is always prolonged when the thrombin time is prolonged

32. The most common cause of familial predisposition to thrombosis is
    A. hemophilia antibodies
    B. protein C deficiency
    C. protein S deficiency
    D. factor V Leiden mutation
    E. antithrombin III deficiency

33. Unexplained anemia in a patient with suspected idiopathic thrombocytopenic purpura should suggest all of the following EXCEPT

A. leukemia
B. drug exposure
C. Evans syndrome
D. hemorrhage
E. tuberculosis
F. SLE

34. Chronic thrombocytopenia in a male with eczema should suggest
    A. infection
    B. malignancy
    C. Evans syndrome
    D. Wiskott-Aldrich syndrome
    E. JRA

35. **Matching:** Regional lymphadenopathy
    1. Rubella   A. Cervical
    2. *Yersinia*   B. Occipital
    3. Kawasaki   C. Mesenteric
    4. Sarcoidosis   D. Mediastinal

PART 21

Neoplastic Diseases and Tumors

The good news is that many childhood cancers are curable. The bad news is that cancer is still a leading cause of disease-based childhood morbidity and mortality. In addition, survivors of childhood malignancies now face the long-term complications of their therapy, including secondary new malignancies. This part has been updated, and chapters on epidemiology, molecular pathogenesis, principles of diagnosis, and principles of treatment have added to our general understanding of childhood malignancies.

Questions in this part do not expect you to be up to date on the latest Children's Cancer Group (CCG) chemotherapeutic protocols. Rather, they are directed at general pediatricians who usually diagnose the malignancy, work with the child and the family, and thankfully monitor the ever-increasing number of survivors of childhood cancer.

1. A 15-year-old white female reports that she has had a fever, weight loss, and night sweats for 3 months. On physical examination, she has painless swelling of the left cervical and supraclavicular lymph nodes. Her liver and spleen are not enlarged. The initial evaluation of the patient should include
   A. bone marrow aspiration
   B. abdominal CT
   C. chest radiograph
   D. head CT
   E. erythrocyte sedimentation rate

2. The chest radiograph of the patient described in Question 1 reveals mediastinal lymphadenopathy. The next appropriate diagnostic test is
   A. abdominal CT
   B. head CT
   C. bone marrow biopsy
   D. lymph node biopsy
   E. thoracic CT

3. **Matching:**
   1. Hypertension
   2. Congenital onset
   3. Aniridia
   4. Opsoclonus
   5. Diarrhea
   6. Ataxia
   7. Leukemic transformation
   8. Favorable prognosis
   9. Denys-Drash syndrome
   10. Pancytopenia
   11. Bilateral disease

   A. Neuroblastoma
   B. Wilms tumor
   C. Both *A* and *B*
   D. Neither *A* nor *B*

4. A 9-year-old previously healthy white female manifests progressive painless proptosis and decreased visual acuity of the left eye during a 2-month period. The most likely diagnosis is
   A. pseudotumor of the orbit
   B. trichinosis
   C. retinoblastoma
   D. rhabdomyosarcoma
   E. orbital cellulitis

5. **Matching:**
   1. All races
   2. Limp
   3. Fever of unknown origin
   4. Differential diagnosis of osteomyelitis

   A. Osteogenic sarcoma
   B. Ewing sarcoma
   C. Both *A* and *B*
   D. Neither *A* nor *B*

5. May be a secondary malignancy
6. Radiosensitive
7. Metastasis to orbit
8. Sunburst radiographic pattern
9. Bone pain
10. Small round cell tumor

6. A mother states that her 14-month-old infant's eye has a "cat's eye" appearance. On routine office ophthalmoscopic examination, you have a hard time seeing the fundus but observe no gross abnormalities. The extraocular muscles and remaining head and neck and general physical findings are normal. You should
   A. reassure the mother that nothing is wrong
   B. obtain toxoplasmosis titers
   C. culture for rubella
   D. refer the patient to an infectious disease specialist
   E. refer the patient to an ophthalmologist for examination under general anesthesia

7. **Matching:** Presentation of malignancy
   1. Diarrhea
   2. Vaginal bleeding
   3. Headache
   4. Night sweats
   5. Leukocoria
   6. Periorbital ecchymosis
   7. Pancytopenia

   A. Rhabdomyo-sarcoma
   B. Cerebellar astrocytoma
   C. Lymphoma
   D. Neuroblastoma
   E. Leukemia
   F. Retinoblastoma

8. Which is not true of the epidemiology of childhood cancer?
   A. Childhood cancer accounts for approximately 15–20% of all cases of cancer.
   B. Cancer is the leading cause of death due to disease between 1 and 15 years of age.

C. Leukemia and central nervous system tumors predominate in children.
D. Chronic leukemia is more common in adults than children.
E. All of the above are true.

9. Match the infectious agent with the associated cancer.
   1. Hepatitis B virus
   2. Epstein-Barr virus
   3. Human herpesvirus type 8
   4. Human papillomaviruses
   5. Polyomavirus (e.g., SV40)
   6. Human T-lymphotropic virus type I

   A. Ependymoma
   B. Kaposi sarcoma
   C. T-Cell lymphoma
   D. Cervical cancer
   E. Burkitt lymphoma
   F. Hepatocellular carcinoma

10. Match the chemical agent with the associated cancer.
    1. Tobacco
    2. Diethylstilbestrol (prenatal)
    3. Asbestos
    4. Aflatoxin
    5. Intramuscular iron
    6. Alkylating agents

    A. Vaginal clear cell adenocarcinoma
    B. Hepatic carcinoma
    C. Lung cancer
    D. Leukemia
    E. Sarcoma
    F. Mesothelioma

11. Which cancer is associated with Epstein-Barr virus?
    A. Hodgkin disease
    B. Burkitt lymphoma
    C. Nasopharyngeal carcinoma
    D. Post-transplantation lymphoma
    E. All of the above

12. Which is not a metabolic complication of anticancer therapy?
    A. Hyperuricemia
    B. Hyperkalemia
    C. Hyperphosphatemia
    D. Hypocalcemia

E. All of the above are metabolic complications of anticancer therapy.

13. A 12-year-old female receives cranial, neck, and spinal irradiation for cancer. Which is not a likely long-term sequela of the irradiation?
    A. Infertility
    B. Scoliosis
    C. Cardiomyopathy
    D. Impaired cognition and intelligence
    E. Pituitary dysfunction

14. A 10-year-old male undergoes bone marrow transplantation with stem cells harvested from his 14-year-old sister. Which term describes this type of transplantation?
    A. Autologous
    B. Syngeneic
    C. Familiogeneic
    D. Allogeneic
    E. Xenogeneic

15. Which is not true concerning childhood lymphocytic and myelogenous leukemias?
    A. Leukemias as a group are the most common childhood cancer.
    B. Acute lymphocytic leukemia accounts for approximately 75% of cases.
    C. The incidence is higher in white children than in black children.
    D. The clinical features at presentation are similar.
    E. The responses to therapy and prognoses are similar.

16. Which is not true concerning acute lymphocytic leukemia (ALL)?
    A. Most cases are derived from B-cell progenitors.
    B. The anatomic staging system correlates better with prognosis than the morphologic staging system.
    C. Chromosomal abnormalities can be identified in most cases.
    D. Terminal deoxynucleotidyltransferase (TdT) is a useful marker for relapse.
    E. All of the above are true.

17. Which is not a frequent presenting symptom or sign of childhood leukemia?
    A. Pallor
    B. Petechiae
    C. Lymphadenopathy
    D. Bone pain
    E. All of the above are common presenting signs

18. Which is an indicator of greater-than-average risk of relapse for childhood ALL?
    A. Age between 1 and 10 years
    B. Presenting white blood cell count under 100,000/mm³
    C. Absence of a mediastinal mass
    D. T-cell immunophenotype
    E. All of the above indicate average risk of relapse.

19. Which is an important extramedullary site of relapse of childhood ALL?
    A. Adrenal glands
    B. Kidney
    C. Lung
    D. Heart
    E. Central nervous system

20. A neonate with Down syndrome experiences transient myeloproliferative syndrome that spontaneously resolves. Which best characterizes the prognosis?
    A. This almost never recurs.
    B. This recurs intermittently during early childhood.
    C. This indicates an increased risk of leukemia.
    D. This invariably develops later into leukemia.
    E. This invariably develops later into malignant histiocytosis.

21. Chromosomal analysis of bone marrow reveals a clonal disorder of stem cells with the specific translocation, t(9;22)(q34;q11), which is also known as the Philadelphia chromosome. What is the diagnosis?
    A. Acute myelocytic leukemia
    B. Acute megakaryocytic leukemia
    C. Chronic myelogenous leukemia

D. Juvenile myelomonocytic leukemia

E. Juvenile chronic myelogenous leukemia

22. A child experiences weight loss and night sweats, with a white blood cell count of 80,000/mm³ and a platelet count of 600,000/mm³. Chromosomal analysis of bone marrow cells reveals a clonal disorder of stem cells with the specific translocation, t(9;22)(q34;q11), which is also known as the Philadelphia chromosome. What is the diagnosis?

A. Acute myelocytic leukemia

B. Acute megakaryocytic leukemia

C. Chronic myelogenous leukemia

D. Juvenile chronic myelogenous leukemia

E. Hodgkin disease

23. A 4-year-old child presents with a hard, fixed abdominal mass that is producing discomfort. Physical examination also shows hypertension. Which is the most likely etiology?

A. Hodgkin disease

B. Ewing sarcoma

C. Nephroblastoma

D. Neuroblastoma

E. Renal clear cell carcinoma

24. Which is a good prognostic factor in neuroblastoma?

A. Age < 1 year

B. Stage 3 or 4

C. Amplified *mycn*

D. Chromosome 1p deletion in 80–90% of cells

E. All of the above are good prognostic factors.

25. A 3-year-old child presents with an abdominal mass with microscopic hematuria. Which tumor is most likely?

A. Hodgkin disease

B. Ewing sarcoma

C. Wilms tumor

D. Neuroblastoma

E. Renal clear cell carcinoma

26. Which age group is associated with the highest incidence of osteosarcoma?

A. Neonates

B. Children < 5 years of age

C. Children 5–10 years of age

D. Adolescents

E. All ages have a similar risk for osteosarcoma.

27. A 15-year-old boy presents with a palpable swelling of the humerus that is associated with pain that awakens him at night. There is a sunburst pattern on x-ray (Fig. 21–1). Which diagnosis is most likely?

A. Ewing sarcoma

B. Osteosarcoma

C. Histiocytosis X

D. Osteochondroma

E. Benign bone cyst

28. Which age group is associated with the highest incidence of retinoblastoma?

A. Infants

B. Children 2–5 years of age

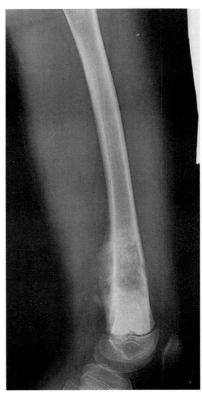

Figure 21-1

C. Children 5–10 years of age

D. Adolescents

E. All ages have a similar risk for retinoblastoma.

29. Which is the most common neoplasm involving the liver in children?

A. Hepatocellular carcinoma

B. Hepatoblastoma

C. Neuroblastoma

D. Wilms tumor

E. Rhabdomyosarcoma

30. A 14-year-old boy presents with a bony, nonpainful mass in the distal femur that has been slowly enlarging. Which tumor is most likely?

A. Ewing sarcoma

B. Osteosarcoma

C. Histiocytosis X

D. Osteochondroma

E. Benign bone cyst

31. An infant has a hemangioma that grows rapidly in size, leading to thrombocytopenia and microangiopathic hemolytic anemia. Which term describes this condition?

A. Kaposi-like form of infantile hemangioma

B. Albright syndrome

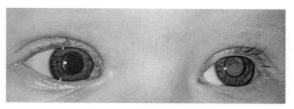

Figure 21-2

C. Kasabach-Merritt syndrome

D. Maffucci syndrome

E. Ollier disease

32. An infant has a hemangioma that grows rapidly in size over the eyelid, obstructing vision. Which systemic therapy is most reasonable?

A. Erythropoietin

B. Heparin

C. Platelet-activating factor

D. Corticosteroids

E. Vitamin A

33. An infant presents with a cat's eye appearance. Which is the most likely tumor of the child in Figure 21–2?

A. Wilms tumor

B. Germ cell tumor

C. Retinoblastoma

D. Rhabdomyosarcoma

E. Leiomyosarcoma

PART 22

Nephrology

This part is particularly valuable in bringing together renal functional anatomy with the disease process in the kidney. Renal physiology, another area in need of curriculum enhancement and better understanding by many house staff and practicing pediatricians, is well integrated into the clinical chapters in this part. Causes of hematuria, proteinuria, tubular dysfunction, and toxic nephropathies are main sections in this part of the *Nelson Textbook*.

Questions for review relate to the parallel chapters in the *Nelson Textbook*. It is hoped that the knowledge gained by answering these questions will contribute to your comfort in diagnosing and managing renal diseases in children.

---

1. The triad of microangiopathic hemolytic anemia, renal failure, and thrombocytopenia is characteristic of which of the following?
   A. Membranous lupus nephritis
   B. Focal glomerulonephritis secondary to septicemia
   C. Hemolytic-uremic syndrome
   D. Acute poststreptococcal glomerulonephritis
   E. Berger disease

2. An infant is admitted to the hospital because of vomiting and lethargy. The child shows evidence of failure to thrive, and physical examination reveals an abdominal mass. Blood and urinary cultures grow *Escherichia coli*. The most likely cause of this disorder is
   A. mesenteric cyst
   B. Wilms tumor
   C. adrenal hemorrhage
   D. obstruction at the ureteropelvic junction
   E. retrocaval ureter

3. **Matching:**
   1. Membranous glomerulonephritis
   2. Goodpasture disease
   3. Rapidly progressive glomerulonephritis
   4. Membranoproliferative glomerulonephritis
   5. Idiopathic nephrotic syndrome

   A. Immune complex deposition
   B. Antiglomerular basement membrane antibody deposition
   C. Both immunologic mechanisms
   D. Neither immunologic mechanism

4. A 4-year-old male experienced an upper respiratory tract infection that was followed in 2 weeks by generalized edema. His blood pressure is normal. Urinalysis reveals 2–5 red blood cells per high-power field and 4+ protein. His BUN is 19 mg/dL, creatinine 0.6 mg/dL, cholesterol 402 mg/dL, serum albumin 0.9 g/dL, antistreptolysin O titer 1:16, and C3 93 mg/dL. The most likely diagnosis is
   A. poststreptococcal glomerulonephritis
   B. membranous glomerulonephritis
   C. minimal lesion nephrotic syndrome
   D. membranoproliferative glomerulonephritis
   E. focal sclerosis

5. A 17-year-old presents with fever, chills, myalgias, and red urine. The examination is unremarkable. Laboratory data reveal a BUN of 30 and a creatinine of 2.5 with a urinalysis demonstrating a positive result for hemoglobin, 3–5 WBCs, and 0–3 RBCs on microscopic examination. This patient most likely has
   A. poststreptococcal glomerulonephritis
   B. lupus nephritis
   C. nephrotic syndrome

D. Goodpasture syndrome

E. none of the above

6. The patient in Question 5 is noted to have tender calf muscles and a CPK of 7,000. The most likely diagnosis is

   A. influenza

   B. aspirin intoxication

   C. Henoch-Schönlein purpura

   D. sickle cell anemia

   E. interstitial nephritis

7. All of the following are true about membranoproliferative glomerulonephritis EXCEPT

   A. age of onset is 15–30 years

   B. rare presentation with nephrotic syndrome

   C. commonly has asymptomatic hematuria

   D. positive antiglomerular basement membrane antibodies

   E. 75% respond to early therapy

8. Recurrent gross hematuria is best characterized by

   A. onset 1–2 days after a viral upper respiratory tract infection

   B. hypertension

   C. high BUN

   D. oliguria

   E. edema

9. All of the following are true about IgA nephropathy (Berger nephropathy) EXCEPT it

   A. recurs in a transplanted kidney

   B. is one cause of recurrent gross hematuria

   C. has a low serum complement level

   D. progresses in 30% of cases

   E. has IgA deposited in the mesangium

10. A 10-year-old male presents with recurrent gross hematuria. Review of symptoms reveals poor vision due to cataracts and poor hearing due to sensorineural hearing loss. The mother's brother has required a renal transplant. The most likely diagnosis is

    A. Berger nephropathy

    B. SLE

    C. Alport syndrome

    D. Fanconi syndrome

    E. Lowe syndrome

11. All of the following are true about idiopathic hypercalciuria EXCEPT

    A. hypercalcemia

    B. possibly autosomal dominant

    C. hematuria

    D. dysuria

    E. nephrolithiasis

12. A 7-year-old had a sore throat 10 days ago. Today she manifests periorbital edema and tea-colored urine. Her blood pressure is 155/95. Her serum complement level is low. The most likely diagnosis is

    A. lupus nephritis

    B. nephrotic syndrome

    C. Berger syndrome

    D. thin basement membrane disease

    E. poststreptococcal glomerulonephritis

13. Early initiation of oral penicillin therapy in the patient in Question 12 would most likely

    A. eliminate the pharyngeal spread to others

    B. prevent the glomerulonephritis

    C. cure the glomerulonephritis

    D. prevent hypertension

    E. none of the above

14. Hemolytic uremic syndrome is characterized by all of the following EXCEPT

    A. microangiopathic hemolytic anemia

    B. disseminated intravascular coagulation

    C. thrombocytopenia

    D. *E. coli* (0157:H7) infection

    E. familial cases

15. *E. coli* organisms responsible for hemolytic uremic syndrome have been recovered from all of the following EXCEPT

    A. fomites

B. meat

C. apple cider

D. swimming pools

E. vegetables

16. The differential diagnosis of hemolytic uremic syndrome includes all of the following EXCEPT

    A. SLE

    B. malignant hypertension

    C. thrombotic thrombocytopenia

    D. renal vein thrombosis

    E. nephrotic syndrome

17. All of the following are true about nephrotic syndrome EXCEPT

    A. elevated serum cholesterol

    B. 85% experience minimal change in disease

    C. reduced sodium reabsorption by the kidney

    D. elevated serum triglycerides

    E. hypoalbuminemia is the cause of the hypoproteinemia

18. Focal segmental sclerosis is characterized by all of the following EXCEPT

    A. presentation with nephrotic syndrome

    B. azotemia occurs in less than 50% of patients

    C. foot process fusion

    D. excellent response to steroids

    E. IgM and C_3 in renal lesions

19. Causes of nephrotic syndrome in the first 3 months of life include all of the following EXCEPT

    A. syphilis

    B. CMV

    C. Finnish-type nephrotic syndrome (autosomal recessive)

    D. minimal change disease

    E. Drash syndrome

20. **Matching:** Renal tubular acidosis

    1. High anion gap acidosis
    2. Interstitial nephritis

    A. Proximal
    B. Distal
    C. Mineralo-corticoid

3. Nephrocalcinosis
4. Galactosemia
5. Pseudohypoaldosteronism
6. Normal anion gap acidosis
7. Wilson disease
8. Elliptocytosis
9. Mitochondrial cytopathies
10. Diabetes mellitus
11. Toluene
12. Fanconi syndrome

D. All of the above
E. None of the above

21. Possible causes of hypernatremia with polyuria and polydipsia in the absence of hyperglycemia include all of the following EXCEPT

    A. hypercalcemia

    B. hypokalemia

    C. lithium

    D. pituitary tumor

    E. X-linked unresponsiveness to ADH

    F. obstructive uropathy

    G. cystic fibrosis

22. **Matching:** Bartter syndrome

    1. Hypokalemia
    2. Normal blood pressure
    3. Tetany
    4. Gene for thiazide-sensitive sodium chloride co-transporter
    5. Hypomagnesemia
    6. Metabolic acidosis

    A. Bartter syndrome
    B. Gitelman syndrome
    C. Both A and B
    D. Neither A nor B

23. **Matching:** Acute renal failure: etiology

    1. High BUN
    2. Myoglobin
    3. Burns
    4. Hyperkalemia

    A. Prerenal
    B. Renal
    C. Both A and B
    D. Neither A nor B

5. Fractional excretion of sodium $> 1\%$
6. Urine sodium <20 mEq/L
7. Hypotension
8. Nephrolithiasis

24. Seizures associated with acute renal failure may be due to all of the following EXCEPT
    A. hyponatremia
    B. hypocalcemia
    C. hypertensive encephalopathy
    D. anemia
    E. cerebral hemorrhage

25. The use of erythropoietin in chronic renal failure is associated with all of the following EXCEPT
    A. iron deficiency
    B. reduced need for blood transfusions
    C. improved appetite
    D. hyperkalemia
    E. hemorrhage
    F. improved sleep

PART 23

Urologic Disorders in Infants and Children

Urinary anomalies, infection, and reflux greatly contribute to end-stage renal disease. This part of the *Nelson Textbook* emphasizes early recognition, intensive evaluation, and comprehensive management and follow-up.

Questions for this part are clinically based and re-emphasize the important principles of early identification and prevention of morbidity.

1. Potter phenotype may be due to
   A. renal agenesis
   B. renal dysplasia
   C. obstructive uropathy
   D. severe amniotic fluid leak
   E. none of the above
   F. all of the above

2. Risk factors for urinary tract infections include all of the following EXCEPT
   A. uncircumcised male infants
   B. sexual activity
   C. reflux nephropathy
   D. double-ureteral systems
   E. chronic use of antibiotics
   F. spina bifida

3. The presence of renal parenchymal scarring due to vesicoureteral reflux is best determined by
   A. DMSA scan
   B. renal ultrasonography
   C. VCUG
   D. CT scan
   E. intravenous pyelography

4. The most common abdominal mass in a neonate is
   A. renal dysplasia—hydronephrosis
   B. Wilms tumor
   C. neuroblastoma
   D. Meckel diverticulum
   E. ovarian teratoma

5. The primary pathology in classic Potter syndrome is best characterized as
   A. oligohydramnios
   B. renal agenesis
   C. pulmonary hypoplasia
   D. facial deformation
   E. skeletal dysplasia

6. Multicystic dysplastic kidneys are characterized by all of the following EXCEPT
   A. usually unilateral
   B. incidence of 1:2,000
   C. autosomal dominant inheritance
   D. most common neonatal abdominal mass
   E. no function

7. A 12-year-old presents with headaches and a blood pressure of 210/110. There is no history of recent infection. The urinalysis is unremarkable. The next step in the evaluation of the patient is to
   A. measure serum complement
   B. perform a renal ultrasound examination
   C. perform a voiding cystourethrogram
   D. measure streptococcal titers
   E. perform a renal arteriogram

8. The most likely diagnosis for the patient in Question 7 is
   A. polycystic renal disease
   B. multicystic renal disease
   C. segmental hypoplasia

D. renal infarction

E. neurofibromatosis

9. Epidemiologic risks for urinary tract infections include all of the following EXCEPT

A. average age in females is 3 years

B. average age in males is less than 1 year

C. circumcision reduces the risk

D. bladder reflux increases the risk

E. *Staphylococcus saprophyticus* is the most common pathogen in male infants

10. Cystitis is associated with all of the following EXCEPT

A. urgency

B. adenovirus

C. fever

D. absence of renal scarring

E. sexual activity in females

11. Risk factors for urinary tract infection include all of the following EXCEPT

A. pinworms

B. constipation

C. pregnancy

D. neurogenic bladder

E. Henoch-Schönlein purpura

12. The imaging studies needed to evaluate a 9-week-old with pyelonephritis include (may choose more than one)

A. intravenous pyelogram

B. CT scan

C. DMSA scan

D. renal ultrasound examination

E. voiding cystourethrogram

F. cystoscopy

13. Vesicoureteral reflux is associated with all of the following EXCEPT

A. contralateral kidney of pair with unilateral dysplasia

B. ureteral duplication

C. familial inheritance

D. ureterocele

E. asymptomatic bacteriuria

14. A 7-month-old white male presents with failure to thrive and a BUN of 75. He has a history of a poor urinary stream. The most likely diagnosis is

A. renal artery stenosis

B. renal hypoplasia

C. urogenic bladder

D. posterior urethral valves

E. nephrolithiasis

15. A 6-year-old girl has a long history of urinary frequency and urgency. She also has nocturnal enuresis. In addition, she has urge incontinence. The most likely diagnosis is

A. unstable bladder

B. Wilms tumor

C. constipation

D. chronic cystitis

E. nephrolithiasis

16. A 10-year-old manifests an acute onset of testicular pain and swelling not relieved by acetaminophen. The next step in management is to

A. apply ice

B. check for a history of *Chlamydia*

C. immediately refer to a urologist

D. perform laparoscopy

E. apply a scrotal support device

PART 24

Gynecologic Problems of Childhood

Traditional gynecologic problems are relatively uncommon before puberty. In the large population of adolescents, many of whom are also sexually active, gynecologic problems become similar to those in young adult women. Pediatricians initially see many young women with gynecologic problems and should carefully study this part of the *Nelson Textbook*.

Questions in this part do not make you an expert in the art of bimanual palpation but help reinforce your understanding of the signs, symptoms, and management of pediatric gynecologic problems.

---

1. A 17-year-old Tanner stage 2 female presents with a history of bilateral spontaneous milky discharge from her breasts for 2 months. Menarche was at age 12 years, and her periods had been regular until 4 months before this visit to your office. In addition, she complains of headache on awakening for the past 2 weeks. The most useful screening test is

   A. urine pregnancy test
   B. serum pregnancy test
   C. serum prolactin level
   D. serum estrogen level
   E. serum luteinizing hormone level

2. The prolactin level of the young woman described in Question 1 is 1000 times higher than normal. The next test in her evaluation should be

   A. cranial MRI
   B. abdominal CT
   C. pelvic ultrasonography
   D. uterine biopsy
   E. mammography

3. **Matching:** Vulvovaginitis

1. Umbilicated pink-white small nodule	A. Enterobiasis (pinworm)
2. Nits on hair shaft	B. Molluscum contagiosum
3. Associated	C. Pediculosis pubis

   bloody mucous stools

   4. Purulent vaginal discharge
   5. Nocturnal perineal pruritus

   D. *Shigella*
   E. Group A *Streptococcus*

4. A 7-year-old female complains of a brown-green discharge on her underwear. She has no fever or labial tenderness and denies sexual contact. Her mother states that for the past 4 months her daughter has been taking ballet classes and frequently sleeps in her leotards. The most likely diagnosis is

   A. nonspecific vaginitis
   B. *Gardnerella vaginalis* vaginitis
   C. gonorrhea
   D. chlamydial vaginitis
   E. *Candida* vaginitis

5. Initial therapy for the girl described in Question 4 should include all of the following EXCEPT

   A. instruction in perineal hygiene
   B. sitz baths
   C. use of mild soaps
   D. avoiding tight clothing
   E. metronidazole

6. Vulvovaginitis in prepubertal girls is characterized by all of the following EXCEPT
   A. exacerbation at puberty
   B. vaginal discharge
   C. erythema
   D. pruritus
   E. masturbation

7. Successful treatment of nonspecific vulvovaginitis includes all of the following EXCEPT
   A. topical estrogen cream
   B. switching from tight-fitting underwear
   C. sitz baths
   D. mild soap
   E. oral tetracycline

8. The treatment of choice for labial adhesions is
   A. topical erythromycin
   B. oral erythromycin
   C. oral estrogens
   D. topical estrogens
   E. topical progesterones

9. Possible causes of vaginal bleeding in a prepubertal female include all of the following EXCEPT
   A. exposure to sex steroids
   B. foreign body
   C. hemorrhagic cystitis
   D. urethral prolapse
   E. neoplasms
   F. ectopic pregnancy

10. *Mastodynia* is best characterized as
    A. dependent on breast size
    B. beginning 18 months after menarche
    C. noncyclical nature
    D. unrelated to menstrual cycle
    E. no response to nonsteroidal anti-inflammatory agents

11. A 16-year-old non–sexually active female has had increasingly severe headaches and a breast discharge for 3 months. Physical examination reveals bitemporal hemianopsia. An important laboratory study in evaluating this patient is a serum level of
    A. estrogen
    B. progesterone
    C. prolactin
    D. cortisol
    E. luteinizing hormone

12. The next diagnostic test for the patient in Question 11 is
    A. abdominal CT
    B. pelvic ultrasound
    C. head CT
    D. breast biopsy
    E. thyroid scan

13. The treatment of choice for the patient in Questions 11 and 12 is
    A. trans-sphenoidal surgery
    B. bromocriptine
    C. Ondansetron
    D. phenothiazine
    E. tricyclic antidepressants

14. The most common ovarian neoplasm in adolescents is
    A. cancer
    B. teratoma
    C. adenoma
    D. sinus endodermal tumors
    E. gonadoblastoma

15. Dysgerminomas of the ovaries are usually associated with
    A. Noonan syndrome
    B. X-Y gonadal dysgenesis
    C. Turner syndrome
    D. prenatal diethylstilbestrol (DES)
    E. radiation therapy

16. Maternal exposure to DES places the female offspring at increased risk for
    A. ovarian cancer
    B. clear cell adenocarcinoma of the vagina
    C. cervical prolapse
    D. sarcoma botryoides
    E. melanoma

PART 25

The Endocrine System

Disorders of the hypothalamus-pituitary gland, thyroid gland, parathyroid glands, adrenal glands, and gonads in addition to diabetes mellitus are well described in this part of the *Nelson Textbook*. These problems, taken together as endocrine-related diseases, are relatively common and are rarely encountered in an inpatient setting but occupy a significant amount of outpatient pediatrics. Tall or short boys, girls with early or delayed menarche, and other common endocrine problems in practice are covered here. In addition to clinical recognition and management, the diagnostic utility of genetic testing and hormone assays or provocative testing is highlighted.

The questions in this part should reinforce your reading of the *Nelson Textbook* chapters and the 1-month rotation in outpatient endocrinology that you probably had as an elective during residency.

---

1. **Matching:** Adrenocortical insufficiency

    1. Holoprosencephaly
    2. Male predominance
    3. Familial glucocorticoid deficiency
    4. Allgrove syndrome
    5. Most common cause of adrenocortical insufficiency

    A. ACTH receptor mutations
    B. ACTH resistance
    C. Corticotropin deficiency
    D. Adrenal hypoplasia congenita
    E. Congenital adrenal hyperplasia

2. A 12-year-old female has a hypoglycemic seizure, weakness, and increased cutaneous pigmentation. She is also noted to have a chronic history of mucocutaneous candidiasis, which is especially severe on her nails. In addition, she has been on thyroid replacement medication since the age of 9 years. The most likely diagnosis is

    A. insulinoma
    B. growth hormone deficiency
    C. AIDS
    D. autoimmune polyendocrinopathy
    E. DiGeorge syndrome

3. **Matching:**

    1. Hypokalemia
    2. Alkalosis
    3. Hyponatremia
    4. Hypochloremia
    5. Hypertension
    6. High renin level
    7. High urinary prostaglandin levels
    8. Growth failure

    A. Primary hyperaldosteronism
    B. Bartter syndrome
    C. Neither *A* nor *B*
    D. Both *A* and *B*

4. A 16-year-old male has a tall stature but no facial, axillary, or pubic hair. His penis and scrotum are obscured by pubic adipose tissue, but they appear infantile. Chromosome analysis reveals XY karyotype. His serum follicle-stimulating hormone (FHS) and luteinizing hormone (LH) levels are elevated. The most likely diagnosis is

    A. galactosemia
    B. primary hypogonadism
    C. adrenal hyperplasia
    D. Noonan syndrome
    E. none of the above

5. A 14-year-old male has unilateral gynecomastia and is Tanner stage 3 in pubertal development. He complains of occasional episodes of breast tenderness, which last less than 30 minutes and occur once a month. His serum estradiol and prolactin levels are normal. The most likely next step in the treatment of this patient is

A. reassurance and explaining the transient nature

B. mammography

C. abdominal CT including the pelvis

D. head CT focusing on the pituitary

E. karyotype

6. **Matching:** Diabetes

1. Autoimmune
2. Obesity
3. Insulin resistance
4. Honeymoon period
5. Glucokinase mutation
6. Antibody to glutamic acid decarboxylase
7. Familial
8. Hypothyroidism
9. Blindness
10. Cure available

A. Insulin-dependent diabetes

B. Non–insulin-dependent diabetes

C. Both *A* and *B*

D. Neither *A* nor *B*

7. A 12-year-old female has muscle cramps and tingling of her hands and feet unrelated to exertion. When she grabs a door handle to open the door, she is unable to release her grasp because her hand is in spasm. The most important laboratory test is

A. serum glucose determination

B. serum calcium determination

C. electromyography (EMG)

D. nerve conduction velocity testing

E. arterial blood gas determination

8. Acquired hypothyroidism is associated with all of the following EXCEPT

A. diabetes mellitus

B. cystinosis

C. hyperparathyroidism

D. lymphocytic thyroiditis

E. Langerhans cell histiocytosis

9. Physical findings in Graves disease include all of the following EXCEPT

A. motor hyperactivity

B. cold intolerance

C. tremor

D. weight loss

E. tachycardia

F. smooth, flushed, warm skin

10. McCune-Albright syndrome is associated with all of the following EXCEPT

A. precocious puberty in females

B. hyperthyroidism

C. diabetes mellitus

D. Cushing syndrome

E. phosphaturic osteomalacia

F. neonatal cholestasis

G. bony fibrous dysplasia

11. Diabetes insipidus is associated with all of the following EXCEPT

A. optic glioma

B. craniopharyngioma

C. diabetes mellitus

D. Langerhans cell histiocytosis

E. encephalitis

F. atypical mycobacteria

12. Constitutional growth delay is characterized by all of the following EXCEPT

A. normal length at birth

B. growth below the third percentile after 1 year of age

C. delayed bone age

D. positive family history

E. insulin resistance

13. A mother and her 14½-year-old daughter come to you because the girl has not begun to menstruate. Findings on her medical history and complete physical examination are normal. Breast development and pubic hair have been present for 18 months and are normal. Which would be the most appropriate?

A. Reassurance that she likely will begin menstruating within the year

B. Laboratory evaluation for systemic disease

C. Urinary estriol determination

D. Buccal smear

E. Referral for psychologic counseling

14. An 8-month-old previously well infant is brought to the emergency room with vomiting, lethargy, dehydration, and failure to thrive. Intravenous administration of fluids is begun. Serum electrolyte values are sodium 124 mEq/L, chloride 88 mEq/L, and potassium 6.8 mEq/L. Serum glucose level is 35 mg/dL. The child is hypotensive and has areas of hyperpigmentation. The most likely diagnosis is
    A. Addison disease
    B. Waterhouse-Friderichsen syndrome
    C. 17-hydroxylase deficiency
    D. Cushing syndrome
    E. adrenoleukodystrophy

15. Treatment for the infant described in Question 14 should include which of the following (choose as many as are appropriate)?
    A. Desoxycorticosterone acetate (DOCA)
    B. Hydrocortisone hemisuccinate
    C. Adrenalectomy
    D. Insulin
    E. Glucagon

16. Holoprosencephaly is associated with all of the following EXCEPT
    A. cyclopia
    B. pituitary hypoplasia
    C. cebocephaly
    D. congenital toxoplasmosis
    E. orbital hypotelorism

17. Hall Pallister syndrome includes all of the following EXCEPT
    A. absent pituitary gland
    B. postaxial polydactyly
    C. nail dysplasia
    D. bifid uvula
    E. maternal DES exposure

18. Conditions associated with growth hormone deficiency include all of the following EXCEPT
    A. cleft palate
    B. midfacial anomalies
    C. solitary maxillary central incisor
    D. optic nerve hypoplasia
    E. VATER syndrome

19. Children with growth hormone deficiency are best characterized by all of the following EXCEPT
    A. low birthweight
    B. delayed epiphyseal closure
    C. short stature by 1 year of age
    D. round-shaped head
    E. hypoglycemia
    F. small hands and feet

20. Suggestive laboratory features of classic growth hormone deficiency include all of the following EXCEPT
    A. low IGF-I
    B. low IGF-BP3
    C. low GH
    D. delayed bone age
    E. low calcium

21. Potential causes of central diabetes insipidus include all of the following EXCEPT
    A. Wolfram syndrome
    B. craniopharyngiomas
    C. septo-optic dysplasia
    D. autosomal dominant DI
    E. Graves disease

22. A 10-year-old presents with 1 year of polyuria and polydipsia. On voiding cystourethrogram, she is noted to have megacystis and hydroureter. Her most diagnosis is
    A. posterior urethral valves
    B. obstructive uropathy
    C. bladder stones
    D. psychogenic polyphagia
    E. central diabetes insipidus

23. Sotos syndrome is characterized by all of the following EXCEPT
    A. macrocrania
    B. large size at birth
    C. tall stature
    D. clumsiness
    E. normal intelligence

24. Precocious puberty is defined by all of the following EXCEPT

A. presence of secondary sexual characteristics in girls by age 8 years

B. presence of secondary sexual characteristics in boys by age 9 years

C. gonadotropin-dependent or central or true

D. gonadotropin-independent or pseudopuberty

E. ectopic gonadotropin production

25. A 6-year-old female presents with breast enlargement and pubic hair development. Otherwise, she is asymptomatic. Her serum LH level is elevated. The most likely diagnosis is

A. hypothyroidism

B. exposure to exogenous estrogen

C. an estrogen-secreting tumor

D. an adrenal tumor

E. central precocious puberty

26. The next best step in the evaluation of the child in Question 25 is to obtain a

A. serum prolactin level

B. head MRI

C. no further testing

D. serum testosterone test

E. adrenal ultrasound test

27. The treatment of the girl in Questions 25 and 26 is best accomplished with

A. leuprolide

B. growth hormone

C. progesterone

D. prednisone

E. cranial irradiation

28. A male infant is thought to have hypothyroidism because of a neonatal screening program that detected a low serum T_4 level. His TSH level is normal. The most likely diagnosis is

A. neonatal goiter

B. congenital goiter

C. maternal Graves disease

D. thyroxine binding globulin deficiency

E. iodine deficiency

29. All of the characteristics of congenital hypothyroidism are true EXCEPT

A. higher incidence in females

B. incidence of 1:4000

C. lower incidence in African-Americans

D. central role of thyroid peroxidase antibodies

E. asymptomatic at birth

30. A 6-week-old infant has gained no weight since birth. She is mottled and has an indirect bilirubin level of 24 mg/dL. Her extremities are cold, and her temperature is 35°C. The most likely diagnosis is

A. kernicterus

B. sepsis

C. galactosemia

D. hypothermia

E. hypothyroidism

31. The evaluation of the child in Question 30 is best accomplished by determining

A. serum TSH

B. serum T_4

C. bone age

D. head CT

E. thyroid scan

32. A 14-year-old presents with poor growth and delayed puberty. She denies headaches or poor school performance. She is physically sluggish and has a small goiter, and her serum cholesterol is 500 mg/dL. The most likely diagnosis is

A. Hashimoto disease

B. Graves disease

C. congenital hypothyroidism

D. familial type II hyperlipidemia

E. pituitary prolactinoma

33. The antimicrosomal antibodies noted in lymphocytic thyroiditis are central to its etiology but have been renamed

A. Graves disease antibodies

B. thyroid antiperoxidase antibodies

C. thyroglobulin antibodies

D. Hashimoto antibodies

E. thyroid autoimmunity globulins

34. Common features of Graves disease include all of the following EXCEPT

A. 5:1 male:female ratio

B. 6-month to 1-year delay in diagnosis

C. emotional disturbances

D. poor school work

E. tremors

F. varacious appetite

G. exophthalmos

35. The initial treatment of choice for Graves disease is

A. surgery

B. radioactive iodine

C. iodine

D. propylthiouracil

E. propranolol (Inderal)

36. All of the following are associated with hypocalcemia EXCEPT

A. maternal hyperparathyroidism

B. Kearns-Sayre syndrome

C. DiGeorge syndrome

D. Magnesium deficiency

E. early vitamin D–deficient rickets

37. A 6-year-old has a chronic rash involving all of the nails of the fingers and toes. Last year she had a seizure and was noted to have a low serum ionized calcium. Currently she has weakness and hypotension, and she presents with a hypoglycemic seizure. The most likely diagnosis causing this seizure is

A. AIDS

B. metachromatic leukodystrophy

C. adrenal leukodystrophy

D. Addison disease

E. panhypopituitarism

38. The underlying disorder affecting the child in Question 37 is most likely

A. type I autoimmune polyendocrinopathy

B. type II autoimmune polyendocrinopathy

C. tuberculosis

D. sarcoidosis

E. adrenoleukodystrophy

39. **Matching:** Congenital adrenal hyperplasia

1. 11β-

2. 21-OH deficiency

3. Lipoid congenital adrenal hyperplasia

4. 3β-HSD deficiency

hydroxylase deficiency

A. Most common

B. Hypertension

C. Male and female pseudohermaphroditism

D. Low levels of all steroid hormones

40. Noonan syndrome is associated with all of the following EXCEPT

A. short stature

B. chromosomal duplication

C. hypogonadism in males

D. web neck

E. leukemia

41. Features of Klinefelter syndrome include all of the following EXCEPT

A. 47XXY chromosomes

B. mental retardation

C. short stature

D. psychiatric disturbances

E. breast cancer

42. Type I diabetes mellitus is most often associated with

A. mumps infection

B. coxsackievirus

C. antibodies to glutamic acid dehydrogenase

D. cow's milk

E. mitochondrial DNA deletions

43. Hyperglycemia during diabetic ketoacidosis may be associated with

A. hypocalcemia

B. hypernatremia

C. hyponatremia

D. hypomagnesemia

E. hypocholesterolemia

44. Hyperkalemia in severe diabetic ketoacidosis is due to

A. renal failure

B. hemolysis

C. hyperglycemia

D. artifact

E. acidosis

PART 26

The Nervous System

This part of the *Nelson Textbook* is an important reminder of the complexities of neurologic disorders. This part has chapters that discuss examination and evaluation, congenital anomalies, seizures, headaches, neurocutaneous syndromes, movement disorders, encephalopathies, coma, brain death, injuries, neurodegenerative disorders, stroke, abscesses, tumors, pseudotumor cerebri, and spinal cord disorders. Previously grouped together with unknown causes or pathophysiologies, many neurologic diseases are being more completely understood today, thus providing rational diagnosis and therapy.

Questions for the nervous system part emphasize the recognition and differential diagnosis of neurologic disorders.

1. A 4-year-old female has experienced progressive loss of ambulation for a 2-year period. On examination, the child is apathetic and uninterested in her surroundings. She has horizontal nystagmus and optic atrophy. Her voice is dysarthric. She is hypotonic, and her deep tendon reflexes are absent. A sibling died at the age of 6 years with a similar history. The motor nerve conduction velocities show marked slowing, and computed tomography (CT) of the head shows diffuse symmetric attenuation of the cerebral and cerebellar white matter. The most likely diagnosis is
   A. multiple sclerosis
   B. metachromatic leukodystrophy
   C. GM_2 gangliosidosis (Tay-Sachs disease)
   D. neuronal ceroid lipofuscinosis
   E. Pelizaeus-Merzbacher disease

2. A 3-year-old female has a 2-week history of fever associated with bifrontal headache, lethargy, and vomiting. She has a history of perioral cyanosis and dyspnea with exertion beginning in infancy. She suddenly has a 10-minute focal tonic-clonic seizure. The child is obtunded and has a temperature of 100.8°F (38.2°C), pulse of 118, and blood pressure of 96/70 mm Hg in her right arm, supine. Perioral cyanosis is noted at rest. A harsh pansystolic murmur is heard best along the left sternal border. Examination of her eye grounds reveals bilateral papilledema. She has right-sided weakness associated with hyperreflexia and an extensor plantar reflex. The most likely cause of the hemiparesis is
   A. moyamoya disease
   B. a brain tumor
   C. an intracranial hemorrhage
   D. methemoglobinemia
   E. a brain abscess

3. **Matching:**
   1. Prevented by folic acid
   2. Detected by antenatal ultrasonography
   3. Elevated maternal serum α-fetoprotein
   4. May be X linked
   5. Valproic acid as teratogen
   6. Radiation exposure

   A. Hydrocephalus
   B. Spina bifida
   C. Both *A* and *B*
   D. Neither *A* nor *B*

4. Causes of megalocephaly include all of the following EXCEPT
   A. thalassemia
   B. chronic subdural effusions
   C. hydrocephalus
   D. Canavan disease
   E. congenital CMV
   F. familial

5. All of the following cause neonatal seizures EXCEPT
   A. pyridoxine deficiency
   B. lissencephaly
   C. hypoglycemia
   D. hypoxia-ischemia
   E. spina bifida
   F. incontinentia pigmentosa

6. **Matching:** Neurocutaneous lesions
   1. Seizures
   2. Facial nevi
   3. *Café au lait* spots
   4. Ash leaf spot
   5. Lisch nodules
   6. Shagreen patch
   7. Glaucoma
   8. Melanoma
   9. Axillary freckling
   10. Kyphoscoliosis

   A. Neurofibromatosis
   B. Tuberous sclerosis
   C. Sturge-Weber
   D. None of the above
   E. All of the above

7. A 12-year-old female experiences acute monocular blindness of 2 days' duration. Past medical history reveals that she has had headaches for the past 3 years that she cannot characterize, one brief episode of diplopia, and one episode of paresthesias of the feet. These episodes were not related in time, did not occur in immediate proximity to the headache, and resolved spontaneously. Physical examination, other than reduced visual acuity, is unremarkable, including the funduscopic examination. The most important diagnostic step is to perform
   A. CT
   B. MRI
   C. an electroencephalogram
   D. peripheral nerve conduction tests
   E. a nerve biopsy

8. **Matching:**
   1. Tay-Sachs disease
   2. Optic atrophy and peripheral neuropathy
   3. Hurler-like facies
   4. Optic atrophy and brown retina
   5. Academic deterioration and gait disturbance
   6. Marked startle response
   7. Spasticity with delayed nerve conduction
   8. Increased caudate densities
   9. Tan skin pigmentation
   10. Unexplained hyperpyrexia
   11. Arylsulfatase A deficiency
   12. Macroglossia

   A. GM_1 gangliosidosis
   B. GM_2 gangliosidosis
   C. Krabbe disease
   D. Metachromatic leukodystrophy
   E. Neuronal ceroid lipofuscinosis
   F. Adrenoleuko-dystrophy

9. A 6-year-old complains of headaches on arising in the morning before school for 2 months. In addition, for the past 2 days the patient has demonstrated head tilt. Physical examination reveals past pointing and difficulty in performing rapid alternating hand movements. The fundi are difficult to visualize. The next part of the evaluation should be
   A. an EEG
   B. a visit to the school psychologist
   C. a CT scan
   D. lumbar puncture
   E. a vision test

10. A 7-year-old with poor dentition has persistent frontal headaches, fever, and irritability of 5 weeks' duration. A lumbar puncture reveals an opening pressure of 250 mm Hg, a white blood cell count of 120 with 75% leukocytes, a glucose level of 80 mg/dL, and a protein level of 95 mg/dL. Results of a Gram stain and culture are negative. The next appropriate step is
    A. CSF culture for tuberculosis

B. cryptococcal antigen determination

C. EEG

D. CT scan

E. dental consultation

11. A 12-year-old presents with a severe headache, a grand mal seizure, and sudden collapse with unresponsive flaccid coma. The patient had a history of intermittent right-sided headaches without an aura and at times without relief with rest. In addition to coma on physical examination, the patient is afebrile and has nuchal rigidity. The most likely diagnosis is

A. bacterial meningitis

B. tuberculous meningitis

C. brain tumor

D. arteriovenous malformation

E. Pott puffy tumor

12. **Matching:** Development

1. Pulls to stand   A. 18 months

2. Two- to three- word sentences   B. 6 months

   C. 9 months

3. Mimics actions   D. 24 months

4. Pincer grasp   E. 3 months

5. Opens hand spontaneously

13. The average time of closure of the anterior fontanel is

A. 12 months

B. 14 months

C. 16 months

D. 18 months

E. 22 months

14. The average time of closure of the posterior fontanel is

A. 2 weeks

B. 2 months

C. 12 months

D. 18 months

E. 20 months

15. Papilledema of acute onset is associated with all of the following EXCEPT

A. reduced visual activity

B. hyperemia of the optic nerve

C. constricted arterioles of the disc

D. dilated disc veins

E. indistinct optic nerve border

16. The Gowers sign demonstrates

A. poor reflexes

B. spinal dysraphism

C. tethered cord

D. proximal motor weakness

E. hysterical paralysis

17. An effective way to screen for fetal neural tube defects is to determine, in the mother,

A. chromosomes

B. α-fetoprotein

C. estriols

D. prolactin

E. fibronectin

18. A method to reduce the incidence of neural tube defects is

A. supplement the diet with folate at 12 weeks' gestation

B. supplement the diet with folate 1 month before conception

C. avoid sexually transmitted diseases

D. chromosomal screening

E. maternal α-fetoprotein levels 1 month before conception

19. **Matching:** Migration disorders

1. Lissencephaly   A. Cerebral clefts

2. Schizencephaly

3. Porencephaly   B. Cerebral cysts

4. Holoprosencephaly   C. Cyclopia

   D. Absent gyri

20. **Matching:** Hydrocephalus

1. Familial   A. Neurofibromatosis

2. *Café au lait* spots   B. X-linked hydrocephalus

3. Sacral hair tuft   C. Vein of Galen arteriovenous malformation

4. Cranial bruit

5. Chorioretinitis   D. Spinal dysraphism

   E. Toxoplasmosis

21. Characteristics of simple partial seizures include all of the following EXCEPT
    A. loss of consciousness
    B. versive seizures
    C. duration of 10–20 seconds
    D. no postictal state
    E. abnormal EEG

22. Rasmussen encephalitis is characterized by all of the following EXCEPT
    A. epilepsia partialis continue
    B. onset before 10 years
    C. no sequelae
    D. abnormal EEG
    E. possible role of CMV

23. Landau-Kleffner syndrome is characterized by all of the following EXCEPT
    A. onset at 5 years of age
    B. more common in girls
    C. aphasia
    D. normal hearing
    E. multiple seizure types

24. The most common cause of neonatal seizures is
    A. febrile seizures
    B. pre-eclampsia/eclampsia
    C. hypocalcemia
    D. hypoxic-ischemic encephalopathy
    E. Aicardi syndrome

25. **Matching:** Seizure mimics
    1. Benign paroxysmal vertigo
    2. Night terrors
    3. Breath-holding spells
    4. Syncope
    5. Prolonged QT syndrome
    6. Pseudoseizures

    A. Nystagmus
    B. Cyanosis
    C. Stage 3–4 sleep
    D. Deafness
    E. Positive tilt test
    F. Normal serum prolactin level

26. Migraine is defined as a recurrent headache with symptom-free intervals and at least three of the following EXCEPT

    A. abdominal pain
    B. nausea or emesis
    C. throbbing quality
    D. unilateral location
    E. absent family history
    F. relief following sleep
    G. aura

27. Migraine variants and complications include all of the following EXCEPT
    A. cluster headaches
    B. cyclic vomiting
    C. amaurosis fugax
    D. alternating hemiplegia
    E. confusional states

28. The drug of choice for migraine in a 7-year-old with mild headaches and infrequent occurrence is
    A. acetaminophen
    B. sumatriptan
    C. aspirin
    D. chlorpromazine
    E. ergotamine

29. Neurofibromatosis type I, an autosomal dominant disorder (gene on chromosome 17), is defined by six or more *café au lait* macules over 5 mm in prepubertal or greater than 15 mm in postpubertal children plus at least one of the following EXCEPT
    A. axillary or inguinal freckling
    B. Lisch nodules of the iris
    C. two or more neurofibromas or one plexiform neurofibroma
    D. ash leaf macule
    E. osseous lesions (sphenoid dysplasia, scoliosis)
    F. optic gliomas
    G. an affected first-degree relative

30. A 19-year-old female presents with headache, unsteadiness, and poor hearing that has progressed over the past 5 years. Her father had some type of brain surgery and has been deaf since the age of 35 years. The most likely diagnosis is
    A. neurofibromatosis type II

B. optic glioma

C. neurofibromatosis type I

D. tuberous sclerosis

E. late-onset congenital deafness

31. A 6-year-old is recovering from chickenpox and becomes ataxic and unable to walk. The rest of the physical examination is normal. The most likely diagnosis is

A. encephalitis

B. cerebral thrombosis

C. cerebellar ataxia

D. an acute demyelinating process

E. chorea

32. Physical features of Sydenham chorea include all of the following EXCEPT

A. hypertonia

B. milkmaid's grip

C. choreic hand

D. darting tongue

E. emotional lability

33. **Matching:** Metabolic encephalopathies

1. Galactosemia
2. Schilder disease
3. Metachromatic leukodystrophy
4. Tay-Sachs
5. Maple syrup urine disease
6. Phenylketonuria
7. Canavan disease
8. MERRF
9. Neuronal ceroid lipofuscinosis
10. Wilson disease

A. Onset < 2 years with hepatomegaly

B. Onset < 2 years without hepatomegaly

C. Onset 2–5 years

D. Onset 5–15 years

PART 27

Neuromuscular Disorders

The differential diagnosis of hypotonia is extensive and intimidating, but if approached in a systematic manner, it is educationally rewarding. This part focuses on the peripheral nervous system and includes the ever-expanding field of myopathies (inherited, endocrine, lipid, glycogenosis, mitochondrial, vitamin deficiency).

The ability to respond to the questions in this part of the *Nelson Review* will test your knowledge of neuroanatomy and neurophysiology as well as your patience and differential diagnostic abilities.

1. A 12-year-old female experienced diarrhea, which lasted for 3 days, 2 weeks before manifesting progressive weakness and inability to walk. She has intermittent tingling of her fingers and toes. Physical examination reveals marked peripheral muscle weakness without atrophy or fasciculations. The deep tendon reflexes are absent in her ankles and 1+ at her knees. Findings on the sensory examination are normal. Motor involvement is symmetric. The most likely diagnosis is
   A. transverse myelitis
   B. Guillain-Barré syndrome
   C. polio
   D. myasthenia gravis
   E. mononeuritis multiplex

2. The patient described in Question 1 is admitted to the hospital and now experiences progressive weakness and areflexia of the knee and ankle reflexes. An important test to perform is
   A. urine specific gravity
   B. electrocardiogram (ECG)
   C. serum CPK determination
   D. muscle biopsy
   E. pulmonary function test

3. A 15-year-old male has lost his ability to walk. On physical examination, his ankle and knee deep tendon reflexes are noted to be diminished. The weakness is greatest in peripheral muscles. Cranial nerves all

are normal. One week before these symptoms arose, he returned from a camping trip. The most likely diagnosis is
   A. myasthenia gravis
   B. Organophosphate poisoning
   C. spinal muscular atrophy
   D. botulism
   E. tick paralysis

4. **Matching:** Neuromuscular disorders
   1. Absent deep tendon reflexes
   2. Proximal weakness
   3. Spasticity
   4. Fatigable weakness
   5. Paresthesias

   A. Polyneuropathy
   B. Myopathy
   C. Neuromuscular junction defect
   D. Upper motor neuron defect

5. **Matching:** Endocrine and metabolic myopathies
   1. Kocher-Debré-Sémélaigne syndrome
   2. Myasthenia gravis–like syndrome
   3. Episodic paralysis
   4. Cardiomegaly
   5. Exercise-induced rhabdomyolysis
   6. External ophthalmoplegia

   A. Hypokalemia
   B. Pompe disease
   C. McArdle disease
   D. Hypothyroidism
   E. MELAS
   F. Hyperthyroidism
   G. Kearns-Sayre syndrome

7. Cerebrovascular accidents

6. A 10-year-old female has had diplopia and ptosis and weakness of her neck flexors for 2 months. Symptoms are worse in the evening and are usually partially improved on awakening in the morning. She has no fasciculations or myalgias, and her deep tendon reflexes are 1–2 + . The most likely diagnosis is
   A. hysterical weakness
   B. muscular dystrophy
   C. spinal muscular atrophy
   D. botulism
   E. myasthenia gravis

7. A 4-year-old has difficulty in climbing stairs, slow motor development, and hypertrophied calf muscles. The most likely diagnosis is
   A. myasthenia gravis
   B. myotonia congenita
   C. Duchenne muscular dystrophy
   D. hypokalemic periodic paralysis
   E. central core disease

8. Which is not true of creatine phosphokinase (CK)?
   A. It is the most useful serum enzyme reflecting damaged muscle fibers.
   B. The MM isozyme is found primarily in skeletal muscle.
   C. The MB isozyme is found primarily in cardiac muscle.
   D. The BB isozyme is found primarily in smooth muscle.
   E. All of the above are true of creatine phosphokinase.

9. Which is not true of congenital neuromuscular disorders?
   A. Most are hereditary.
   B. Most are nonprogressive conditions.
   C. The definitive diagnosis is best made by electromyography (EMG).
   D. Diagnosis for some disorders may be confirmed by genetic analyses of lymphocytes.
   E. Hypotonia is a common feature.

10. Which is not true of muscular dystrophies?
    A. They are a primary myopathy.
    B. They have a genetic basis.
    C. The course is progressive.
    D. Degeneration and death of muscle fibers occur at some stage of disease.
    E. All of the above are true of muscular dystrophies.

11. Which is not true of Duchenne muscular dystrophy?
    A. It is the most common hereditary neuromuscular disease.
    B. It is inherited as an autosomal dominant trait.
    C. Symptoms are rarely present at birth or in early infancy.
    D. The serum creatine phosphokinase (CK) is consistently greatly elevated.
    E. It is most common in males.

12. Which is a characteristic clinical manifestation of Duchenne muscular dystrophy?
    A. Cardiomyopathy
    B. Intellectual impairment
    C. Weakness of respiratory muscles
    D. Scoliosis
    E. All of the above are common clinical manifestations of Duchenne muscular dystrophy.

13. Which is not associated with constant muscle weakness?
    A. Hypothyroidism
    B. Hyperparathyroidism
    C. Corticosteroids
    D. Hyperaldosteronism (Conn syndrome)
    E. All of the above may be associated with muscle weakness.

14. Which is not true of malignant hyperthermia?
    A. It is inherited as an autosomal dominant trait.
    B. Acute episodes are typically precipitated by intravenous administration of dyes for radiographic studies.

C. Myoglobinuria may result in tubular necrosis and acute renal failure.

D. Attacks may be prevented by administration of dantrolene sodium.

E. Metabolic acidosis may be severe.

15. Which is the etiology of most cases of myasthenia gravis?
    A. Inheritance as a recessive trait
    B. Inheritance as an X-linked trait
    C. Postinfectious, usually after either influenza or chickenpox
    D. Autoimmune disorder
    E. Idiopathic

16. Which is the earliest and most consistent sign of myasthenia gravis?
    A. Positive Gower sign
    B. Trendelenburg gait
    C. Ptosis and extraocular muscle weakness
    D. Respiratory muscle weakness
    E. Head lag

17. Which is the best means for diagnosis of myasthenia gravis?
    A. Anti-ACh antibodies
    B. Nerve conduction velocity (NCV) studies
    C. Electromyogram (EMG)
    D. Nerve biopsy
    E. Muscle biopsy

18. Which is a common clinical manifestation of myasthenia gravis?
    A. Cardiomyopathy
    B. Intellectual impairment
    C. Weakness of respiratory muscles
    D. Scoliosis
    E. Headache

19. A one-day-old newborn born to a myasthenic mother has generalized hypotonia and weakness. What is the prognosis?
    A. Greatly increased risk of the complete picture of myasthenia gravis
    B. Small but increased risk of the complete picture of myasthenia gravis

C. No increased risk of myasthenia gravis

D. Some residual weakness until puberty but no increased risk of myasthenia gravis

E. Episodes of diminishing severity of muscle weakness until puberty

20. A 4-year-old child with a history of poor sucking and swallowing as an infant recently experienced excessive sweating and blotchy erythema, especially when excited. Walking is clumsy. There has been new onset of episodes of cyclic vomiting lasting 24–27 hours, with retching and vomiting every 15–20 minutes with profuse sweating, blotchy erythema, apprehension, and irritability. Which is the most likely diagnosis?
    A. Duchenne muscular dystrophy
    B. Fabry disease
    C. Chronic organophosphate intoxication
    D. Familial dysautonomia (Riley-Day syndrome)
    E. Guillain-Barré syndrome

21. A 4-year-old child presents with symmetric weakness that began in the lower extremities and subsequently progressed over 10–14 days to involve the trunk and upper limbs. Deep tendon reflexes are absent. There are no sensory deficits or bowel or bladder dysfunction. Nerve conduction velocity test results are abnormal. The cerebrospinal fluid shows protein of 78 mg/dL and 5 white blood cells/μL. Which is the most likely diagnosis?
    A. Duchenne muscular dystrophy
    B. Fabry disease
    C. Familial dysautonomia (Riley-Day syndrome)
    D. Bell palsy
    E. Guillain-Barré syndrome

22. A 9-year-old presents with paresis of the upper and lower portions of the face, and loss of taste on the right side of the anterior portion of the tongue. On physical examination, the corner of the mouth droops, and he is unable to

close the right eye tightly. The remainder of the physical examination is normal. Which is the most likely diagnosis?

A. Duchenne muscular dystrophy

B. Fabry disease

C. Familial dysautonomia (Riley-Day syndrome)

D. Bell palsy

E. Guillain-Barré syndrome

PART 28

Disorders of the Eye

Ocular manifestations of systemic illnesses often provide clues to the underlying disease. Of equal importance are primary ophthalmologic problems that are congenital, inherited, or acquired and that affect the vision of children. This part appropriately emphasizes early detection and treatment to avoid preventable visual impairment or blindness.

Questions in this part of the *Nelson Review* reinforce the concepts of early detection and treatment to prevent blindness. Nonetheless, answering these questions will unfortunately not enable you to decipher the many Latin-based notations of our ophthalmology colleagues.

1 **Matching:** Pupils
   1. Abnormal pupil position
   2. Inequality of pupil size
   3. Abnormal pupil shape
   4. Absence of dilator pupillae muscle
   5. Ocular trauma

   A. Dyscoria
   B. Corectopia
   C. Anisocoria
   D. Fixed, dilated pupil
   E. Microcoria

2. The differential diagnosis of leukocoria includes all of the following EXCEPT
   A. retinoblastoma
   B. endophthalmitis
   C. larval granulomatosis
   D. cataract
   E. retinal artery occlusion
   F. Coats disease
   G. persistent hyperplastic primary vitreous
   H. retinal detachment

3. Delayed removal of a congenital and complete unilateral cataract may lead to
   A. amblyopia
   B. glaucoma
   C. uveitis
   D. strabismus
   E. nyctalopia

4. **Matching:** Strabismus
   1. Inward deviation

   A. Heterophoria
   B. Heterotropia

   2. Latent tendency to malalignment
   3. Outward deviation
   4. Misalignment at all times
   5. Downward deviation
   6. Upward deviation

   C. Esophoria
   D. Exophoria
   E. Hyperdeviation
   F. Hypodeviation

5. **Matching:** Papilledema—optic neuritis
   1. Blurring of optic disk margin
   2. Acute vision loss
   3. Chronic vision loss
   4. Elevation of optic nerve head
   5. Engorgement of optic nerve veins
   6. May be unilateral
   7. Nerve fiber layer hemorrhage
   8. Pain on movement of globe
   9. Normal-appearing nerve head
   10. Occurs after an epileptic seizure

   A. Papilledema
   B. Optic neuritis
   C. Neither *A* nor *B*
   D. Both *A* and *B*

6. Cataracts are noted in all of the following EXCEPT

A. rubella (congenital)

B. galactosemia

C. galactokinase deficiency

D. neonatal hypoglycemia

E. hypocalcemia

F. Lowe syndrome

G. hyperoxygenation

H. steroid therapy

I. child abuse

7. An 18-month-old manifests pendular nystagmus, head nodding, and torticollis. Findings on a cranial MRI scan are normal. This child most likely has

A. epilepsy

B. congenital blindness

C. neuroblastoma

D. dysmetria

E. spasmus nutans

8. A 7-year-old female experiences fullness of the right upper eyelid and downward displacement of the eye over a 2-month period. The right eye also appears to be proptotic. What is the most likely diagnosis?

A. Myasthenia gravis

B. Right superior oblique palsy

C. Chalazion

D. Rhabdomyosarcoma

E. Hypothyroidism

9. Which is not true of normal development of the eye?

A. The cornea may have an opalescent appearance in premature infants.

B. Superficial retinal hemorrhages may be observed in normal infants after birth.

C. The iris is light blue or gray at birth and undergoes progressive color change for the first 6 months of life.

D. The visual acuity of newborns is approximately 20/100 but is usually 20/20 by 3–6 months of age.

E. Tears often are not present with crying until 1–3 months of age.

10. Which of the following is not true of amblyopia?

A. Younger children are more susceptible to amblyopia than older children.

B. Amblyopia is reversed more rapidly in younger children than older children.

C. Amblyopia occurs only after the cortex becomes visually mature.

D. Amblyopia is usually asymptomatic.

E. All of the above are true of amblyopia.

11. Which is the most common cause of aniridia?

A. Trauma

B. Congenital infection

C. Wilms tumor

D. Inheritance as an autosomal dominant trait

E. Idiopathic

12. Which of the following is associated with aniridia?

A. Optic nerve hypoplasia

B. Poor visual acuity

C. Lens and corneal abnormalities

D. Wilms tumor

E. All of the above are associated with aniridia.

13. A 4-month-old infant presents with unilateral overflow of tears that have a clear appearance. Which is the recommended initial treatment?

A. Topical antibiotics appropriate for dacryocystitis

B. Oral antibiotics appropriate for dacryocystitis

C. Warm compresses

D. Nasolacrimal massage 2–3 times each day

E. Referral for surgical repair

14. Which is not true of ophthalmia neonatorum caused by *Chlamydia trachomatis*?

A. Conjunctivitis usually develops at 5–14 days of age.

B. Chlamydial conjunctivitis is a self-limiting disease with no sequelae.

C. Ten to 20% of infants exposed to *Chlamydia trachomatis* will also experience pneumonia.

D. Recommended treatment is cefotaxime or ceftriaxone.

E. Topical erythromycin is not recommended.

15. Which is the most common presenting sign of retinoblastoma?
    A. Heterophoria
    B. Hypopyon
    C. Leukocoria
    D. Coloboma
    E. Red reflex

16. A 17-year-old female on oral contraceptives presents with headache, nausea, and vomiting. Physical examination reveals papilledema. Which is the most appropriate action?
    A. Discontinue the oral contraceptives and re-evaluate in 7–14 days.
    B. Discontinue the oral contraceptives and administer promethazine (Phenergan) as needed for nausea and vomiting.
    C. Discontinue the oral contraceptives and administer oral corticosteroids.
    D. Computed tomography (CT) or magnetic resonance imaging (MRI) of the head
    E. Lumbar puncture for determination of cerebrospinal fluid pressure

17. A 1-year-old child presents with increased size of the cornea. Review of systems reveals history of increased tearing and apparent sensitivity to light. The cornea appears cloudy. Which is the most likely diagnosis?
    A. Retinoblastoma
    B. Glaucoma
    C. Chorioretinitis
    D. Aniridia
    E. Coloboma

18. Which is the most appropriate initial treatment for the child in Question 17?
    A. Topical glaucoma medications
    B. Oral glaucoma medications
    C. Corticosteroids
    D. Surgery
    E. Medications and surgery

19. A 12-year-old boy has a small corneal abrasion detected by Wood lamp examination. Which is the most appropriate treatment?
    A. Topical antibiotic ointment
    B. Topical antibiotic ointment and a semipressure patch
    C. Topical antibiotic ointment, a semipressure patch, and a topical cycloplegic agent
    D. Topical antibiotic ointment, a semipressure patch, and a topical anesthetic as necessary for pain
    E. Topical antibiotic ointment, a topical cycloplegic agent, and a topical anesthetic as necessary for pain

PART 29

The Ear

Deafness and otitis media are two fundamentally important problems that affect children. Hearing loss has significant implications for the development of hearing-impaired children. Poor speech development should always suggest hearing loss. Otitis media is an extremely common disorder with potentially serious acute and chronic sequelae. Expert pediatricians should never miss the diagnosis of either of these disorders.

Questions in this part are designed for general pediatricians and focus on important aspects of the ear from a preventive, diagnostic, and therapeutic perspective.

1. Which of the following are associated with conductive hearing loss?
   A. Cholesteatoma
   B. Otosclerosis
   C. Otitis media with effusion
   D. Foreign body in the external canal
   E. Impacted cerumen
   F. All of the above

2. A hearing deficit of moderate loss is associated with an average sound threshold of 30–50 dB and which of the following?
   A. Misses most speech sounds at normal conversational levels
   B. Language retardation
   C. Misses unvoiced consonant sounds
   D. Inattention
   E. All of the above

3. Common features of external otitis include all of the following EXCEPT
   A. itching
   B. edema
   C. green otorrhea
   D. perforation of the tympanic membrane
   E. regional lymphadenopathy
   F. pain on movement of the pinna and tragus

4. **Matching:**
   1. Bulging eardrum
   2. Pain on movement of auricle
   3. Lymphadenitis
   4. Periauricular edema
   5. Sinusitis
   6. Obliteration of posterior auricular fold

   A. External otitis
   B. Mastoiditis
   C. Both *A* and *B*
   D. Neither *A* nor *B*

5. Which is least likely to be associated with sensorineural hearing loss?
   A. Family history of sensorineural hearing loss
   B. In utero infection (e.g., cytomegalovirus, rubella, syphilis)
   C. Otitis media
   D. Bacterial meningitis
   E. Apgar scores of 0–4 at 1 minute or 0–6 at 5 minutes

6. Which organism is not a common cause of otitis media?
   A. *Staphylococcus aureus*
   B. *Streptococcus pneumoniae*
   C. Nontypable *Haemophilus influenzae*
   D. *Moraxella catarrhalis*

7. Which of the following is the most reliable finding associated with acute otitis media?
   A. Otalgia (ear pain)
   B. Visual inspection showing a thickened tympanic membrane
   C. Hyperemia of the tympanic membrane

D. Decreased mobility of the tympanic membrane by pneumatic otoscopy

8. Which is the drug of choice for empirical treatment of a first episode of acute otitis media?
   A. Amoxicillin
   B. Trimethoprim-sulfamethoxazole
   C. Amoxicillin-clavulanate
   D. Ceftriaxone
   E. Any of the above

9. Which factor is associated with increased risk for otitis media caused by resistant *Streptococcus pneumoniae*?
   A. Recent antimicrobial exposure
   B. Young age (<2 years)
   C. Daycare attendance
   D. All of the above
   E. None of the above

10. Which is not true of examination of the tympanic membrane?
    A. The normal tympanic membrane has a translucent, ground-glass, or waxed paper appearance.
    B. A red tympanic membrane can be normal.
    C. A retracted tympanic membrane usually indicates negative middle-ear pressure.
    D. Prominent short process and foreshortened long process of the malleus are typical of a bulging tympanic membrane.
    E. Middle-ear effusion with little or no air in the middle ear results in severely decreased or absent responses to both applied positive and negative pressures.

11. Which is not associated with sensorineural hearing loss?
    A. Family history of hereditary hearing loss
    B. In utero infection (e.g., cytomegalovirus, rubella, syphilis)
    C. Otitis media
    D. Bacterial meningitis
    E. Apgar scores of 0–4 at 1 minute or 0–6 at 5 minutes

12. The American Academy of Pediatrics has endorsed that hearing loss be detected by which age?
    A. At birth
    B. 3 months
    C. 2 years
    D. 4–5 years (at school entry)
    E. 12 years

13. Which of the following does not indicate the need for referral for audiologic assessment?
    A. No differentiated babbling or vocal imitation at 12 months of age
    B. No use of single words at 18 months of age
    C. Single-word vocabulary of ≤10 words at 24 months of age
    D. Fewer than a 100-word vocabulary, or no evidence of two-word combinations at 30 months of age
    E. All of these indicate the need for referral for audiologic assessment.

14. An admittance tympanogram of a 7-year-old child reveals the following (Fig. 29–1). Which is the most likely interpretation?
    A. Normal
    B. Middle-ear effusion
    C. Obstruction of the auditory duct

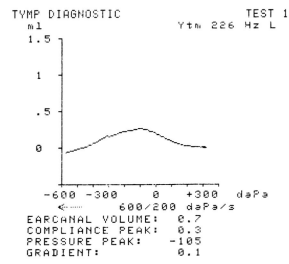

Figure 29-1

D. Not interpretable, probably because of operator error

15. A 4-year-old child that is new to your clinic has a small pit-like depression anterior to the helix and above the tragus. There are no symptoms. Which is the recommended initial management?
    A. Observation only
    B. Exploration by probing
    C. Computed tomography (CT) or magnetic resonance imaging (MRI) to evaluate for possible branchial cleft cyst
    D. Referral for surgical excision
    E. Referral for chromosome analysis

16. A 12-year-old child has recurrent bouts of otitis externa that are associated with swimming. Which is the recommended method for preventing recurrences?
    A. Advise against all swimming, even when asymptomatic
    B. Instillation of trolamine polypeptide oleate-condensate (Cerumenex) or carbamide peroxide (Debrox) after swimming
    C. Instillation of dilute alcohol or acetic acid (2%) solution after swimming
    D. Instillation of otic neomycin and hydrocortisone drops, otic ciprofloxacin and hydrocortisone, or otic acetic acid (2%) and hydrocortisone drops after swimming
    E. There is no recognized prophylaxis to minimize risk for otitis externa.

17. Which is a common bacterial cause of otitis media?
    A. *Staphylococcus aureus*
    B. Group A *Streptococcus*
    C. *Haemophilus influenzae* type b

D. *Moraxella catarrhalis*
E. *Pseudomonas aeruginosa*

18. Which of the following is the most reliable finding associated with acute otitis media?
    A. Otalgia (ear pain)
    B. Visual inspection showing a thickened tympanic membrane
    C. Hyperemia of the tympanic membrane
    D. Decreased mobility of the tympanic membrane by pneumatic otoscopy
    E. Tugging at the ears

19. Which is the drug of choice for empirical treatment of a first episode of acute otitis media?
    A. Amoxicillin
    B. Trimethoprim-sulfamethoxazole
    C. Axomicillin-clavulanate
    D. Ceftriaxone
    E. Any of the above

20. Which factor is associated with increased risk for otitis media caused by resistant *Streptococcus pneumonia*?
    A. Recent antimicrobial exposure
    B. Young age (<2 years)
    C. Daycare attendance
    D. All of the above
    E. None of the above

21. Which is not a sign of temporal bone fracture?
    A. Bleeding from a laceration of the external canal
    B. Hemotympanum (blood behind the tympanic membrane)
    C. Cerebrospinal fluid otorrhea
    D. Conductive hearing loss
    E. Hemiplegia

PART 30

The Skin

Most pediatricians feel like full-time but amateur dermatologists. Rashes are common at all ages. Because of their obvious appearance, rashes often prompt parents to bring their child to a pediatrician's office for evaluation. This part concentrates on diseases of the skin, hair, and nails that may be congenital, neoplastic, infectious, inflammatory, or of unknown cause. The treatments are well described.

Questions in this part enhance the amateur dermatologist in all of us and reinforce our diagnostic skills.

1. Giant congenital pigmented nevi are associated with all of the following EXCEPT
   A. an incidence of less than 1 in 20,000 births
   B. leptomeningeal involvement
   C. malignant melanoma
   D. hydrocephalus
   E. male predominance

2. Incontinentia pigmenti is associated with all of the following EXCEPT
   A. lethality in females
   B. erythematous linear streaks and vesicles
   C. alopecia
   D. hypodontia
   E. microphthalmos
   F. seizures

3. Stevens-Johnson syndrome (erythema multiforme major) is associated with all of the following EXCEPT
   A. a good response to prednisone
   B. involvement of two mucous membranes
   C. esophageal stricture
   D. corneal scarring
   E. infectious causes
   F. drug-related causes

4. A rash that is visible but not palpable consists of small solitary lesions of 0.5–1 cm in diameter. Which term best describes these lesions?
   A. Macules
   B. Papules
   C. Patch
   D. Plaques
   E. Wheals

5. A child with eczema experiences ulcerated lesions inflicted by scratching. Which term best describes these lesions?
   A. Fissures
   B. Erosions
   C. Ulcers
   D. Excoriations
   E. Crusts

6. Match the condition with the appearance under the Wood lamp (ultraviolet light)
   1. *Tinea corporis*
   2. *Tinea versicolor*
   3. Erythrasma
   4. *Pseudomonas aeruginosa*
   5. Hypopigmented lesions

   A. Pink-orange fluorescence
   B. Golden fluorescence
   C. No fluorescence but lesions appear lighter than surrounding skin
   D. No fluorescence and without distinction from surrounding skin
   E. Yellow-green fluorescence

7. Which is not true of topical corticosteroids?

A. Topical corticosteroids are potent antipruritic agents.

B. Fluorinated corticosteroids are more potent than nonfluorinated corticosteroids.

C. Fluorinated corticosteroids have more local and systemic adverse effects than nonfluorinated corticosteroids.

D. Fluorinated corticosteroids have equivalent potency and differ primarily in their formulation and delivery vehicle.

E. All of the above are true.

8. Which is not true of sunscreens?

A. Some sunscreens permit tanning without burning.

B. A minimum SPF of 15 is recommended for fair-skinned persons to prevent sunburn.

C. Effective sunscreens reflect all wavelengths of both UV and visible spectrums.

D. Even effective sunscreens do not give complete protection against all harmful UV wavelengths.

E. All of the above are true.

9. A well-appearing newborn has a lacy, reticulated, red and/or blue cutaneous pattern over most of the body, which is prominent when the neonate is in a cool environment. What is the diagnosis?

A. Mongolian spots

B. Salmon patch

C. Cutis marmorata

D. Harlequin color change

E. Erythema toxicum

10. A 2-day-old full-term neonate experiences multiple firm, yellow-white, 1- to 2-mm papules or pustules with a surrounding erythematous flare on the trunk (Fig. 30–1). Wright stain of the lesions shows numerous eosinophils. Which is the most likely diagnosis?

A. Erythema toxicum

B. Pustular melanosis

C. Acropustulosis

D. Eosinophilic pustular folliculitis

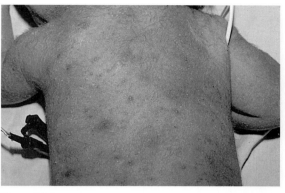

Figure 30-1

E. Herpes simplex virus infection

11. Which therapy is recommended for port-wine nevus?

A. Tattooing

B. Excision and skin-grafting

C. Cryosurgery

D. Laser therapy

E. Interferon-γ

12. An 8-year-old girl presents with large *café au lait* spots with irregular borders and precocious puberty. X-ray shows polyostotic fibrous dysplasia of bone. Which is the most likely diagnosis?

A. Neurofibromatosis

B. McCune-Albright syndrome

C. Tuberous sclerosis

D. Maffucci syndrome

E. Normal child

13. A 3-year-old boy is found to have two small, 0.5- to 1-cm *café au lait* spots that were not present during infancy. Which is the most likely diagnosis?

A. Neurofibromatosis

B. McCune-Albright syndrome

C. Tuberous sclerosis

D. Maffucci syndrome

E. Normal child

14. A 10-year-old girl experiences multiple hyperpigmented scaly plaques without a raised border (Fig. 30–2). Which is the recommended treatment?

A. Tar compounds

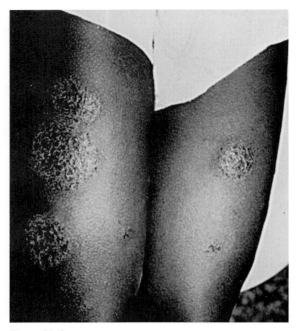

Figure 30-2

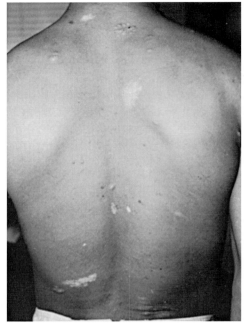

Figure 30-3

B. A fluorinated topical corticosteroid

C. Mupirocin

D. A topical antifungal agent

E. griseofulvin

15. A 9-year-old boy has a history of a seizure disorder and multiple white macules that first appeared in early infancy. A large, skin-colored, irregularly thickened plaque with an orange-peel or cobblestone texture has developed on the back in the lumbosacral area (Fig. 30–3). Which is the most likely diagnosis?

A. Psoriasis

B. Tuberous sclerosis

C. Partial albinism

D. Pityriasis rosea

E. Lichen striatus

16. A 13-year-old boy experiences a single 8-cm annular lesion with a raised border with fine, adherent scales. Approximately 5–7 days later, he experiences a widespread, symmetric eruption involving the trunk with multiple, ovoid, maculopapular lesions less than 1 cm in diameter that are pink to brown (Fig. 30–4). Which is the most likely diagnosis?

A. Psoriasis

B. Eczema

C. Pityriasis rosea

D. Lichen striatus

E. Tinea versicolor

17. A black teenager presents with a sharply demarcated, dense, firm, rubbery growth on the face at the site of a previous,

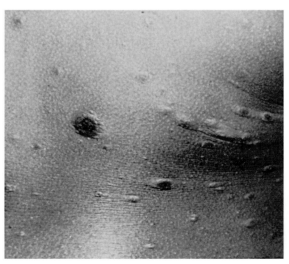

Figure 30-4

smaller laceration that occurred long ago. Which is the most likely diagnosis?

A. Granuloma annulare

B. Keloid

C. Necrobiosis lipoidica

D. Anetoderma

E. Mastocytosis

18. A young child has gradually experienced unusual skin hyperelasticity and joint hypermobility. The skin snaps back into place when pulled. Which diagnosis is most likely?

A. Cutis laxa

B. Ehlers-Danlos syndrome

C. Anetoderma

D. Pseudoxanthoma elasticum

E. Elastosis perforans serpingosa

19. Which is the most common cause of angular cheilitis?

A. Impetigo

B. Thrush

C. Herpes simplex virus

D. Dryness and chapping

E. Sjögren syndrome

20. Which is the most common cause of impetigo?

A. *Corynebacterium minutissimum*

B. *Staphylococcus aureus*

C. Group A β-hemolytic *Streptococcus*

D. Herpes simplex virus

E. Coxsackieviruses

21. Which is not recommended for impetigo?

A. 3% Hexachlorophene soap

B. Topical mupirocin

C. Oral erythromycin

D. Oral dicloxacillin

E. Oral clindamycin

22. Which is the etiology of tinea versicolor?

A. *Staphylococcus aureus*

B. *Malassezia furfur*

C. *Corynebacterium minutissimum*

D. *Trichophyton*

E. Herpes simplex virus

23. Which of the following is a recommended treatment of tinea unguium?

A. Oral ketoconazole

B. Oral itraconazole

C. Topical miconazole

D. Topical terbinafine

E. All of the above are recommended treatments of tinea unguium.

24. A child presents with multiple, discrete, skin-colored, 1- to 3-mm dome-shaped smooth papules on the face with central umbilication (Fig. 30–5). Which is the most likely diagnosis?

A. Verruca vulgaris (common warts)

B. Verruca plana (flat warts)

C. Condylomata acuminata

D. Molluscum contagiosum

E. Keloid

25. Which is the cause of the lesions pictured in Question 21 (see Fig. 30–5)?

A. Herpes simplex virus type 1

B. Herpes simplex virus type 2

C. Coxsackieviruses

D. Human papillomaviruses

E. Molluscum contagiosum virus

26. Which is the recommended treatment of scabies?

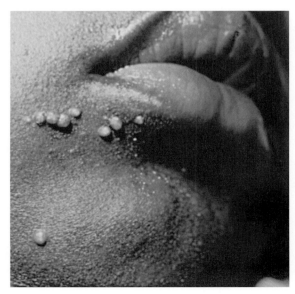

Figure 30-5

A. Permethrin 5%

B. Crotamiton

C. Griseofulvin

D. Itraconazole

E. Ivermectin

27. Which is the recommended treatment of pediculosis capitis (head lice)?

A. Permethrin

B. Lindane

C. Crotamiton

D. Itraconazole

E. Ivermectin

28. Which is the hallmark symptom of pediculosis?

A. Low-grade fever

B. Wheals

C. Lichenification

D. Pruritus

E. Id reaction

29. What is the most serious adverse event associated with isotretinoin?

A. Hepatitis

B. Cardiomyopathy

C. Pseudotumor cerebri

D. Teratogenicity

E. Carcinogenicity

30. A 2-year-old child presents with symmetric psoriasiform skin lesions distributed in the perioral, acral, and perineal areas and on the cheeks, knees, and elbows. There is mild alopecia and a history of chronic diarrhea. Which is the most likely diagnosis?

A. Psoriasis

B. Juvenile xanthogranuloma

C. Acrodermatitis enteropathica

D. Scurvy

E. Pellagra

PART 31

Bone and Joint Disorders

Limps, bumps, pain, disuse, and poor function are common orthopedic problems of childhood. These are due to congenital, inherited, infectious, anatomic, inflammatory, and neoplastic lesions. This extensive part of the *Nelson Textbook* includes sections on general basic orthopedics (including fractures and sports medicine), genetic skeletal dysplasias, and metabolic bone disease.

These questions help clarify definitions (varus vs. valgus) and identify common bone and joint diseases. Management of simple and complex disorders is also covered.

1. An adolescent female who is a cheerleader comes to you with a painful bump below her right knee. She denies fever or trauma. Which is the most likely diagnosis?
   A. Legg-Calvé-Perthes disease
   B. Osteoid osteoma
   C. Osgood-Schlatter disease
   D. Osteochondritis dissecans
   E. Osteomyelitis of the tibial tubercle

2. The best treatment for the patient described in Question 1 is
   A. decreased activity of the knee
   B. anti-inflammatory drugs
   C. antibiotics
   D. excisional biopsy
   E. casting for 6–8 weeks

3. Which is the best initial treatment for dislocated, unrelocatable, congenitally dysplastic hips first discovered at 7 months of age?
   A. Triple diapers
   B. von Rosen splint or other rigid device
   C. Plaster spica case
   D. Traction
   E. Open (surgical reduction)

4. An overweight adolescent male complains of pain in the medial aspect of his knee. He denies trauma, and he has not had a fever. The most likely diagnosis is
   A. Toxic synovitis
   B. Legg-Calve-Perthes disease
   C. Medial collateral ligament (knee) strain
   D. Slipped capital femoral epiphysis
   E. Avulsion of the gastrocnemius muscle

5. A 2-year-old child is brought to you because he refuses to use his right arm. Any attempt to touch it is met with a cry, and the child will not hold objects in his right hand. The mother denies trauma, but she did pull the child by the arm recently when he refused to go into an elevator. The most likely diagnosis is
   A. nonaccidental trauma (child abuse)
   B. fracture of the radius
   C. muscle strain of the right pronator
   D. dislocated radial head
   E. osteomyelitis

6. Plans for the child described in Question 5 should include (choose one or more)
   A. radiograph of the arm, thin casting or splinting
   B. supination of the forearm
   C. antibiotics
   D. alerting the parents to the cause of the problem
   E. reporting the case to a child welfare agency

7. **Matching:** Bone and joint orthopedic terminology

1. Angulation of the vertex of bone or joint toward midline	A. Varum
	B. Cavus
	C. Valgum
2. Plantar-flexed foot	D. Equinus
	E. Arthrotomy

167

3. Angulation of bone or joint away from midline

4. High-arched foot

5. Incision into a joint

8. A 12-year-old male sustains a nail puncture of the high right foot through an old sneaker. Two days later, he limps and complains of pain and swelling in that area. The most likely diagnosis is

A. tetanus

B. osteochondritis

C. foreign body reaction

D. toxic shock syndrome

E. ecthyma gangrenosum

9. The most likely organisms causing the problem described in Question 8 include (choose one or more)

A. *Clostridium perfringens*

B. *Staphylococcus aureus*

C. *Staphylococcus epidermidis*

D. *Pseudomonas aeruginosa*

E. *Serratia marcescens*

10. The most appropriate important first therapeutic approach for the boy described in Questions 8 and 9 is

A. piperacillin-tazobactam

B. ciprofloxacin

C. incision, drainage, debridement

D. tetanus toxoid

E. warm soaks

11. **Matching:**

1. Talipes equinovarus
2. Congenital vertical talus
3. Flexible flatfeet
4. Tarsal coalition
5. Cavus feet

A. Soft tissue surgical release required

B. Usually painless

C. Peripheral neuropathy

D. Responds to serial casting

E. Fusion or failure of segmentation

12. **Matching:** Match the disorder with the laboratory values

1. Hyperphosphatasia
2. X-linked hypophosphatemic rickets
3. Hypophosphatasia
4. Vitamin D–dependent rickets type 1
5. Vitamin D deficiency rickets

Serum Chemistry Values

	Calcium (mg/dL)	Phosphate (mg/dL)	Alkaline Phosphatase (IU/L)	25(OH)D (ng/mL)	1,25(OH)$_2$D$_3$ (pg/mL)
A.	9.2	1.9	754	28	31
B.	12.2	4.5	74	28	31
C.	9.3	4.8	8700	28	43
D.	6.1	2.4	1070	3	21
E.	6.1	2.4	1070	28	4

13. An infant has the physical findings shown in Figure 31–1. What is the diagnosis?

A. Normal

B. Calcaneovalgus

C. Metatarsus adductus

D. Talipes equinovarus

E. Pes planus

14. Match the following terms with the common names.

1. Genu varum
2. Genu valgum
3. Pes planus
4. Talipes equinovarus
5. Tarsal coalition
6. Kyphosis
7. Torticollis
8. Subluxation of the radial head

A. Wryneck

B. Clubfoot

C. Bowlegs

D. Pigeon breast

E. Knock-knees

F. Peroneal spastic flatfoot

G. Funnel chest

H. Round-back

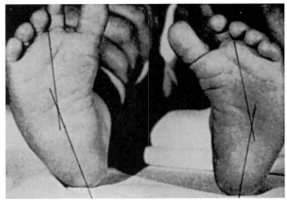

Figure 31-1

9. Pectus excavatum
10. Pectus carinatum

I. Nursemaid's elbow
J. Flatfeet

15. Which is the most common cause of in-toeing in children 2 years of age and older?
    A. Patellar subluxation
    B. External tibial torsion
    C. Internal femoral torsion
    D. Slipped capital femoral epiphysis
    E. Legg-Calvé-Perthes disease

16. A 17-year-old adolescent is found to have a leg length discrepancy of 1 cm, which is confirmed by radiographic evaluation. There is no limp. Which is the recommended treatment?
    A. No treatment is indicated.
    B. Heel lift for the shortened leg
    C. Epiphysiodesis
    D. Tibial diaphyseal lengthening
    E. Femoral diaphyseal lengthening and contralateral epiphysiodesis

17. An adolescent has vague knee pain. With the knee fully flexed, there is a discrete tender area on the lateral portion of the articular cartilage of the medial femoral condyle. Which is the most likely diagnosis?
    A. Idiopathic adolescent anterior knee pain syndrome
    B. Patellar subluxation
    C. Osgood-Schlatter disease
    D. Osteochondritis dissecans
    E. Baker cyst

18. An adolescent has vague knee pain. There is tenderness and increased prominence of the tibia tubercle. Which is the most likely diagnosis?
    A. Idiopathic adolescent anterior knee pain syndrome
    B. Patellar subluxation
    C. Osgood-Schlatter disease
    D. Osteochondritis dissecans
    E. Baker cyst

19. Which is the recommended treatment for the patient in Question 18?

A. Rest, restriction of activities, and a knee immobilizer if necessary
B. Oral nonsteroidal anti-inflammatory agents
C. Oral corticosteroids
D. Injection of corticosteroids
E. Surgical repair of the insertion of the patellar tendon

20. The Barlow test is used to diagnose which condition?
    A. Patellar subluxation
    B. Legg-Calvé-Perthes disease
    C. Developmental dysplasia of the hip
    D. Slipped capital femoral epiphysis
    E. Scoliosis

21. Which is the recommended management of a newborn with an unstable hip examination indicating developmental dysplasia of the hip?
    A. Observation alone
    B. Pavlik harness or use of double- or triple-diapering
    C. Serial spica casts
    D. Surgical closed reduction
    E. Open surgical reduction with pelvic or femoral osteotomy

22. Which is the most serious complication of developmental dysplasia of the hip?
    A. Femoral shortening
    B. Avascular necrosis of the capital femoral epiphysis
    C. Joint instability
    D. Fat embolism
    E. Myelokathexis

23. An 8-year-old child with mild, intermittent right hip pain and a limp undergoes radiography of the hip (Fig. 31–2). What is the diagnosis?
    A. Slipped capital femoral epiphysis
    B. Legg-Calvé-Perthes disease
    C. Osgood-Schlatter disease
    D. Developmental dysplasia of the hip
    E. Salter-Harris type III fracture

24. Which is a suspected contributing factor

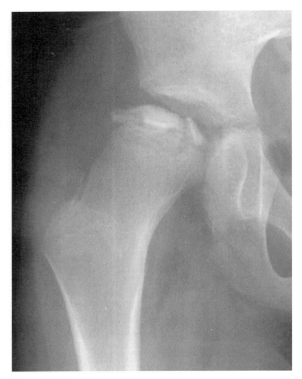

Figure 31-2

for development of slipped capital femoral epiphysis?

A. Hypocalcemia

B. Rapid alterations of growth hormone and sex hormones

C. Eating disorders (e.g., bulimia)

D. Vitamin C deficiency

E. Repeated, minor trauma associated with strenuous physical exercise

25. Which is not true of scoliosis?

A. The most common cause is idiopathic, but there appears to be a genetic component.

B. The incidence is much higher in girls than in boys (4:1 ratio).

C. Scoliosis is more likely to progress and require treatment in girls than in boys.

D. The age of onset is most commonly in adolescence.

E. All of the above are true of scoliosis.

26. Which is the most common bacterial cause of diskitis?

A. *Haemophilus influenzae* type b

B. Group A *Streptococcus*

C. *Pneumococcus*

D. *Staphylococcus aureus*

E. *Salmonella* spp.

27. A child presents after a fall, which occurred while running. While falling, the child attempted to brace against the fall using his hands in dorsiflexion. There is tenderness over the wrist. Which is the most likely diagnosis?

A. Subluxation of the radial head

B. Torus fracture of the distal radial metaphysis

C. Torus fracture of the distal ulnar metaphysis

D. Spiral fracture of the radius

E. Avulsion of the navicular

28. Which defines toddler fractures?

A. Subluxation of the radial head

B. Salter-Harris type 3 fracture of the distal fibular epiphysis

C. Fracture of the distal radius

D. Spiral fracture of the tibia

E. Any fracture occurring in a toddler

29. Which type of injury does not require immediate attention and orthopedic consultation?

A. Fracture with vascular or nerve compromise

B. Open fracture

C. Deep laceration over a joint

D. Grade III (complete) tear of a muscle-tendon unit

E. All of the above require immediate orthopedic consultation.

30. An adolescent who regularly engages in strenuous physical activity has mild pain along the medial tibia, which is now developing earlier in the exercise period. The pain is over a 5- to 15-cm area of the posterior tibialis muscle body, just medial to the medial tibia, but not over the bone. Which is the most likely diagnosis?

A. Slipped capital femoral epiphysis

B. Legg-Calvé-Perthes disease

C. Osgood-Schlatter disease

D. Stress fracture of the lower leg

E. Shin splints

31. Which is not true of the skeletal dysplasias?

A. Manifestations are restricted to the skeleton.

B. Some skeletal dysplasias are lethal in utero.

C. Some skeletal dysplasias have mild features that may go unnoticed.

D. Skeletal dysplasia result from mutations of a relatively small number of genes.

E. There are more than 100 distinct skeletal dysplasias.

32. Which is not a principal feature of osteogenesis imperfecta?

A. Fragile bones

B. Blue sclerae

C. Deafness

D. Microcephaly

E. All of the above are features of osteogenesis imperfecta.

33. Which is the diagnosis of the patient pictured in Figure 31–3?

A. Thanatophoric dysplasia

B. Osteogenesis imperfecta type I

C. Osteogenesis imperfecta type IV

D. Marfan syndrome

E. Cleidocranial dysplasia

34. Which is not true of rickets?

A. Rickets results from poor mineralization at the growth plate.

B. All patients with rickets have osteomalacia.

C. All patients with osteomalacia have rickets.

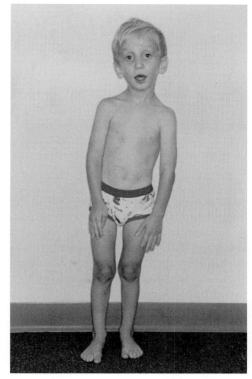

Figure 31-3

D. Rickets is found only in growing children before fusion of the epiphyses.

E. Rickets may result from calcium deficiency or phosphate deficiency.

35. Which is not a stimulus for production of $1,25(OH)_2D_3$?

A. Low serum calcium

B. Low serum phosphate

C. Thyroid hormone

D. Parathyroid hormone

E. All of the above stimulate production of $1,25(OH)_2D_3$.

PART 32

Unclassified Diseases

This part includes sudden infant death syndrome (SIDS), sarcoidosis, progeria, and chronic fatigue syndrome. Slowly but surely, these will eventually be reclassified into other chapters as their causes become more apparent. Nonetheless, other new diseases of unknown cause or classification are likely to appear soon and take their place.

Questions in this part help readers identify many of these unclassified disorders.

---

1. Prone sleep position has been identified as an apparently important epidemiologic risk factor for SIDS. Suggested likely mechanisms include an interaction with all of the following biologic risk factors EXCEPT
   A. impaired temperature regulation
   B. deficient ventilatory responsiveness
   C. impaired arousal responsiveness
   D. gastroesophageal reflux
   E. none of the above

2. A 5-month-old infant is admitted to the hospital 15 minutes after being discovered apneic, blue, and limp by the baby sitter during an afternoon nap. The baby had been placed down for sleep in the supine position. The baby was seen in the emergency room 1 day previously for nasal congestion and a low-grade temperature; because no immunizations had yet been given, the first DTaP and IPV were administered. Findings on physical examination on admission were normal. A five-channel cardiorespiratory recording performed during the first night in the hospital was unremarkable. The most likely diagnosis is
   A. reaction to pertussis component of DTaP
   B. sepsis and/or meningitis
   C. child abuse

   D. apnea of infancy
   E. congenital fatty acid metabolic abnormality

3. Which is the characteristic immune abnormality of chronic fatigue syndrome?
   A. Hypergammaglobulinemia
   B. Immunoglobulin G (IgG) subclass deficiencies
   C. Elevated circulating immune complexes
   D. Increased CD4/CD8 ratio
   E. None of the above

4. Which is the most likely etiology of chronic fatigue syndrome?
   A. *Candida albicans*
   B. Epstein-Barr virus
   C. Influenza virus
   D. Human herpesvirus type 7 (HHV-7)
   E. None of the above

5. Which is a recognized long-term complication of chronic fatigue syndrome?
   A. Hepatocellular carcinoma
   B. Lymphoma
   C. Autoimmune disease
   D. Opportunistic infections
   E. None of the above

PART 33

Environmental Health Hazards

After this part, the test is finally over. This part includes important chapters on the ever-increasing number of intoxicants or pollutants to which children are exposed. Their proper identification and treatment are emphasized.

Questions in this part help identify the im-portant aspects about environmental health hazards. Good luck with this test. We hope that you were appropriately challenged and that in being challenged you were able to continue to learn.

---

1. A 2-year-old child presents with a peeling, erythematous rash on the hands and feet. The mother reports that he has become ill tempered and refuses to walk about, preferring to lie in bed. Physical examination reveals an irritable, pale child with photophobia. Temperature is 98.5°F, heart rate is 80/minute, and respiratory rate is 23/minute. Tremor of the tongue is evident. Further history and follow-up evaluation reveal that the child's elder brothers have been playing with liquid mercury. Which is the most likely diagnosis?
   A. Measles
   B. Fifth disease
   C. Kawasaki disease
   D. Acrodynia
   E. Photosensitivity

2. Laboratory confirmation of the diagnosis in Question 1 can best be obtained by measuring the toxic compound's concentration in which of the following?
   A. Urine
   B. Blood
   C. Hair
   D. Saliva
   E. Feces

3. A 3-year-old child from a suburban community presents with vomiting, diarrhea, and blurred vision. Physical examination reveals an afebrile child with pinpoint pupils, salivation, and muscular fasciculations. The child's lawn was treated yesterday for insects. Which of the following tests will establish the correct diagnosis?
   A. Blood-lead level
   B. 24-hour urine mercury level
   C. Plasma cholinesterase level
   D. Urine malathion level
   E. Urine morphine level

4. Deteriorating insulation is found in the ceilings of a local school built in 1958. Parents and teachers are extremely concerned that it may be asbestos, and they call on you, the local pediatrician, to give advice in an open meeting. What advice would you give?
   A. Immediately remove all of the insulation.
   B. Confirm the presence of asbestos by laboratory evaluation, and do nothing further.
   C. Confirm the presence of asbestos by laboratory evaluation. If asbestos is confirmed, call a certified engineer for expert assessment.
   D. Reassure the parents that the hazards of asbestos have been overstated.
   E. Obtain chest x-rays from all of the students and teachers.

5. **Matching:** Chemical pollutants
   1. Cerebral palsy
   2. Dark skin pigmentation (transient)
   3. Neuroblastoma
   4. Chloracne
   5. Hypocalcemia

   A. Polychlorinated biphenyls
   B. Methylmercury
   C. Dioxin
   D. Phenytoin
   E. Fluoride

173

6. Potential sources of mercury include all of the following EXCEPT
   A. swordfish
   B. old teething powders
   C. quicksilver
   D. milk
   E. pesticides
   F. latex paint
   G. folk remedies

7. The most serious manifestation of lead intoxication is
   A. peripheral neuropathy
   B. mental retardation
   C. anemia
   D. cerebral edema
   E. lead lines

8. A 2-year-old is noted to be drinking from a container filled with kerosene. He immediately coughs, becomes tachypneic, and is brought to the hospital. The best approach to his treatment is to
   A. induce emesis
   B. perform nasogastric tube lavage
   C. instill mineral oil
   D. administer steroids
   E. do none of the above

9. **Matching:** Drug intoxication—antidotes
   1. Carbon monoxide
   2. Cyanide
   3. Heroin
   4. Methemoglobinemia
   5. Organophosphate insecticides
   6. Ethylene glycol
   7. Acetaminophen

   A. Sodium nitrate and sodium thiosulfate
   B. Narcan
   C. Oxygen
   D. Atropine
   E. Methylene blue
   F. *N*-acetylcysteine
   G. Ethanol

10. **Matching:** Spider bites
    1. Orange hourglass marking
    2. Lives in dark, undisturbed areas
    3. Neurotoxin

    A. Black widow
    B. Brown recluse
    C. Both *A* and *B*
    D. Neither *A* nor *B*

    4. Bite may be unnoticed initially
    5. Severe muscle spasms
    6. Hypertension
    7. Acute abdomen
    8. Fiddle marking on back
    9. Bite becomes hemorrhagic blister
    10. Laryngospasm
    11. Hemolysis
    12. Disseminated intravascular coagulation

11. **Matching:** Plant intoxications
    1. Dieffenbachia
    2. Jimson weed
    3. Castor bean
    4. Foxglove
    5. Hemlock

    A. Atropine-like
    B. Oxalates
    C. Hyperkalemia
    D. Hemolytic anemia
    E. Similar to nicotine

12. A child with which of the following diseases may suffer a severe acute reaction to radiotherapy?
    A. Chédiak-Higashi syndrome
    B. Neurofibromatosis
    C. Chronic mucocutaneous candidiasis
    D. Ataxia-telangiectasia
    E. Wiskott-Aldrich syndrome

13. About 500 children have just been exposed to radiation from a nuclear power plant accident. The most appropriate first step in your treatment of these children should be to
    A. prescribe potassium iodide to protect the thyroid
    B. order thyroid function tests
    C. order complete blood counts (CBCs)
    D. do nothing acutely; evaluate in 4–6 weeks
    E. look for signs or symptoms of acute radiation sickness

14. Antivenins should be considered in the treatment of all of the following EXCEPT
    A. rattlesnake envenomations
    B. scorpion envenomations
    C. black widow envenomations
    D. stonefish envenomations
    E. Hymenoptera envenomations

15. A 2-year-old child is found playing with a can of crystalline drain cleaner. There are several crystals in the mouth, which you have the mother wash out. Treatment should be to
    A. have the mother administer lemon juice or orange juice to neutralize the alkaline crystals and come to your office
    B. have the mother administer water or milk and call you back in 2 hours
    C. have the mother administer water or milk and bring the child in for esophagoscopy
    D. simply observe the child because the crystals are so bitter that the child was trying to spit them out when the mother called, and therefore no problems should occur
    E. administer ipecac at home and bring the child in to see you

16. A 16-year-old, 165-pound patient reports consuming 20–40 325-mg capsules containing acetaminophen 1 hour ago. You should
    A. measure the plasma level and determine potential toxicity from the level on the nomogram
    B. wait until 4 hours after ingestion to measure the plasma level and do nothing else
    C. administer activated charcoal immediately and measure the plasma level of acetaminophen 4 hours after ingestion
    D. send the patient home because an ingestion of this magnitude is not toxic
    E. administer N-acetylcysteine at a dose of 140 mg/kg

Answers

1 *The Field of Pediatrics*

1. **B.** Injuries, congenital anomalies, and malignancy are the three leading causes of death in children 1–4 years old. Homicide is the fourth most prevalent cause of death in this group. (See Chapter 1 in *Nelson Textbook of Pediatrics*, 16th ed.)

2. **D.** Injuries, homicide, and suicide all are potentially preventable. (See Chapter 5 in *Nelson Textbook of Pediatrics*, 16th ed.)

3. **D.** If a decision is based on reliable data and is in the best interest of a patient, the act of withholding life support is no different from withdrawing such futile therapy. (See Chapter 2 in *Nelson Textbook of Pediatrics*, 16th ed.)

4. **D.** If a child is not initially crying, the cardiac examination is potentially the least disturbing to an infant or toddler. (See Chapter 6 in *Nelson Textbook of Pediatrics*, 16th ed.)

5. **D.** Basic principles applied to any geographic region—urban, rural, or international—have helped improve child health in the United States and abroad. (See Chapter 4 in *Nelson Textbook of Pediatrics*, 16th ed.)

6. **A.** Breast-feeding is the best way to prevent various infectious and nutritional disorders in developing countries. (See Chapter 4 in *Nelson Textbook of Pediatrics*, 16th ed.)

7. **B.** The American Academy of Pediatrics recommends oral rehydration therapy for diarrhea in the United States. (See Chapter 5 in *Nelson Textbook of Pediatrics*, 16th ed.)

8. **C.** In 1996, the black infant mortality rate was 2–3 times greater than that for whites, which had a rate equal to Hispanics. Native Americans had an intermediate rate. (See Chapter 1 in *Nelson Textbook of Pediatrics*, 16th ed.)

9. **E.** In the under-1-year-old grouping, deaths from congenital anomalies exceed that for SIDS and is second to perinatal problems (RDS, asphyxia). In the 1- to 4-year age group, it is second to injuries.

(See Chapter 1 in *Nelson Textbook of Pediatrics*, 16th ed.)

10. **E.** Autonomy is a conceptual ethical issue based on the principle that competent patients have an almost absolute right to decide what is to be done to them. (See Chapter 2 in *Nelson Textbook of Pediatrics*, 16th ed.)

11. **B.** A competent person should be able to understand the consequences of his or her choices and to understand the available alternatives. (See Chapter 2 in *Nelson Textbook of Pediatrics*, 16th ed.)

12. **B.** Autonomy is the overriding principle for competent patients. Such patients may chose to refuse beneficial therapy if they are competent and over 18 years. In neonates, beneficence "do no harm—do good" is a stronger principle because we do not know the child's choice, only the surrogate choice of the parent. (See Chapter 2 in *Nelson Textbook of Pediatrics*, 16th ed.)

13. **E.** Unfortunately, health care today is often rationed on the ability to pay. The grave inequity in access contributes to the twofold or higher differences in morbidity and mortality between different socioeconomic groups. (See Chapter 2 in *Nelson Textbook of Pediatrics*, 16th ed.)

14. **A.** In developing countries, economic and social issues are closely related and inseparable from health. (See Chapter 4 in *Nelson Textbook of Pediatrics*, 16th ed.)

15. **G.** Indeed, breast-feeding is recommended as the safest from a biologic and environmental public health perspective. (See Chapter 4 in *Nelson Textbook of Pediatrics*, 16th ed.)

16. **A.** The pathogens are similar to those of the developed world, although secondary infections—usually bacterial (with the same organisms as in the United States)—are more common. (See Chapter 4 in *Nelson Textbook of Pediatrics*, 16th ed.)

17. **C.** In third-world settings, parasites often cause malnutrition and not acute diarrhea. (See Chapter 4 in *Nelson Textbook of Pediatrics*, 16th ed.)

18. **C.** Teens should be seen every year. Each developmental stage of adolescents requires targeted preventions. (See Chapter 5 in *Nelson Textbook of Pediatrics,* 16th ed.)

19. **B.** Its peak incidence is 9–12 months. (See Chapter 5 in *Nelson Textbook of Pediatrics,* 16th ed.)

20. **D.** Rash, fever, or diarrhea is not associated with teething. (See Chapter 5 in *Nelson Textbook of Pediatrics,* 16th ed.)

21. **C.** Juice bottles at the time of sleep is a terrible habit that reinforces the relationship between sleep and food but also produces severe caries once teeth appear. (See Chapter 5 in *Nelson Textbook of Pediatrics,* 16th ed.)

22. **D.** The range is up to 3–4 years. (See Chapter 5 in *Nelson Textbook of Pediatrics,* 16th ed.)

23. **B.** Young children have a poor concept of time. Removal of privileges and time out are two proven and safe methods; parents need to be clear about expectations and what is correct behavior. (See Chapter 5 in *Nelson Textbook of Pediatrics,* 16th ed.)

24. **E.** Glasgow Coma Scales have been adapted to infants and toddlers. A → D are correct. (See Chapters 6 and 64 in *Nelson Textbook of Pediatrics,* 16th ed.)

25. **E.** The reflex is developmentally regulated and should have disappeared by 2 years of age. Its presence at this age is a frontal cortex release phenomenon and is indicative of CNS injury. (See Chapter 6 in *Nelson Textbook of Pediatrics,* 16th ed.)

26. **D.** This is a critical part of well child care throughout childhood. Growth parameters must be documented for each child. (See Chapter 6 in *Nelson Textbook of Pediatrics,* 16th ed.)

27. **B.** Anticipatory guidance is the best way to prevent accidents and avoid ill health, especially when it is based on the child's developmental stages. (See Chapter 6 in *Nelson Textbook of Pediatrics,* 16th ed.)

2 Growth and Development

1. 1. **C**
   2. **E**
   3. **D**
   4. **A**
   5. **B**

2. **D.** Newborn infants have six characteristic organizational behavioral states. (See Chapter 9 in *Nelson Textbook of Pediatrics,* 16th ed.)

3. **B.** The formula in choice **A** is used for 7- to 12-year-old children; **C,** for 3- to 12-month-old infants; **D,** for 1- to 6-year-olds in pounds; and **F,** for 7- to 12-year-olds in pounds. (See Chapter 15 in *Nelson Textbook of Pediatrics,* 16th ed.)

4. **D.** Crying may or may not be in response to obvious stimuli (e.g., need for a diaper change). (See Chapter 10 in *Nelson Textbook of Pediatrics,* 16th ed.)

5. **D.** Demand feedings prevent periods of hunger and episodes of being fed while not being hungry for a child with an irregular rhythm. (See Chapter 11 in *Nelson Textbook of Pediatrics,* 16th ed.)

6. **A.** Out of sight, out of mind is the characteristic response of a 2-month-old. Object permanence appears at approximately 8 months of age. This is also called *object constancy.* (See Chapter 10 in *Nelson Textbook of Pediatrics,* 16th ed.)

7. **D.** The pincer grasp, which is noted at 8–9 months, along with increasing mobility, enables an infant to explore the environment. (See Chapter 10 in *Nelson Textbook of Pediatrics,* 16th ed.)

8. **D.** Each pediatrician should learn key developmental milestones such as these. (See Chapter 10 in *Nelson Textbook of Pediatrics,* 16th ed.)

9. **D.** Transitional objects help toddlers (18–24 months) cope with separation (e.g., at nighttime for sleep, baby sitter, daycare). (See Chapter 11 in *Nelson Textbook of Pediatrics,* 16th ed.)

10. **E.** Handedness should not be attempted to be modified because this leads to frustration. After 4 years of age, a spontaneous change in handedness should lead to the suspicion of a central nervous system lesion. (See Chapter 12 in *Nelson Textbook of Pediatrics,* 16th ed.)

11. **D.** It is impossible to rationalize away a preschool child's fear of monsters. (See Chapter 12 in *Nelson Textbook of Pediatrics,* 16th ed.)

12. **C.** Waking up at night (if in fact the baby had already slept through the night) at

6–8 months is common behavior. Whether this is related to separation anxiety or something else (teething?) is not clear (edentulous babies wake up, too). Choice **A** would be highly unlikely, because 6½-month-old circumcised boys who have grown normally rarely contract urinary tract infections. Choice **B** would be unnecessary because increased food intake does not improve night fussiness. **D** is wrong because DTP reactions occur 4–36 hours after the shot, not 2 weeks. (See Chapter 10 in *Nelson Textbook of Pediatrics,* 16th ed.)

13. **E.** In general, all other socioeconomic factors held constant, both means of infant feeding are equally effective. Nonetheless, in less advantaged environments, breast milk has specific biologic advantages. The biopsychosocial model helps combine the nature vs. nurture aspects of previous theories of development. (See Chapter 7 in *Nelson Textbook of Pediatrics,* 16th ed.)

14. **A.** Temperament is only moderately stable over time, and a mellow 2-year-old does not always equate to a mellow 22-year-old. (See Chapter 7 in *Nelson Textbook of Pediatrics,* 16th ed.)

15. **B.** The seven characteristics of temperament have a wide range of responsiveness; the seven are activity level, rhythmicity, approach and withdrawal, adaptability, threshold of responsiveness, intensity of reaction, quality of mood, distractibility, attention span, and persistence. (See Chapter 7 in *Nelson Textbook of Pediatrics,* 16th ed.)

16. 1. **B**
    2. **D**
    3. **A**
    4. **E**
    5. **C**
    (See Chapter 7 in *Nelson Textbook of Pediatrics,* 16th ed.)

17. **B.** The near-sighted neonate has a fixed focal length of 8–12 inches. The newborn also has a visual preference for faces. (See Chapter 9 in *Nelson Textbook of Pediatrics,* 16th ed.)

18. **C.** This normal sleep after a 40-minute period of social interaction wakefulness is a great time to continue the bonding process. (See Chapter 9 in *Nelson Textbook of Pediatrics,* 16th ed.)

19. **E.** Colic is not a neonatal state and does not even occur during the neonatal period. (See Chapter 9 in *Nelson Textbook of Pediatrics,* 16th ed.)

20. **A.** B is best for 9-month-olds in pounds. (See Chapter 10 in *Nelson Textbook of Pediatrics,* 16th ed.)

21. **B.** A is in inches. (See Chapter 10 in *Nelson Textbook of Pediatrics,* 16th ed.)

22. **E.** Colostrum has a high protein content. Mature milk has a higher fat and lower protein content than colostrum. (See Chapter 10 in *Nelson Textbook of Pediatrics,* 16th ed.)

23. **A.** Teething doesn't occur until approximately 5–6 months. (See Chapter 10 in *Nelson Textbook of Pediatrics,* 16th ed.)

24. **B.** These milestones correspond respectively to visuomotor coordination, exploration labeling, and symbolic thought. (See Chapter 10 in *Nelson Textbook of Pediatrics,* 16th ed.)

25. **A.** These milestones correspond respectively to control of exploration, exploration of small objects, response to tone, and comparison of objects. (See Chapter 10 in *Nelson Textbook of Pediatrics,* 16th ed.)

26. **C.** This is a normal response that does not cause the child to cross growth percentiles in a growth chart. (See Chapter 10 in *Nelson Textbook of Pediatrics,* 16th ed.)

27. **A.** Indeed, stranger anxiety may start to set in at this time. (See Chapter 10 in *Nelson Textbook of Pediatrics,* 16th ed.)

28. **E.** This is normal, appropriate motor, language, and social development. (See Chapter 11 in *Nelson Textbook of Pediatrics,* 16th ed.)

29. **D.** More active types tend to walk early. The other choices are not true. (See Chapter 11 in *Nelson Textbook of Pediatrics,* 16th ed.)

30. **B.** A 2-year-old has two-word sentences, such that language is dependent on the environment and verbal interactions with adults. (See Chapter 12 in *Nelson Textbook of Pediatrics,* 16th ed.)

31. **C.** Language plays a critical part in the regulation of behavior as children internalize speech. (See Chapter 12 in *Nelson Textbook of Pediatrics,* 16th ed.)

32. **A.** 3.5 kg (7 lb) and 6 cm (2.5 in) per year are the average increments in this time period. (See Chapter 13 in *Nelson Textbook of Pediatrics,* 16th ed.)

33. **D.** Language-based classes produce difficulties for children with word-finding difficulties. (See Chapter 13 in *Nelson Textbook of Pediatrics,* 16th ed.)

34. 1. **B** or **A**
    2. **D**
    3. **A**
    4. **C**
    5. **E**

3 *Psychologic Disorders*

1. **D.** Common complications of neuroleptic antipsychotic agents include extrapyramidal symptoms (Parkinson-like syndrome), sedation, and anticholinergic symptoms. Neuroleptic malignant syndrome (malignant hyperthermia) and tardive dyskinesia are rarer complications. (See Chapter 27 in *Nelson Textbook of Pediatrics,* 16th ed.)

2. **D.** Autism is a disease of unknown cause and is more common in males. It is characterized by the symptoms noted in this patient, with onset usually before 30 months of age. (See Chapter 27 in *Nelson Textbook of Pediatrics,* 16th ed.)

3. 1. **C**
   2. **B**
   3. **A**
   4. **D**

4. **A.** The belief that choice **B** is correct leads to repeated attempts to "break" children (a distressing term and concept), probably in effect reinforcing the behavior. (See Chapter 21 in *Nelson Textbook of Pediatrics,* 16th ed.)

5. **A.** Gilles de la Tourette syndrome, which has a lifetime prevalence rate of 0.5 per 1000 persons, is a rare condition in children. It is characterized by multiple tics, compulsive barking, and shouting obscene words (coprolalia). It is more common in first-degree relatives of patients with Tourette syndrome than in the general population and affects boys three to four times more than girls. The cause is uncertain, but research has shown that drugs that increase dopaminergic action precipitate or worsen both tics and Gilles de la Tourette syndrome. Many environmental precipitants have been noted to serve as emotional stress sources. The syndrome can be fairly well managed with haloperidol, a dopaminergic antagonist. Anecdotal reports in the literature suggest that the serotonin reuptake inhibitors are also efficacious in its treatment. (See Chapter 21 in *Nelson Textbook of Pediatrics,* 16th ed.)

6. **D.** Night terrors most commonly occur during stage IV, deep sleep. Neither the use of antipsychotic medications nor overeating after 7:00 P.M. has ever been shown to be associated with night terrors. They usually begin in the preschool years. A child having night terrors is confused and disorientated and shows signs of intense autonomic activity (labored breathing, dilated pupils, sweating, tachypnea, tachycardia). Sleepwalking may occur during night terrors and may put a child at risk for injury. The incidence of night terrors is said to be between 1% and 4% and is greater in boys. There is a familial pattern in the development of the symptoms, and febrile illnesses may serve as precipitating factors. (See Chapter 20.5 in *Nelson Textbook of Pediatrics,* 16th ed.)

7. **E.** Conduct disorder is a distinct clinical entity manifested by several different antisocial behaviors: stealing, lying, fire setting, truancy, property destruction, cruelty to animals, rape, use of weapons while fighting, armed robbery, physical cruelty to others, and repeated attempts to run away from home. Many argue that conduct disorder is not a unitary illness but instead comprises three different syndromes characterized primarily by aggression, intermittent antisocial behaviors, and delinquency. Little is known about the antecedents of each of these subtypes or the outcome of patients suffering from them. Risk factors associated with the development of

conduct disorders include antisocial behavior within family members, criminality in the father, physical abuse within the home, and marital discord within the home. Many different approaches have been used in the treatment of children and adolescents with aggressive behavior, antisocial behavior, and delinquency. The most effective results have been obtained with parent training management, in which parents are trained directly to promote prosocial behaviors within the home and to place reasonable limits on unwanted, destructive behaviors. (See Chapter 25 in *Nelson Textbook of Pediatrics,* 16th ed.)

8. **E.** Previous suicide attempts, substance abuse, easy access to firearms, and a family history of depression and suicide are all closely related to both suicide attempts and completed suicides in both children and adolescents. Fifteen to 40% of completed suicides are preceded by other suicide attempts. In more than one third of suicides, a parent, a sibling, or another first-degree relative has previously shown overt suicidal behavior. Firearms served as the major method of death in adolescent suicide. Among preadolescents, jumping from heights is the most common method. Although perfectionism in the classroom has been shown to be associated with specific types of anxiety, no correlation has been shown between perfectionism and suicidal ideation or suicidal behavior. (See Chapter 24 in *Nelson Textbook of Pediatrics,* 16th ed.)

9. **C.** The question offers a classic example of a language problem, particularly in a child with partial understanding. Many children or parents do not admit to this problem. (See Chapter 29 in *Nelson Textbook of Pediatrics,* 16th ed.)

10. **E.** Simultaneous retrieval memory defects are depicted by the history of the child described in the question. (See Chapter 29 in *Nelson Textbook of Pediatrics,* 16th ed.)

11. **B.** Asthma may be exacerbated by psychologic factors and is therefore a psychophysiologic disorder. (See Chapter

19 in *Nelson Textbook of Pediatrics,* 16th ed.)

12. **C.** In the Munchausen by proxy syndrome, patients' symptoms disappear if the parent goes home. Manifestations reappear when the involved parent returns to the hospital. (See Chapter 35 in *Nelson Textbook of Pediatrics,* 16th ed.)

13. 1. **A**
   2. **B**
   3. **A**
   4. **B**
   5. **A**
   6. **A**
   7. **D**
   8. **C**

14. **D.** Children may be frightened and react to fear with a personal manner of withdrawal or poor cooperation. (See Chapter 17 in *Nelson Textbook of Pediatrics,* 16th ed.)

15. **A.** Parents often hold back questions that are highly charged or that may appear "stupid." They may be angry, ashamed, or uncomfortable in asking these questions. (See Chapter 17 in *Nelson Textbook of Pediatrics,* 16th ed.)

16. **F.** Noncompliance is a complicated issue and is influenced by many factors: hearing, understanding, physical ability to do the treatment, and competing social and financial forces. Neglect is an unusual cause of poor compliance. (See Chapter 17 in *Nelson Textbook of Pediatrics,* 16th ed.)

17. 1. **B**
   2. **C**
   3. **A**
   4. **E**
   5. **D**
(See Chapter 17 in *Nelson Textbook of Pediatrics,* 16th ed.)

18. 1. **B**
   2. **A**
   3. **F**
   4. **C**
   5. **D**
   6. **E**
(See Chapter 17 in *Nelson Textbook of Pediatrics,* 16th ed.)

19. **E.** Disturbances may manifest as such conditions as depression, anxiety, aggression, and learning problems. (See

Chapter 27 in *Nelson Textbook of Pediatrics,* 16th ed.)

20. **A.** An important aspect of these conditions is the capacity of the parents to adjust and cope. (See Chapter 18 in *Nelson Textbook of Pediatrics,* 16th ed.)

21. **F.** The loss or alteration of function without a demonstrable organic cause defines a conversion reaction, a type of somatoform disorder. (See Chapter 19 in *Nelson Textbook of Pediatrics,* 16th ed.)

22. **A.** Alternately, if it produces clinically significant distress for the child. (See Chapter 20 in *Nelson Textbook of Pediatrics,* 16th ed.)

23. **D.** There is no higher rate of emotional disturbances in age-matched enuretic and nonenuretic children. (See Chapter 20 in *Nelson Textbook of Pediatrics,* 16th ed.)

24. **E.** Repeated waking may be beneficial for a few children but creates added stress and hostility. (See Chapter 20 in *Nelson Textbook of Pediatrics,* 16th ed.)

25. **B.** Polysomnography reveals episodes of apnea and hypoxia. (See Chapter 20 in *Nelson Textbook of Pediatrics,* 16th ed.)

26. **C.** OSAS commonly presents with airway obstruction during sleep with resultant sleep disturbances at night and daytime sleepiness. (See Chapter 20 in *Nelson Textbook of Pediatrics,* 16th ed.)

27. **A.** Removal of the hypertrophied tissue relieves the symptoms of OSAS. (See Chapter 20 in *Nelson Textbook of Pediatrics,* 16th ed.)

28. **E.** All of the answers are risk factors as well as the more obvious such as Pierre Robin syndrome and Prader-Willi syndrome. (See Chapter 20 in *Nelson Textbook of Pediatrics,* 16th ed.)

29. **D.** Stuttering is often discussed with habit disorders; however, it is probably not a true habit in that it is not regarded as a tension-relieving activity. (See Chapter 21 in *Nelson Textbook of Pediatrics,* 16th ed.)

30. **B.** This would be more compatible with a minor seizure. (See Chapter 21 in *Nelson Textbook of Pediatrics,* 16th ed.)

31. **E.** Both drugs provide a fair degree of relief. (See Chapter 21 in *Nelson Textbook of Pediatrics,* 16th ed.)

32. **D.** Parents often consciously or unconsciously encourage this intense fear of separation because of a fear that something will happen to the caregiver. (See Chapter 22 in *Nelson Textbook of Pediatrics,* 16th ed.)

33. **E.** Positron emission tomography may reveal excessive metabolic activity in the frontal lobes and basal ganglia. (See Chapter 22 in *Nelson Textbook of Pediatrics,* 16th ed.)

34. **F.** Major depression may also include manifestations of fatigue, loss of interest or pleasure (dysphoria), agitation or retardation, excessive guilt, feelings of worthlessness, and poor concentration. (See Chapter 23 in *Nelson Textbook of Pediatrics,* 16th ed.)

35. **A.** Twin studies show a strong genetic component to major depression. (See Chapter 23 in *Nelson Textbook of Pediatrics,* 16th ed.)

36. **C.** SSRIs have proven efficacy and have a reasonable safety profile. (See Chapter 23 in *Nelson Textbook of Pediatrics,* 16th ed.)

37. **D.** Alcohol use and other drugs are associated epidemiologically to suicide. (See Chapter 24 in *Nelson Textbook of Pediatrics,* 16th ed.)

38. **G.** These are all helpful in discharge planning and assessing recurrence risks. (See Chapter 24 in *Nelson Textbook of Pediatrics,* 16th ed.)

39. **A.** Caregiver anger reinforces the child's behavior and teaches a vicious cycle of oppositional behavior. (See Chapter 25 in *Nelson Textbook of Pediatrics,* 16th ed.)

40. **E.** Lying is common at every developmental age and has reasons at each level of development. It may include fantasy, avoidance of punishment, and fear. Pathologic repeated chronic lying often occurs in combination with other antisocial behavior. At any time, lying should be approached calmly with an understanding of the fears of the child. Nonetheless, honesty must be reinforced. (See Chapter 25 in *Nelson Textbook of Pediatrics,* 16th ed.)

41. **B.** Overemphasis may create an excitement to repeat the offense. (See Chapter 25 in *Nelson Textbook of Pediatrics,* 16th ed.)

42. **D.** Autism begins before 30 months of age and has a 4:1 male:female ratio. It is characterized by impaired verbal and nonverbal communication, imaginative activity, and reciprocal social interaction. (See Chapter 27 in *Nelson Textbook of Pediatrics*, 16th ed.)

43. **A.** Lack of social relations and absent empathy are typical of children with autism. (See Chapter 27 in *Nelson Textbook of Pediatrics*, 16th ed.)

44. 1. **D**
    2. **A**
    3. **B**
    4. **C**
    (See Chapter 27 in *Nelson Textbook of Pediatrics*, 16th ed.)

45. 1. **D**
    2. **A**
    3. **E**
    4. **B**
    5. **C**
    (See Chapter 28 in *Nelson Textbook of Pediatrics*, 16th ed.)

46. **D.** Comorbidity includes oppositional defiant disorder in 50%, conduct disorders in 30–50%, anxiety disorder in 20–25%, mood disorders in 15–20%, and learning disorders in 10–25%. (See Chapter 29 in *Nelson Textbook of Pediatrics*, 16th ed.)

47. **E.** Anorexia is common; this affects growth. (See Chapter 29 in *Nelson Textbook of Pediatrics*, 16th ed.)

4 *Social Issues*

1. **E.** In the classic shaken baby syndrome, a computed tomography scan of the head reveals diffuse cerebral edema and hemorrhage. CPR in young children does not usually produce retinal hemorrhages and rarely, if ever, produces rib fractures. (See Chapter 35 in *Nelson Textbook of Pediatrics*, 16th ed.)

2. 1. **B**
   2. **C**
   3. **A**
   4. **E**
   5. **D**
   (See Chapter 35 in *Nelson Textbook of Pediatrics*, 16th ed.)

3. **B.** Many young children continue in the daily activities and use denial and magical wishful thoughts for reunion and reappearance. (See Chapter 33 in *Nelson Textbook of Pediatrics*, 16th ed.)

4. **C.** Statements such as "stop it or you'll give me a headache" may cause a child to suffer significant and unrealistic guilt, especially of the parent leaves for some time or is hospitalized. (See Chapter 33 in *Nelson Textbook of Pediatrics*, 16th ed.)

5. **B.** Five percent of adoptions are from overseas. (See Chapter 30 in *Nelson Textbook of Pediatrics*, 16th ed.)

6. **D.** Early prevention screening and developmental testing programs are underutilized in the foster care system. (See Chapter 31 in *Nelson Textbook of Pediatrics*, 16th ed.)

7. **D.** Sibling rivalry and aggression may not be affected as much as the cognitive issues. (See Chapter 32 in *Nelson Textbook of Pediatrics*, 16th ed.)

8. **C.** It is not unusual for the young child to keep asking for the missing parent, to wait at the door or window, or to go outside to look for the parent. (See Chapter 33 in *Nelson Textbook of Pediatrics*, 16th ed.)

9. **E.** Indeed, most children fantasize about the possibility that their parents will remarry. (See Chapter 33 in *Nelson Textbook of Pediatrics*, 16th ed.)

10. **C.** All the rest are true as well as poor appetite, decreased exploration of the environment in toddlers, and poor school performance with hyperactivity in older children. (See Chapter 34 in *Nelson Textbook of Pediatrics*, 16th ed.)

11. **D.** Parents often deny their involvement in inducing symptoms in their children and will rapidly change doctors if it is discussed with them. (See Chapter 35 in *Nelson Textbook of Pediatrics*, 16th ed.)

12. **E.** Each is a risk factor. Of note, abuse has been reported in all communities and from all socioeconomic levels. (See Chapter 35 in *Nelson Textbook of Pediatrics*, 16th ed.)

13. **C.** Often, relatives do not know the nature or the cause of the injury, nor do they readily know or admit to the person

who did the trauma. (See Chapter 35 in *Nelson Textbook of Pediatrics,* 16th ed.)

14. **B.** Retinal hemorrhages and broken ribs rarely follow CPR. The nature of rib fractures is also different in abuse. (See Chapter 35 in *Nelson Textbook of Pediatrics,* 16th ed.)

15. **B.** This is sexual play and is usually normal exploratory behavior if there is no force or coercion and the children are not more than 4 years different in age. (See Chapter 35 in *Nelson Textbook of Pediatrics,* 16th ed.)

16. **C.** Pedophiles often seek out positions and opportunities to be around children. Children may be particularly vulnerable, such as those with mental and physical handicaps. (See Chapter 35 in *Nelson Textbook of Pediatrics,* 16th ed.)

17. **A.** By DNA typing, the blood turned out to be the mother's. The mother has diabetes and employs home glucose monitoring and would purposely put blood on her daughter's underwear. (See Chapter 35 in *Nelson Textbook of Pediatrics,* 16th ed.)

18. **E.** Munchausen by proxy brings attention to the child and caregiver. Often, the perpetrator has some medical background. (See Chapter 35 in *Nelson Textbook of Pediatrics,* 16th ed.)

5 *Children with Special Health Needs*

1. **B.** The pattern of abnormalities described in the question is most compatible with a congenital TORCH (*t*oxoplasmosis, *o*ther, *r*ubella, *c*ytomegalovirus, *h*erpes *s*implex) infection. In addition, intrauterine and postnatal growth retardation may be evident. (See Chapter 37.2 in *Nelson Textbook of Pediatrics,* 16th ed.)

2. **E.** Many children with common chronic diseases of childhood (e.g., asthma, seizures, diabetes, arthritis, cystic fibrosis, sickle cell anemia) attend high school and graduate. (See Chapter 37 in *Nelson Textbook of Pediatrics,* 16th ed.)

3. **C.** Parents who are not able to see their deformed neonate may greatly exaggerate the severity of any anomaly and may have excessive feelings of guilt. Most

parents benefit from seeing their child with anomalies and often identify aspects of beauty or normalcy with the help of a nurse or physician. (See Chapter 37 in *Nelson Textbook of Pediatrics,* 16th ed.)

4. **D.** The child described in the question demonstrates important educational and social milestones that are partially predictive of future achievements. (See Chapter 37.2 in *Nelson Textbook of Pediatrics,* 16th ed.)

5. **B.** Neurogenic bladder is not typically encountered in Down syndrome, but Hirschsprung disease may occur. (See Chapter 37.2 in *Nelson Textbook of Pediatrics,* 16th ed.)

6. **C.** Cranial computed tomography is not indicated until other evaluations are completed unless a patient has macrocephaly, microcephaly, abnormal neurologic signs, or significant dysmorphology. (See Chapter 37.2 in *Nelson Textbook of Pediatrics,* 16th ed.)

7. **C.** Forced feeding exacerbates abnormal psychosocial tension between a child and his or her caregiver. (See Chapter 36 in *Nelson Textbook of Pediatrics,* 16th ed.)

8. **A** and **B.** Corrected age rather than chronologic age is one solution. A 24-week premature infant who is now 20 weeks old is "really" 44 weeks' gestation (1 month corrected age may also be valuable). (See Chapter 36 in *Nelson Textbook of Pediatrics,* 16th ed.)

9. **A.** Formula fed in sufficient amounts that is not malabsorbed is not a cause of failure to thrive. (See Chapter 36 in *Nelson Textbook of Pediatrics,* 16th ed.)

10. **B.** All must be considered, but **B** is No. 1. (See Chapter 36 in *Nelson Textbook of Pediatrics,* 16th ed.)

11. **C.** Adenoid hypertrophy or poor oropharyngeal motility (possible CP) can cause failure to thrive from obstructive sleep apnea. Mononucleosis is rare in infants. (See Chapter 36 in *Nelson Textbook of Pediatrics,* 16th ed.)

12. **D.** AIDS usually presents with failure to thrive and recurrent infections. Lymphadenopathy, parotitis, and hepatosplenomegaly are classic features of AIDS in infants. (See Chapter 36 in *Nelson Textbook of Pediatrics,* 16th ed.)

13. **A.** Indeed, most survive to be adults. (See Chapter 37 in *Nelson Textbook of Pediatrics*, 16th ed.)

14. **C.** Labeling depersonalizes the child and marks the child for life. A disease should not define a child. (See Chapter 37 in *Nelson Textbook of Pediatrics*, 16th ed.)

15. **B.** Supplemental security income programs provide cash support for people of all ages with disabilities. (See Chapter 37 in *Nelson Textbook of Pediatrics*, 16th ed.)

16. 1. **D**
    2. **A**
    3. **B**
    4. **E**
    5. **C**
    6. **G**
    7. **F**
    (See Chapter 37 in *Nelson Textbook of Pediatrics*, 16th ed.)

17. **A.** At this age, germ theory is an easily comprehended but unfortunately not always accurate view of chronic illness. Nonetheless, it does help with compliance of taking medicines. (See Chapter 37 in *Nelson Textbook of Pediatrics*, 16th ed.)

18. **D.** This functional approach places the child's needs for support into the context of the environment. (See Chapter 37 in *Nelson Textbook of Pediatrics*, 16th ed.)

19. **E.** Cystic fibrosis itself does not cause mental retardation. **A → D** is common; hypothyroid-induced retardation is preventable by early screening and rapid therapy. (See Chapter 37 in *Nelson Textbook of Pediatrics*, 16th ed.)

20. **B.** Mild retardation is related to low SES, whereas more severe retardation is equally distributed in all classes. (See Chapter 37 in *Nelson Textbook of Pediatrics*, 16th ed.)

21. **B.** Sports per se are not an adaptive skill but could be categorized into leisure activities. (See Chapter 37 in *Nelson Textbook of Pediatrics*, 16th ed.)

22. **D.** Fragile X syndrome manifests in males with mental retardation, large ears, and large testes. It is relatively common. (See Chapter 37 in *Nelson Textbook of Pediatrics*, 16th ed.)

23. **B.** Congenital rubella was once a common cause of mental retardation. Thanks to active immunization programs, congenital rubella is rare. (See Chapter 37 in *Nelson Textbook of Pediatrics*, 16th ed.)

24. 1. **C**
    2. **A**
    3. **B**
    4. **D**
    (See Chapter 38 in *Nelson Textbook of Pediatrics*, 16th ed.)

25. **D.** Causality is a late developmental state of understanding. P.S.—Don't reinforce the immature child's belief that death is like sleep because the child will be fearful of sleeping lest he or she may die. (See Chapter 38 in *Nelson Textbook of Pediatrics*, 16th ed.)

26. **C.** Separation from loved ones is the dominant and often only concern of young children. (See Chapter 38 in *Nelson Textbook of Pediatrics*, 16th ed.)

27. **E.** Most chronically ill children have a sense of impending death and need to articulate this with parents or caregivers who can discuss fears and provide some reassurance (at least for comfort). (See Chapter 38 in *Nelson Textbook of Pediatrics*, 16th ed.)

28. **A.** Population-based statistics are poor about predicting the time of death of an individual child. (See Chapter 38 in *Nelson Textbook of Pediatrics*, 16th ed.)

6 *Nutrition*

1. **C.** A strict vegan diet contains no eggs, meat, or milk products and is thus deficient in vitamin B_{12}.
   (See Chapters 40.7 and 44 in *Nelson Textbook of Pediatrics*, 16th ed.)

2. 1. **C**
   2. **A**
   3. **D**
   4. **E**
   5. **C**
   6. **D**
   7. **B or E**
   8. **F**
   9. **G**
   10. **H**
   11. **I**
   (See Chapters 40.7 and 44 in *Nelson Textbook of Pediatrics*, 16th ed.)

3. 1. **B**
    2. **D**
    3. **A**
    4. **C**
    5. **F**
    6. **A**
    7. **E**
    8. **H**
    9. **G**
    (See Chapter 40.6 in *Nelson Textbook of Pediatrics*, 16th ed.)

4. 1. **B**
    2. **D**
    3. **A**
    4. **C**
    5. **E**
    (See Chapter 44 in *Nelson Textbook of Pediatrics*, 16th ed.)

5. 1. **C**
    2. **A**
    3. **C**
    4. **A**
    5. **B**
    6. **A**
    7. **A**
    8. **A**
    The bottom line is that breast milk is best for babies, and except in unusual circumstances, cow's milk should be reserved for calves. (See Chapter 41 in *Nelson Textbook of Pediatrics*, 16th ed.)

6. **D.** Although breast milk contains relatively less iron by weight, the iron is more bioavailable than the iron in cereals. Fruits, yellow vegetables, and cow's milk are poor sources of iron. (See Chapter 40.6 in *Nelson Textbook of Pediatrics*, 16th ed.)

7. **B.** In rickets, parathyroid hormone level is elevated and results in low serum phosphate levels. Low serum phosphate levels result in abnormal osteoblastic activity, which may result in craniotabes and a rachitic rosary with enlargement at the costochondral junctions. Even though osteoid of the legs is uncalcified, bowing does not occur until weight is borne on the legs. (See Chapter 44.10 in *Nelson Textbook of Pediatrics*, 16th ed.)

8. **C.** The EAR is one form of nutrient evaluation. The RDA (answer **B**) is the daily dietary intake sufficient to meet individual nutrient needs of 97–98% in age and gender groups. The RDA $= +2$ SD_{EAR}. (See Chapter 40 in *Nelson Textbook of Pediatrics*, 16th ed.)

9. **D.** The AI is one component of the DRI (dietary reference intakes). The DRI also considers the EAR, RDA, and tolerable upper level (UL). (See Chapter 40 in *Nelson Textbook of Pediatrics*, 16th ed.)

10. 1. **C**
    2. **A**
    3. **B**
    4. **E**
    5. **D**
    6. **F**
    (See Chapter 40 in *Nelson Textbook of Pediatrics*, 16th ed.)

11. 1. **E**
    2. **A**
    3. **C**
    4. **F**
    5. **B**
    6. **D**
    (See Chapter 40 in *Nelson Textbook of Pediatrics*, 16th ed.)

12. **E.** Vitamin K must be given (intramuscularly at birth) to all infants. Breast-fed infants who are not supplemented with vitamin K are at risk for bleeding. (See Chapter 41 in *Nelson Textbook of Pediatrics*, 16th ed.)

13. **E.** Antibodies in mother's milk are inactivated in the infant's intestines and do not contribute to intravascular hemolysis. (See Chapter 41 in *Nelson Textbook of Pediatrics*, 16th ed.)

14. **E.** Colic usually recurs in the early evening. (See Chapter 41 in *Nelson Textbook of Pediatrics*, 16th ed.)

15. **D.** Baby bottle caries syndrome is a significant problem because the milk bathes the teeth, setting up multiple caries. (See Chapter 41 in *Nelson Textbook of Pediatrics*, 16th ed.)

16. **B.** The rash of kwashiorkor is in areas of irritation. Sun-exposed dermatitis is typical of pellagra. (See Chapter 42 in *Nelson Textbook of Pediatrics*, 16th ed.)

17. **A.** Ketonuria is present early but does not persist into the later stages. (See Chapter 42 in *Nelson Textbook of Pediatrics*, 16th ed.)

18. **A.** Obese children don't necessarily eat more food or more junk food than leaner

children. (See Chapter 43 in *Nelson Textbook of Pediatrics*, 16th ed.)

19. **A.** Although hyperlipidemia secondary to obesity may be present, coronary artery disease does not manifest in children. (See Chapter 43 in *Nelson Textbook of Pediatrics*, 16th ed.)

20. 1. **B**
    2. **E**
    3. **A**
    4. **C**
    5. **D**
    (See Chapter 44 in *Nelson Textbook of Pediatrics*, 16th ed.)

21. **A.** Bitot spots are seen in vitamin A deficiency (dry plaques on the bulbar conjunctiva). (See Chapter 44 in *Nelson Textbook of Pediatrics*, 16th ed.)

22. **E.** **A** → **C** often occurs in patients with malabsorption. **D** has been reported in premature infants. (See Chapter 44 in *Nelson Textbook of Pediatrics*, 16th ed.)

7 *Pathophysiology of Body Fluids and Fluid Therapy*

1. **E.** Adrenal deficiency may cause renal salt wasting and usually does not affect free water excretion. (See Chapter 45 in *Nelson Textbook of Pediatrics*, 16th ed.)

2. **E.** Nephrogenic diabetes insipidus is a sex-linked recessive disorder due to deficient binding of ADH to the renal tubular cell. Exogenous administration of ADH is therefore ineffective. (See Chapter 45 in *Nelson Textbook of Pediatrics*, 16th ed.)

3. **B.** Hyponatremia due to feeding diluted formula or excessive amounts of sodium-free fluids (especially water) is relatively and unfortunately common among poor families who run out of formula. (See Chapter 46 in *Nelson Textbook of Pediatrics*, 16th ed.)

4. **E.** Metabolic alkalosis produces hypokalemia. (See Chapters 47 and 52 in *Nelson Textbook of Pediatrics*, 16th ed.)

5. **B.** Renal tubular acidosis with renal bicarbonate loss or diarrhea-induced stool losses of bicarbonate are the common causes of a normal anion gap acidosis. (See Chapter 55.8 in *Nelson Textbook of Pediatrics*, 16th ed.)

6. **C.** Dehydration of 6–9% represents moderate dehydration and early shock. Tachycardia reflects the intravascular volume loss, and deep respirations represent the pulmonary response to metabolic acidosis. (See Chapter 53 in *Nelson Textbook of Pediatrics*, 16th ed.)

7. **B.** Cerebral edema occurs if free water is given in excessive amounts, if the serum sodium falls more than 10 mEq/L/day, and if idiogenic osmols remain in neurons during rehydration. Cerebral thrombosis may occur before therapy is started and may be associated with inherited hypercoagulable conditions. (See Chapter 46 in *Nelson Textbook of Pediatrics*, 16th ed.)

8. **E.** Kayexalate, a potassium-binding resin, and dialysis are the only methods to remove potassium from the body. Other methods shift potassium from the extracellular to the intracellular space. (See Chapter 47 in *Nelson Textbook of Pediatrics*, 16th ed.)

9. **B.** Marked potassium depletion is more likely, although laboratory error is possible. When in doubt, repeat laboratory tests, but such a repeat in this case would confirm the finding. (See Chapter 47 in *Nelson Textbook of Pediatrics*, 16th ed.)

10. **C and D.** Insensible water losses usually occur independently of total body water homeostasis. (See Chapter 45 in *Nelson Textbook of Pediatrics*, 16th ed.)

11. **C.** All the others may stimulate ADH release. (See Chapter 45 in *Nelson Textbook of Pediatrics*, 16th ed.)

12. **A.** Indeed, hyperglycemia may produce pseudohyponatremia. (See Chapter 46 in *Nelson Textbook of Pediatrics*, 16th ed.)

13. **C.** The WIC syndrome in families receiving formula from the Women's, Infant's, and Children's nutritional supplementation program occurs when families run out of formula toward the end of the month and begin to dilute the formula with water. Another common cause is feeding excess amounts of pure water in general. (See Chapter 46 in *Nelson Textbook of Pediatrics*, 16th ed.)

14. 1. **C**
    2. **A**

3. **D**
4. **E**
5. **B**
(See Chapter 46 in *Nelson Textbook of Pediatrics,* 16th ed.)

15. **E. A → D** are noted in hyperkalemia. The first ECG change is peak T waves. Lengthening of the PR and QRS complexes occurs later. (See Chapter 47 in *Nelson Textbook of Pediatrics,* 16th ed.)

16. **D.** Beta-agonists often cause hypokalemia. (See Chapter 47 in *Nelson Textbook of Pediatrics,* 16th ed.)

17. **B.** RTA produces a non-anionic gap acidosis due to loss of bicarbonate by the kidney and not due to net gain of new acid in the circulation. (See Chapter 48 in *Nelson Textbook of Pediatrics,* 16th ed.)

18. **A, B,** and **C** would be helpful in the management of these immediate problems. A CBC would be of some use if anemia or infection were suspected. (See Chapter 50 in *Nelson Textbook of Pediatrics,* 16th ed.)

19. **A, B,** and **C** are correct, although with supportive care and time, most patients do quite well. (See Chapter 50 in *Nelson Textbook of Pediatrics,* 16th ed.)

20. **A.** Indeed, hypercalcemia is more common as a compensatory mechanism to release phosphate from bone. (See Chapter 51 in *Nelson Textbook of Pediatrics,* 16th ed.)

8 *The Acutely Ill Child*

1. **E.** Lack of immunization against tetanus may be managed with tetanus toxoid and, if a wound is large or dirty, with tetanus immune globulin. The other responses are high risk and require hospitalization. (See Chapter 70 in *Nelson Textbook of Pediatrics,* 16th ed.)

2. **C.** All other statements in the question are serious misconceptions. (See Chapter 74 in *Nelson Textbook of Pediatrics,* 16th ed.)

3. **E.** Age is usually not as predictive of the prognosis after near drowning as the other risk factors listed in the question. The best predictive factors are the initial signs of improvement within 24 hours of the episode. In addition, normal

cardiopulmonary function and alertness at the scene are favorable prognostic features. (See Chapter 69 in *Nelson Textbook of Pediatrics,* 16th ed.)

4. **A.** Control of the airway is essential in the gravely ill and unstable patient described in the question. Prevention of hypoxia and hypercarbia is critical to avoid secondary injury to vital tissues. (See Chapter 64.7 in *Nelson Textbook of Pediatrics,* 16th ed.)

5. **A.** Hyperventilation is the fastest method to relieve intracranial hypertension (increased intracranial pressure), which in this patient may be due to cerebral edema or a bleed. Dexamethasone is ineffective in treating this type of cerebral edema, and furosemide may acutely reduce central nervous system perfusion. (See Chapter 64.7 in *Nelson Textbook of Pediatrics,* 16th ed.)

6. **B.** Now is the time to perform a head CT scan. After this patient was stabilized, the CT scan revealed an epidural hematoma, which was surgically evacuated. (See Chapter 64.7 in *Nelson Textbook of Pediatrics,* 16th ed.)

7. 1. **E**
   2. **A**
   3. **B**
   4. **C**
   5. **D**
   (See Chapter 71 in *Nelson Textbook of Pediatrics,* 16th ed.)

8. **C.** Apnea does not respond to any drug (other than the reversal of opioid overdose by naloxone). Apnea is treated with bag and mask or mouth-to-mouth ventilation, or with endotracheal intubation and mechanical ventilation. (See Chapter 64.1 in *Nelson Textbook of Pediatrics,* 16th ed.)

9. **C.** Motor vehicle accidents are the leading cause of death among children 4–15 years old, although firearm-related injury and death are becoming increasingly common in childhood and adolescence. (See Chapter 57 in *Nelson Textbook of Pediatrics,* 16th ed.)

10. **D.** Placement of an intraosseous line is indicated in the emergency situation described in the question. If the child is in cardiopulmonary arrest, certain

medications (epinephrine, lidocaine) may be given by the endotracheal route. This patient requires fluid and blood replacement, which must be given by intraosseus line at this time. (See Chapter 60 in *Nelson Textbook of Pediatrics,* 16th ed.)

11. 1. **C**
    2. **A**
    3. **B**
    4. **C**
    5. **D**
    6. **C**
    7. **B**
    (See Chapter 69 in *Nelson Textbook of Pediatrics,* 16th ed.)

12. **C.** Home ownership of guns poses a greater threat to members of the family or to friends than to any unlawful intruder. (See Chapter 57 in *Nelson Textbook of Pediatrics,* 16th ed.)

13. **C.** Hot food or drinks from the microwave or more often from pots and pans that extend over the top of stoves are the most common causes of burn injury resulting in hospitalization in young children. Beware of the possible telltale signs of child abuse or neglect. (See Chapter 70 in *Nelson Textbook of Pediatrics,* 16th ed.)

14. **D.** Because of large third-space losses in burn victims, urine output as an assessment of intravascular volume and cardiac output is the best determinant of adequate fluid resuscitation. (See Chapter 70 in *Nelson Textbook of Pediatrics,* 16th ed.)

15. **C.** Burns on both hands and wrists in a glove distribution suggest that the child has been forcibly placed in hot water (bathtub). Most children jump out or do not enter a hot bathtub. (See Chapter 70 in *Nelson Textbook of Pediatrics,* 16th ed.)

16. **G.** Choices **A** through **F** are high-risk situations for an associated cervical spine injury. (See Chapter 60 in *Nelson Textbook of Pediatrics,* 16th ed.)

17. **E.** Group B streptococcal meningitis followed by bacteremia, osteomyelitis, septic arthritis, and cellulitis is the most common of the bacterial infections encountered in the first few months of life. Also consider *Escherichia coli* in the context of pyelonephritis. Nonetheless, many febrile episodes during this age period are viral. Unfortunately, it is frequently difficult to differentiate viral from serious bacterial illnesses in infants between birth and 2 months of age. (See Chapter 64 in *Nelson Textbook of Pediatrics,* 16th ed.)

18. **D.** Postoperative severe apnea can occur in former prematures up to roughly 50–55 weeks post conception, even after their apnea of prematurity has resolved and even among prematures who experienced no apnea of prematurity. The risk of postoperative apnea decreases with age. Anemia is an independent risk factor for apnea, but preoperative transfusion is not recommended for this hematocrit. Former premature infants up to perhaps 50–60 weeks' postconceptual age should be monitored for at least 12–18 hours after anesthesia. If apnea does not occur in the first 12 hours, it is unlikely to occur thereafter. Retrospective analysis of anesthetic risk supports delaying elective surgery in the first 1–2 months of life. These risks must be balanced against other studies that suggest that the delay in repairing inguinal hernias may result in incarceration that cannot be reduced and additional complications associated with more emergent surgery. Although apnea is reported to be much less common after spinal anesthesia for inguinal surgery in former prematures, current practice is still to monitor in hospital for apnea for at least 12 hours after a spinal anesthetic. (See Chapter 73 in *Nelson Textbook of Pediatrics,* 16th ed.)

19. **A.** Postoperative behavioral changes, including irritability, hostility, and sleep disturbance, are common in otherwise normal children after surgery. Traumatic induction of anesthesia and inadequate postoperative pain management may predispose to these changes. In the majority of cases, these behaviors resolve over several weeks. Intraoperative awareness during general anesthesia is not rare in adults, and estimates suggest that it may occur in 1–2% of cases. Stable intraoperative vital signs can occur even when there is awareness and recall of

painful events during surgery. The incidence of intraoperative awareness in children is not known but it clearly can occur, and the content of this child's dreams is suggestive that awareness under anesthesia could have occurred. It does appear that the events were traumatic to the child; she may benefit from short-term counseling and reassurance. (See Chapter 73 in *Nelson Textbook of Pediatrics,* 16th ed.)

20. **C.** Atelectasis is the most common cause of fever immediately after surgery, but the severity of the fever, the degree of tachypnea, and the "color isn't too good" description (whether reflecting cyanosis or impaired circulation) are atypical for ordinary postoperative atelectasis. Malignant hyperthermia is an inherited muscle disorder that produces acute hypermetabolism, increased CO_2 production, rhabdomyolysis, and fever.

    Clinically significant aspiration pneumonitis is comparatively uncommon in children after anesthesia and surgery but should be suspected if there is tachypnea, hypoxemia, and fever postoperatively. Although a rapid sequence induction may reduce the likelihood of aspiration, it does not completely prevent aspiration of gastric contents. Aspiration may occur as often on emergence as on induction. Auscultation of the chest would most probably show rales, rhonchi, or wheezes, and chest radiograph would (eventually) show infiltrates. (See Chapter 73 in *Nelson Textbook of Pediatrics,* 16th ed.)

21. **E.** The combination of fever, tachypnea, hypercarbia, hyperkalemia, and presumed myoglobinuria in this setting should evoke immediate treatment of malignant hyperthermia. The hyperkalemia is often immediately life threatening and should be treated immediately with calcium and sodium bicarbonate. The diffuse hypermetabolism and muscle injury process can be stopped in most cases by immediate IV infusion of dantrolene. The ongoing rhabdomyolysis releases myoglobin into the circulation, which can cause acute tubular necrosis; this risk can be reduced by aggressive hydration, diuresis, and alkalinization. Although there is some mild hypoxemia and moderate hypercarbia, endotracheal intubation does not appear immediately necessary at present from the information at hand; the other interventions are of higher priority at present. Supplemental oxygen should be given, and respiratory status should be monitored closely because his condition may deteriorate. Transfer to a PICU should be arranged. (See Chapter 73 in *Nelson Textbook of Pediatrics,* 16th ed.)

22. **D.** The presence of a recent upper and lower respiratory viral infection is predictive of an increased incidence of intraoperative problems, including laryngospasm, coughing, bronchospasm, and desaturation, as well as postoperative respiratory difficulties, including pneumonitis. This risk is greatest in the young, who have narrow airways and do not tolerate edema or increased mucus production. Airway reactivity is increased for several weeks after viral respiratory infections. Although endotracheal intubation may contribute to increased upper airway edema and decreased mucociliary elevator function, it is not possible to stipulate that only mask anesthesia be used. Parental smoking increases the risk of children having airway problems during anesthesia, including coughing, bronchospasm, laryngospasm, and desaturation. Intubation may become necessary because of either the procedure or because of difficulties encountered with mask ventilation. (See Chapter 73 in *Nelson Textbook of Pediatrics,* 16th ed.)

23. **E.** Most infant bathtub drowning occurs in the 7- to 15-month age group. Drowning in normal children above this age should raise suspicion of possible child abuse. Child abuse by drowning is difficult to diagnose, requires an understanding of the normal developmental capabilities of children, and necessitates a high index of suspicion. (See Chapter 69 in *Nelson Textbook of Pediatrics,* 16th ed.)

24. **A.** Neurologic examination at 24–72 hours is probably the most accurate

prognostic indicator after near drowning. Initial blood glucose > 300 mg/dL or submersion duration > 10 minutes is associated with poor outcomes in almost 80% of children. Normal ICP and head CT scan are not reassuring, as many of these children may have significant hypoxic-ischemic injury. (See Chapter 69 in *Nelson Textbook of Pediatrics,* 16th ed.)

25. **B.** Positive end-expiratory pressure is more effective at correcting hypoxemia than is increased inspired oxygen concentration alone. Intracranial pressure monitoring and treatment in victims of drowning or near drowning does not improve outcome. Most victims are in shock and require intravenous fluids to restore adequate perfusion; restoration of oxygenation, ventilation, and perfusion are the most critical features of cerebral resuscitation. Insulin is not recommended to treat hyperglycemia after near drowning. Most victims aspirate only a small quantity of fluid. (See Chapter 69 in *Nelson Textbook of Pediatrics,* 16th ed.)

26. **A.** Because pool covers are often cumbersome, they are unlikely to be replaced immediately after swim time and therefore are not likely to be an effective barrier. Lightweight covers should be discouraged because they do not prevent the child from entering the pool and may obscure visualization of the submerged child. Pool covers should be approved by the American Society for Testing Materials. Door alarms and automatically closing and locking doors are untested in efficacy. Swimming pool alarms cannot be recommended at this time: In all alarms tested, a significant number of false alarms and failure to alarm were noted. All the other aforementioned measures likely play a role in reducing the number of drowning victims. (See Chapter 69 in *Nelson Textbook of Pediatrics,* 16th ed.)

27. **E.** Children 10–14 years of age have the lowest death rate of pediatric age group; older adolescents (15–19 years) have twice this group's risk. The groups **A** through **D** are at increased risk for drowning. Toddlers have the highest drowning rate and children younger than 5 years of age account for 40% of all drowning victims. Black and American Indian children have 2–3 times the drowning rate of white children. The male:female drowning ratio ranges from 2:1 to 10:1 in all age groups. Epilepsy increased drowning risk by 4 to 10 times compared with nonepileptic children. (See Chapter 69 in *Nelson Textbook of Pediatrics,* 16th ed.)

28. **E.** Postoperative opioid dosing must be individualized to account for disease states that alter clearance or increase opioid sensitivity. This patient probably had a multifactorial etiology of his respiratory depression despite an infusion rate that would be effective and safe for the "average" patient.

Morphine is metabolized in the liver by glucuronidation and sulfation to active metabolites, especially morphine 6-glucuronide, or M6G. M6G produces analgesia and respiratory depression similar to morphine. With renal impairment, M6G and other metabolites accumulate and produce delayed narcosis.

Pain is a respiratory stimulant, and opioids produce greater respiratory depression when given to patients with minimal pain. Hip surgery involves dermatomes from roughly T12–L4, depending on the approach. Because this patient was insensitive from L1 caudad, he would be expected to have much less pain than most patients with intact sensation and thereby less respiratory stimulus.

Uremia produces sedation and may intensify the CNS depressant effects of analgesics and sedatives. This was a large operation with significant blood loss and increased potential for fluid shifts and electrolyte disturbances, including hyponatremia, which may depress sensorium.

Patients with myelomeningocele have been shown to have diminished respiratory reflexes to hypoxemia and hypercarbia.

In general, respiratory drive and respiratory sensitivity to opioids mature rapidly over the first few months of life and are normally mature by 6 months. Drug clearance is also mature by this time. Most healthy 14-month-old children receiving a morphine infusion at this rate after hip surgery would probably have had a minimal risk of respiratory depression. (See Chapter 73 in *Nelson Textbook of Pediatrics*, 16th ed.)

29. **B.** Addiction is best defined as a behavioral syndrome of compulsive drug seeking. It is not equivalent to tolerance or physical dependence, and it is extremely rare among patients receiving opioids for pain. Although continued administration can produce tolerance, that is not the same as addiction and does not imply drug-seeking behavior. The rate of opioid dose escalation in oncology patients is extremely variable. In adults with cancer, dose escalation appears to be related more to spread of tumor to more painful sites rather than tolerance per se.

A common error in opioid prescribing is to fail to increase dosing on conversion from intravenous to oral routes to account for the lesser potency of oral dosing. Regular dosing of oral morphine results in an oral/intravenous potency ratio of about 1:3. Average starting morphine doses for cancer pain are roughly 0.3 mg/kg orally every 4 hours, which is comparable to 0.1 mg/kg intravenously every 4 hours. This gives roughly $0.3 \times 6 = 1.8$ mg/kg/day for oral morphine dosing. This child weighs 40 kg and would be expected to require roughly 72 mg/day of oral morphine. Instead, he is getting 6 mg every 6 hours, or only 36 mg/day.

Morphine is effective for the overwhelming majority of children with cancer pain, including that due to bone involvement. Although some patients with neuropathic pain due to tumor involvement of spinal cord, epidural space, roots, or plexus may require very large dose escalation, the majority of these patients can also be made comfortable with opioids.

Depressed affect, sadness, and grief are common among patients with widespread cancer. Nevertheless, many children and adults with cancer appear more sad and withdrawn when they experience unrelieved pain and when they receive inadequate social support. A first step is to aggressively relieve their pain with opioids and to provide comfort and emotional support. In many cases, patients will become less withdrawn and sad. For example, studies have shown that when adults with cancer who initially express suicidal wishes are given appropriate opioid dosing and support from a palliative care team, the overwhelming majority no longer attempt suicide or seek physician-assisted suicide. (See Chapter 74 in *Nelson Textbook of Pediatrics*, 16th ed.)

30. **D.** Brain tumors can be preceded by headaches of increasing frequency as well as nausea with vomiting, but the history and physical examination here suggests a high likelihood of migraine and a comparatively low risk of brain tumor or other worrisome intracranial pathology. Migraine is common in adolescent girls; brain tumors are comparatively rare. A detailed history and thorough physical examination are required in evaluation of children with headache, but low-risk children do not require imaging studies.

Cognitive-behavioral programs often include relaxation training, with or without biofeedback training, and some structured counseling regarding coping with headache episodes and stress management. A number of outcome studies suggest a robust effect on the frequency and severity of migraine episodes; their benefit is not limited to tension/muscle contraction headaches.

Ibuprofen and other NSAIDs have shown benefit relative to placebo in blinded controlled trials for acute migraine episodes in children. The molecular events that lead to constriction and dilatation of dural vessels are complex but involve a number of mediators of neurogenic inflammation, including prostanoids, serotonin, and neurokinin peptides.

Sumatriptan and other selective antagonists of subgroups of serotonin receptors have been shown to abort a high percentage of migraine episodes in adults. Data in pediatric migraine are equivocal. In a recent study in Finland, sumatriptan produced pain scores and response rates indistinguishable from placebo, though, in a cross-over design, children rated their preference for sumatriptan above placebo. Injected sumatriptan often produces a subjective sense of chest tightness or chest pain in both children and adults. In adults, the chest tightness can occur without evidence of either bronchoconstriction or coronary vasospasm. (See Chapter 74 in *Nelson Textbook of Pediatrics,* 16th ed.)

31. **D.** The clinical observation of young patients is critical to help you evaluate and distinguish the degree of risk of infection and physiologic impairment. In addition to observing color, tone, grunting, or a bulging fontanel, the response to social stimuli is valuable. This 3-month-old had pneumococcal meningitis. (See Chapter 56 in *Nelson Textbook of Pediatrics,* 16th ed.)

32. **E.** Paradoxical irritability is present when a child becomes anxious and cries during attempts to cuddle and hold the patient. Movement of a painful extremity, abdomen, or neck may elicit this response. (See Chapter 56 in *Nelson Textbook of Pediatrics,* 16th ed.)

33. **A.** Homicide (infanticide) as child abuse is unfortunately a major problem in children under 5 years of age and is the leading cause of injury death under 1 year. It is the second leading cause of injury death among teens 15–19 years old. (See Chapter 57 in *Nelson Textbook of Pediatrics,* 16th ed.)

34. **C.** Product design modification such as child-proof caps and air bags has been the most successful means to reduce injuries, albeit in a passive way. (See Chapter 57 in *Nelson Textbook of Pediatrics,* 16th ed.)

35. **E.** Pupillary changes and Alert response to Voice or Pain or Unresponsive are sometimes all you may be able to assess after serious head trauma. (See Chapter 58 in *Nelson Textbook of Pediatrics,* 16th ed.)

36. **E.** Despite an uncertain etiology, the physiologic condition is that of shock. The circulation needs to be re-established to perfuse vital organs.

37. **D.** Hemorrhagic shock encephalopathy syndrome may look like heat stroke but is a distinct disorder characterized by encephalopathy, shock, fever, disseminated intravascular coagulopathy, and other organ failures (heart, hepatic). It has a high mortality rate and morbidity. (See Chapter 64 in *Nelson Textbook of Pediatrics,* 16th ed.)

38. **D.** Although somewhat controversial, CPR should be started in an apneic, pulseless, cold patient. The remote theoretical risks of initiating ventricular fibrillation are outweighed by the rarity of this event and the need to perfuse vital organs. (See Chapter 69 in *Nelson Textbook of Pediatrics,* 16th ed.)

39. **A.** Unless mineral oil is needed to remove hot tar, such substances, especially butter, are of no value. (See Chapter 70 in *Nelson Textbook of Pediatrics,* 16th ed.)

40. **E.** This defines a full-thickness burn (also known as third degree). (See Chapter 70 in *Nelson Textbook of Pediatrics,* 16th ed.)

41. **C.** Prophylactic penicillin or tetanus booster (in an immunized patient) is unnecessary in the treatment of minor burns. (See Chapter 70 in *Nelson Textbook of Pediatrics,* 16th ed.)

42. **C.** Because of the high risk of delayed cardiac or visceral injury, all patients should be admitted to the hospital for observation and monitoring. (See Chapter 70 in *Nelson Textbook of Pediatrics,* 16th ed.)

43. **E.** Cold-induced fat necrosis (panniculitis) is probably more common than reported. This Wisconsin pediatrician has seen multiple children with cold-induced panniculitis. (See Chapter 72 in *Nelson Textbook of Pediatrics,* 16th ed.)

44. 1. **D**
    2. **A**
    3. **E**
    4. **B**
    5. **C**
    (See Chapter 73 in *Nelson Textbook of Pediatrics,* 16th ed.)

45. **E.** Latex allergy is common in children with multiple surgical procedures and those who have required catheterization for urinary retention. The presentation includes urticaria, wheezing, and

hypotension. Bananas may cross-react with latex. (See Chapter 73 in *Nelson Textbook of Pediatrics,* 16th ed.)

46. 1. **B**
    2. **C**
    3. **A**
    4. **E**
    5. **D**

    (See Chapter 73 in *Nelson Textbook of Pediatrics,* 16th ed.)

47. **C.** All NSAIDs produce reversible transient platelet dysfunction. The new cyclo-oxygenase inhibitors (COX-2) may reduce the risk of bleeding without altering the analgesic effects.

48. **D.** Neuropathic pain is often very painful and unfortunately difficult to treat. **A, B, C** and **E** are all false.

49. **E.** Although children with hyperactivity may have accidents, they all don't. The accident-prone child may not exist but, more important to prevent accidents, products and the environment should be made safer. (See Chapter 57 in *Nelson Textbook of Pediatrics,* 16th ed.)

50. **D.** Splash burns from boiling water over the stove do not suggest abuse but may be associated with poor education or neglect. (See Chapter 57 in *Nelson Textbook of Pediatrics,* 16th ed.)

51. **B.** The child described in the question is severely ill and may suffer arrest at any moment. (See Chapter 60 in *Nelson Textbook of Pediatrics,* 16th ed.)

52. **A.** Oropharyngeal airways are recommended only for unconscious patients because they may cause gagging and vomiting in conscious patients. (See Chapter 64 in *Nelson Textbook of Pediatrics,* 16th ed.)

53. **C.** The preferred method for opening the airway in a potentially traumatized victim is the jaw thrust, which results in less movement of the cervical spine. (See Chapter 64 in *Nelson Textbook of Pediatrics,* 16th ed.)

9 *Human Genetics*

1. **E.** Fragile X is a common chromosomal cause of mental retardation in boys. Affected boys have allelic expansion of trinucleotide repeats to over 200 (normal is 6–54). (See Chapter 76 in *Nelson Textbook of Pediatrics,* 16th ed.)

2. **D.** Y chromosome material is present in 5–10% of girls with Turner syndrome. Gonadoblastoma may develop in the ovary, thus necessitating bilateral oophorectomy as a preventive measure. (See Chapter 78 in *Nelson Textbook of Pediatrics,* 16th ed.)

3. 1. **A**
   2. **B**
   3. **A**
   4. **D**
   5. **C**
   6. **D**
   7. **C**
   8. **E**
   9. **C**
   10. **C**

   (See Chapter 78 in *Nelson Textbook of Pediatrics,* 16th ed.)

4. **B.** Mitochondrial inheritance of the diseases listed in the question involves mutation of the mitochondrial genome, which originated solely from the ovum. (See Chapter 77 in *Nelson Textbook of Pediatrics,* 16th ed.)

5. 1. **B**
   2. **A**
   3. **A**
   4. **C**
   5. **C**
   6. **B**
   7. **D**
   8. **B**
   9. **A**
   10. **C**
   11. **C**
   12. **C**

   (See Chapter 77 in *Nelson Textbook of Pediatrics,* 16th ed.)

6. **D.** Mitochondria in an offspring are derived from the ovum because sperm have no mitochondria. Mitochondria have their own DNA that encodes mitochondrial proteins. Such inheritance affects both males and females equally. (See Chapter 75 in *Nelson Textbook of Pediatrics,* 16th ed.)

7. **D.** This autosomal recessive disorder, due to a defect in the protein hexosaminidase A, has a degree of genetic heterogenicity in that the defect in Ashkenazi Jews is a

frameshift mutation, whereas that in French Canadians is due to a missing gene segment. (See Chapter 75 in *Nelson Textbook of Pediatrics,* 16th ed.)

8. **D.** Homeobox genes instruct tissue to become a particular anatomic site (e.g., head, abdomen). Once acted on during development, the tissue is destined to a very specific line of development. (See Chapter 76 in *Nelson Textbook of Pediatrics,* 16th ed.)

9. **E.** All the given anatomic anomalies (**A–D**) are due to homeobox gene mutations. (See Chapter 76 in *Nelson Textbook of Pediatrics,* 16th ed.)

10. **D.** Fluorescent in situ hybridization to a chromosome region with a deletion or mutated gene is a powerful new tool in genetic diagnosis. (See Chapter 76 in *Nelson Textbook of Pediatrics,* 16th ed.)

11. **B.** This powerful tool is helpful in genetic research and diagnosis. It also has been valuable in the rapid diagnosis of infectious diseases such as HSV and TB. (See Chapter 76 in *Nelson Textbook of Pediatrics,* 16th ed.)

12. **B.** Multiple repeats of trinucleotides in the coding region and the untranslated or translated region of these genes produce significant disease in the other answers. (See Chapter 76 in *Nelson Textbook of Pediatrics,* 16th ed.)

13. **A.** Myotonic dystrophy, a disorder due to CTG trinucleotide repeats, is characterized by increasing disease severity in successive generations. (See Chapter 76 in *Nelson Textbook of Pediatrics,* 16th ed.)

14. **B.** Autosomal dominance wherein both sexes are affected and 50% of offspring have the disorder. (See Chapter 77 in *Nelson Textbook of Pediatrics,* 16th ed.)

15. **E.** X-linked recessive inheritance classically occurs in hemophilia; carrier females are usually asymptomatic. (See Chapter 77 in *Nelson Textbook of Pediatrics,* 16th ed.)

16. **C.** Carrier detection is difficult because the multiple genes involved in these disorders (e.g., pyloric, stenosis, spina bifida, cleft lip) remain undetermined. Obligate carriers are asymptomatic. (See Chapter 77 in *Nelson Textbook of Pediatrics,* 16th ed.)

17. **C.** Patients with translocation 21 have an identical phenotype to other children with trisomy 21 due to nondisjunction. Offspring of subsequent pregnancies to a normal phenotype translocation carrier either have a normal phenotype and genotype, have a normal phenotype and are a carrier of the translocation, or are affected with trisomy 21. (See Chapter 78 in *Nelson Textbook of Pediatrics,* 16th ed.)

18. 1. **B**
    2. **D**
    3. **C**
    4. **E**
    5. **A**
    (See Chapter 78 in *Nelson Textbook of Pediatrics,* 16th ed.)

19. 1. **B**
    2. **C**
    3. **D**
    4. **A**
    5. **E**
    (See Chapter 78 in *Nelson Textbook of Pediatrics,* 16th ed.)

20. **D.** Y chromosome material places women with Turner syndrome (45,X) at very high risk for gonadoblastoma in the underdeveloped gonads. If Y chromosome material is present, gonadectomy should be considered. (See Chapter 78 in *Nelson Textbook of Pediatrics,* 16th ed.)

21. **E.** Indeed, skin fibroblasts karyotyping is the best method to identify the mosaic. Lymphocytes have a high false-negative rate. (See Chapter 78 in *Nelson Textbook of Pediatrics,* 16th ed.)

22. **B.** Inheritance of two copies of the same affected chromosome from the mother is the best explanation. Although the mother is an obligate carrier, two copies of the affected chromosome are transmitted to the offspring; the normal chromosome was not transmitted. (See Chapter 78 in *Nelson Textbook of Pediatrics,* 16th ed.)

23. **C.** Lack of paternal gene influence or imprinting in this disease results in Prader-Willi syndrome. (See Chapter 78 in *Nelson Textbook of Pediatrics,* 16th ed.)

24. **E.** Trisomy 21, or Down syndrome, is also associated with other cardiac, gastrointestinal, and skeletal problems.

(See Chapter 78 in *Nelson Textbook of Pediatrics*, 16th ed.)

25. **D.** Duodenal atresia is common in neonates with trisomy 21 and may produce polyhydramnios. After birth, intestinal obstruction requires that the child be NPO and undergo intestinal decompression prior to surgery. (See Chapter 78 in *Nelson Textbook of Pediatrics*, 16th ed.)

10 *Metabolic Diseases*

1. 1. **C**
   2. **E**
   3. **A**
   4. **D**
   5. **B**
   6. **F**
   (See Chapter 82 in *Nelson Textbook of Pediatrics*, 16th ed.)

2. **B.** The mechanism for this self-destructive behavior is unknown but is not necessarily thought to be an inability to feel pain. (See Chapter 86 in *Nelson Textbook of Pediatrics*, 16th ed.)

3. **B.** The combination of hypoglycemia, jaundice, elevated liver enzyme values, and *E. coli* sepsis is classic for early-onset severe galactosemia. A white blood cell defect may predispose to *E. coli* sepsis, and the toxic effects of galactose-1-phosphate explain the hepatotoxicity. In this child, who was fed cow's milk–based formula, the urine-reducing substances (galactose) were positive. (See Chapter 84.2 in *Nelson Textbook of Pediatrics*, 16th ed.)

4. **D.** The acute or subacute presentation of hereditary fructose intolerance is very similar to that of galactosemia. The inability to metabolize fructose can produce shock, hypoglycemia, hepatic dysfunction, and emesis. In the child described in the question, the urine-reducing substance was fructose. Before the initiation of fructose (sucrose)-containing foods (e.g., fruit juices), such a child will be asymptomatic. (See Chapter 84.3 in *Nelson Textbook of Pediatrics*, 16th ed.)

5. **C.** Biotinidase levels may reflect enzymatic deficiencies affecting carbohydrate and amino acid (organic acid) metabolism. Both enzymatic pathways require biotinidase; deficiencies produce manifestations, as noted in this case. Treatment with oral biotin may overcome this defect in some affected patients. (See Chapter 82 in *Nelson Textbook of Pediatrics*, 16th ed.)

6. **D.** Muscle biopsy may confirm the diagnosis of Pompe disease (glycogen storage disease type II). Deficiency of acid α-glucosidase results in marked lysosomal glycogen accumulation and primarily affects the heart and skeletal muscle. Death in the infantile form is due to respiratory muscle failure. (See Chapter 84.1 in *Nelson Textbook of Pediatrics*, 16th ed.)

7. 1. **E**
   2. **A**
   3. **D**
   4. **C**
   5. **B**
   (See Chapter 83 in *Nelson Textbook of Pediatrics*, 16th ed.)

8. **C.** All five diseases listed in the question are prevalent among Ashkenazi Jews. Niemann-Pick A and Gaucher type I are the only two diseases that present with a very large spleen. Children with Niemann-Pick A disease are likely to be retarded, but this patient is not. Anemia, leukopenia, and thrombocytopenia are typically found in Gaucher disease. Patients with Canavan disease, Tay-Sachs disease, and mucolipidosis IV are neurologically impaired, but this patient is not. (See Chapter 83 in *Nelson Textbook of Pediatrics*, 16th ed.)

9. **A.** Nonketotic hypoglycemia with or without hyperammonemia in a patient of this age is often due to this relatively common cause. In addition to hypoglycemia, MCAD is associated with a Reye-like syndrome, and some cases are initially diagnosed as SIDS. (See Chapter 83 in *Nelson Textbook of Pediatrics*, 16th ed.)

10. **C.** Acute intermittent porphyria is characterized by neurovisceral symptoms but no photosensitivity reactions. (See Chapter 87 in *Nelson Textbook of Pediatrics*, 16th ed.)

11. **A.** Zellweger syndrome is the prototypic neonatal peroxisomal disorder. (See Chapter 83.2 in *Nelson Textbook of Pediatrics,* 16th ed.)
12. **B.** In rhizomelic chondrodysplasia punctata, plasma levels of phytanic acid and erythrocyte plasmalogens are elevated. (See Chapter 83.2 in *Nelson Textbook of Pediatrics,* 16th ed.)
13. **D.** The Achilles tendon is a first site for the development of xanthomas, an area that most of us do not usually examine other than to test deep tendon reflexes. (See Chapter 83.3 in *Nelson Textbook of Pediatrics,* 16th ed.)
14. **C.** These disorders affect multiple organ systems with many manifestations. Unfortunately, enzyme replacement has not been available or successful to date. (See Chapter 84.6 in *Nelson Textbook of Pediatrics,* 16th ed.)
15. **E.** Many patients may be asymptomatic in the newborn period but, as storage of mucolipids increases, symptoms appear at various later stages of the disease. Many survive until adolescence or young adulthood. (See Chapter 83.5 in *Nelson Textbook of Pediatrics,* 16th ed.)
16. **A.** Chorionic villus cells allow accelerated prenatal diagnosis, revealing results much sooner than the traditional amniocentesis. The recurrence risk is 25% for this autosomal recessive disorder. (See Chapter 83 in *Nelson Textbook of Pediatrics,* 16th ed.)
17. **A.** Tay-Sachs disease classically presents with these clinical features about this time of infancy. A cherry-red spot on the fundi would also be present. (See Chapter 83 in *Nelson Textbook of Pediatrics,* 16th ed.)
18. **E.** This is especially true in patients with this form of Gaucher disease. Started early, enzyme replacement therapy may reverse symptoms and prevent other complications. (See Chapter 83 in *Nelson Textbook of Pediatrics,* 16th ed.)
19. **B.** Liver biopsy is helpful, but as more research comes to the forefront and becomes routine, DNA diagnosis may become the next approach. (See Chapter 83 in *Nelson Textbook of Pediatrics,* 16th ed.)
20. **D.** PKU presents with these symptoms gradually. All children appear normal at birth. (See Chapter 81 in *Nelson Textbook of Pediatrics,* 16th ed.)
21. **E.** Appropriate treatment lowers the serum level of the essential amino acid phenylalanine. Too severe restriction of this amino acid produces lethargy, anorexia, rash, diarrhea, and death. (See Chapter 81 in *Nelson Textbook of Pediatrics,* 16th ed.)
22. **B.** Excessive levels of phenylalanine in affected mothers during pregnancy adversely affect the genetically unaffected heterozygotic carrier fetus. If maternal dietary restoration is not followed, a potentially normal fetus will be severely affected. (See Chapter 82 in *Nelson Textbook of Pediatrics,* 16th ed.)
23. **A.** The acute hepatic crisis of tyrosinemia is heralded by signs of hepatic dysfunction, DIC, and, if severe, death. (See Chapter 82.2 in *Nelson Textbook of Pediatrics,* 16th ed.)
24. **B.** Tyrosinemia is due to a deficiency of fumarylacetoacetate hydrolyase determined in fibroblasts or liver. (See Chapter 82.2 in *Nelson Textbook of Pediatrics,* 16th ed.)
25. **C.** NTBC, an inhibitor of 4-hydroxyphenylpyruvate, has resulted in clinical and biochemical improvement in initial studies. Dietary restriction of phenylalanine, methionine, and tyrosine may be of small benefit but does not usually stop the progression of the disease. (See Chapter 82.2 in *Nelson Textbook of Pediatrics,* 16th ed.)
26. **A.** Cataracts are unusual in tyrosinemia; they are common in galactosemia. (See Chapter 82.2 in *Nelson Textbook of Pediatrics,* 16th ed.)
27. **E.** Nail hypoplasia is not observed in albinism, but **A–D** are common features or potential complications. (See Chapter 82.2 in *Nelson Textbook of Pediatrics,* 16th ed.)
28. 1. **B**
    2. **C**
    3. **E**
    4. **D**
    5. **A**

(See Chapter 82.2 in *Nelson Textbook of Pediatrics*, 16th ed.)

29. **D.** Homocystinuria is due to a deficiency of cystathionine synthase. (See Chapter 82.3 in *Nelson Textbook of Pediatrics*, 16th ed.)

30. **E.** **A–D** are all correct. The hypercoagulable state may even be present if homocysteine levels are elevated without any other signs of homocystinuria. (See Chapter 82.3 in *Nelson Textbook of Pediatrics*, 16th ed.)

31. **A.** After high-dose folate treatment, the patient responds to the primary therapy of high-dose vitamin B_6. (See Chapter 82.3 in *Nelson Textbook of Pediatrics*, 16th ed.)

32. **E.** These neurologic manifestations, together with severe metabolic acidosis with a very high anion gap, suggest an organic acidemia. (See Chapter 82.6 in *Nelson Textbook of Pediatrics*, 16th ed.)

33. **D.** This would be most appropriate if virilizing adrenal hyperplasia was suspected. The other answers are all appropriate. (See Chapter 82.6 in *Nelson Textbook of Pediatrics*, 16th ed.)

34. **A.** MSUD is due to a deficiency of decarboxylation of these amino acids. (See Chapter 82.6 in *Nelson Textbook of Pediatrics*, 16th ed.)

35. 1. **B**
    2. **C**
    3. **D**
    4. **E**
    5. **A**
    6. **F**
    (See Chapter 82.6 in *Nelson Textbook of Pediatrics*, 16th ed.)

36. **C.** MMA presenting like this in a newborn has a poor prognosis even if the child survives the acute episode. (See Chapter 82.6 in *Nelson Textbook of Pediatrics*, 16th ed.)

37. **A.** Some cases of MMA are responsive to large doses (1–2 mg/24 hours) of vitamin B_{12}. (See Chapter 82.6 in *Nelson Textbook of Pediatrics*, 16th ed.)

38. **C.** In neonatal nonketotic hyper-glycinemia, the CSF glycine level is markedly elevated and a CSF:plasma ratio of glycine of > 0.8 is diagnostic of this disorder of glycine metabolism. (See

Chapter 82.7 in *Nelson Textbook of Pediatrics*, 16th ed.)

39. **B.** Trimethylaminuria from metabolism of choline or ingested trimethylamine creates the odor; oxidation to the oxide normally produces an odorless compound. (See Chapter 82.7 in *Nelson Textbook of Pediatrics*, 16th ed.)

40. **B.** The absence of an anion gap and high ammonia rules out organic acidemia. The clinical picture is most compatible with urea cycle defect. (See Chapter 82.11 in *Nelson Textbook of Pediatrics*, 16th ed.)

41. **E.** OTC deficiency is characterized by elevated urinary excretion of orotic acid. (See Chapter 43.11 in *Nelson Textbook of Pediatrics*, 16th ed.)

42. **B.** Initially proteins, especially albumin, are not needed during an acute exacerbation of hyperammonemia from a urea cycle defect. (See Chapter 82.11 in *Nelson Textbook of Pediatrics*, 16th ed.)

43. **A.** Only 20% have moderate mental retardation. Most are mentally normal, but many have hypotonia. (See Chapter 82.13 in *Nelson Textbook of Pediatrics*, 16th ed.)

44. **E.** Canavan disease due to excessive amounts of brain *N*-acetylaspartate acid produces leukodystrophy with macrocephaly and loss of milestones. Alexander disease is similar but progresses at a slower rate. (See Chapter 82.14 in *Nelson Textbook of Pediatrics*, 16th ed.)

45. **A.** MCAD is a relatively common cause of nonketotic hypoglycemia. (See Chapter 83.1 in *Nelson Textbook of Pediatrics*, 16th ed.)

46. **A.** Fasting should not exceed 10–12 hours, and carbohydrate-rich diets should be provided in times of illness. (See Chapter 83.1 in *Nelson Textbook of Pediatrics*, 16th ed.)

47. 1. **D**
    2. **D**
    3. **B**
    4. **E**
    5. **A**
    6. **C**
    7. **D**
    8. **D**
    9. **E**

10. **C**
(See Chapter 83.2 in *Nelson Textbook of Pediatrics*, 16th ed.)

48. **D.** ALD, a peroxisomal disorder, presents with progressive dementia, seizures, MRI cerebral white matter lesions (symmetric periventricular sites), and adrenal insufficiency (as determined by a poor cortisol response to intravenous ACTH). (See Chapter 83.2 in *Nelson Textbook of Pediatrics*, 16th ed.)

49. **C.** VLCFA are elevated in patients with X-linked adrenoleukodystrophy. (See Chapter 83.3 in *Nelson Textbook of Pediatrics*, 16th ed.)

50. **E.** Achilles tendon xanthomas are the most common site. Flexor tendons of the digits of the hand are another common site. (See Chapter 83.3 in *Nelson Textbook of Pediatrics*, 16th ed.)

51. **A.** Patients with just severe homozygous familial hypercholesterolemia do not have high triglycerides. (See Chapter 83.3 in *Nelson Textbook of Pediatrics*, 16th ed.)

52. **B.** LDL apheresis is the treatment of choice. **A** and **C** have some value, but liver transplantation carries considerable risks. Gene therapy is a hopeful future therapy. (See Chapter 83.3 in *Nelson Textbook of Pediatrics*, 16th ed.)

53. 1. **A**
    2. **C**
    3. **C**
    4. **C**
    5. **C**
(See Chapter 83.4 in *Nelson Textbook of Pediatrics*, 16th ed.)

54. **E.** Although leukemia is of concern, there are no blasts in the CBC or bone marrow, and the course is somewhat protracted for acute leukemia. (See Chapter 83.4 in *Nelson Textbook of Pediatrics*, 16th ed.)

55. **B.** Gaucher disease is due to a deficiency of enzyme with the resultant build-up of glucocerebrosides in the reticuloendothelial system and subsequent dysfunction or enlargement of the respective organs. (See Chapter 83.4 in *Nelson Textbook of Pediatrics*, 16th ed.)

56. **B.** Enzyme replacement therapy has been very effective in reducing extraskeletal symptoms. Future hope in recombinant enzyme replacement therapy will eliminate the small risk of infection. (See Chapter 83.4 in *Nelson Textbook of Pediatrics*, 16th ed.)

57. **C.** Ocular manifestations include nystagmus and optic atrophy. (See Chapter 83.4 in *Nelson Textbook of Pediatrics*, 16th ed.)

58. 1. **B**
    2. **C**
    3. **A**
    4. **E**
    5. **D**
(See Chapter 84 in *Nelson Textbook of Pediatrics*, 16th ed.)

59. **B.** This group of disorders includes olivopontocerebellar atrophy and many other neurologic disorders. Diagnosis is confirmed by isoelectric focusing studies to demonstrate abnormalities of carbohydrate-deficient transferrin. (See Chapter 84 in *Nelson Textbook of Pediatrics*, 16th ed.)

11 *The Fetus and Neonatal Infant*

1. 1. **C**
   2. **A**
   3. **E**
   4. **B**
   5. **D**
   6. **F**
   7. **F**
   8. **F**
(See Chapter 104 in *Nelson Textbook of Pediatrics*, 16th ed.)

2. **C.** One point in the Apgar score is taken off for color. (See Chapter 90 in *Nelson Textbook of Pediatrics*, 16th ed.)

3. **B.** The other three choices listed in the question are pathologic, not physiologic. (See Chapter 98.3 in *Nelson Textbook of Pediatrics*, 16th ed.)

4. **D.** No treatment is necessary for the infant described in the question, assuming normal growth and development. (See Chapter 98.3 in *Nelson Textbook of Pediatrics*, 16th ed.)

5. **E.** (See Chapter 99.4 in *Nelson Textbook of Pediatrics*, 16th ed.)

6. **E.** (See Chapter 99.4 in *Nelson Textbook of Pediatrics*, 16th ed.)

7. **C.** (See Chapter 99.4 in *Nelson Textbook of Pediatrics*, 16th ed.)

8. **A.** The infant described in Questions 5–8 has a case of severe vitamin K deficiency—hemorrhagic disease of the newborn. The next most likely diagnosis is child abuse; most infants in coma with retinal hemorrhages have been shaken, and a skeletal survey thus is appropriate. The combination of home delivery (no AquaMEPHYTON administered), breast-feeding (low vitamin K content), and the amoxicillin treatment that eliminated normal intestinal bacterial synthesis of vitamin K led to the tragic demise of an otherwise normal infant. Of all possible preventive measures, administration of vitamin K at birth would have been the most effective. (See Chapter 99.4 in *Nelson Textbook of Pediatrics,* 16th ed.)

9. **E.** Intubate the trachea and apply negative-pressure suction to help clear residual meconium from the airway, preventing meconium from moving more distally and initiating meconium aspiration pneumonia. Stimulating the infant to breathe is potentially dangerous if meconium is present in the airway. Administer epinephrine at a later time if the infant does not respond. Initially providing positive-pressure bag-and-mask ventilation is also dangerous if meconium is in the airway. Intubating the trachea and providing positive-pressure ventilation is dangerous for the same reason. (See Chapter 97.6 in *Nelson Textbook of Pediatrics,* 16th ed.)

10. **D.** The infant described in the question had severe oligohydramnios, which may cause reduced fetal lung growth and may or may not be associated with renal anomalies (Potter syndrome). Pulmonary hypoplasia places the patient at increased risk for a pneumothorax after resuscitation and during mechanical ventilation. IVH would be a consideration in a very premature infant (this patient is 36 weeks' gestation but is small for gestational age). Furthermore, IVH is unusual at 1 hour of age. (See Chapter 97.8 in *Nelson Textbook of Pediatrics,* 16th ed.)

11. **D.** Hypothyroidism was confirmed by the late arrival of the newborn screening results, indicating high TSH and low T_4 levels. Treatment with thyroxine improved the jaundice and the other signs. The hyperbilirubinemia is indirect (unconjugated). Crigler-Najjar syndrome is a possibility and is either autosomal dominant or recessive (check the family history). However, there are signs other than jaundice that suggest another disease. Biliary atresia is always a concern in infants with delayed clearance of jaundice or worsening jaundice after 2 weeks of life. The hyperbilirubinemia is predominantly direct (conjugated). Galactosemia should be considered, especially in the presence of hypoglycemia, direct-reacting jaundice, hepatomegaly, or ascites. (See Chapter 98.3 in *Nelson Textbook of Pediatrics,* 16th ed.)

12. **E.** Jaundice usually resolves in all infants with hyperbilirubinemia due to ABO incompatibility in the first week of life. Nonetheless, the hemolysis continues without evidence of jaundice because the liver can now excrete the bilirubin load. Late-onset anemia must be watched for and treated with a packed red blood cell transfusion if the infant is symptomatic. Hereditary spherocytosis is a possibility but is relatively rare. A well-taken family history and examination of the child's and parents' blood smear are helpful (most are inherited as an autosomal dominant trait). Sickle cell anemia hemolytic crisis is not encountered this early in life because a considerable amount of fetal hemoglobin remains; thus, there are few sickle β-chains to sickle. (See Chapter 99.2 in *Nelson Textbook of Pediatrics,* 16th ed.)

13. **C.** The fetus described in the question has been slowly losing blood by a chronic fetal to maternal hemorrhage. The Kleihauer-Betke test detects fetal cells circulating in the mother's blood by identifying acid stable fetal erythrocytes in the blood smear. (See Chapter 99.1 in *Nelson Textbook of Pediatrics,* 16th ed.)

14. **B.** TORCH titers are overall not of great value in diagnosing a congenital infection. In addition, TORCH infections do not produce congenital heart disease except the PDA associated with

congenital rubella syndrome (which does not produce a cleft palate or lip). (See Chapter 104 and 105 in *Nelson Textbook of Pediatrics,* 16th ed.)

15. 1. **G**
    2. **D**
    3. **A**
    4. **B**
    5. **C**
    6. **E**
    7. **F**
    (See Chapter 106 in *Nelson Textbook of Pediatrics,* 16th ed.)

16. **B.** After an arterial blood gas determination that demonstrates hypoxia on an Fio$_2$ of 1.0, surfactant should be administered by direct endotracheal installation, *not* by aerosol. In addition, the patient described in the question demonstrates severe hypotension, which should be treated first with intravenous fluids such as normal saline and then by inotropic agents such as dopamine. (See Chapter 106 in *Nelson Textbook of Pediatrics,* 16th ed.)

17. **C.** Severe hypoxia, hypotension, prolonged rupture of the membranes, neutropenia, and thrombocytopenia suggest early-onset sepsis and congenital pneumonia. (See Chapter 106 in *Nelson Textbook of Pediatrics,* 16th ed.)

18. **B.** Dermal erythropoiesis is necessary if TORCH (usually cytomegalovirus [CMV] or rubella) infection damages the bone marrow and traditional extramedullary sites of erythropoiesis (liver, spleen). (See Chapter 105 in *Nelson Textbook of Pediatrics,* 16th ed.)

19. **B.** Most LBW infants in the United States are premature. In developing countries, IUGR is a more predominant factor in producing LBW infants (<2500 g at birth). (See Chapter 89 in *Nelson Textbook of Pediatrics,* 16th ed.)

20. **D.** This sign manifests as the body (from head to toe) being divided evenly into a pale side and a red side and is transient and harmless. (See Chapter 90 in *Nelson Textbook of Pediatrics,* 16th ed.)

21. **D.** Conjunctival and retinal hemorrhages are normal after a vaginal delivery and are usually benign and without sequelae.

(See Chapter 90 in *Nelson Textbook of Pediatrics,* 16th ed.)

22. **C.** Although previously thought to be of more value for predicting long-term outcome, most children with low Apgar scores do well, and most children with cerebral palsy have normal Apgar scores. (See Chapter 90 in *Nelson Textbook of Pediatrics,* 16th ed.)

23. **D.** At least two successful feedings are reassuring, whereas these other issues raise concern and need further evaluation or therapy. (See Chapter 90 in *Nelson Textbook of Pediatrics,* 16th ed.)

24. 1. **A**
    2. **B**
    3. **A**
    4. **B**
    5. **A**
    (See Chapter 91 in *Nelson Textbook of Pediatrics,* 16th ed.)

25. 1. **E**
    2. **A**
    3. **F**
    4. **B**
    5. **C**
    6. **D**
    (See Chapter 92 in *Nelson Textbook of Pediatrics,* 16th ed.)

26. 1. **A**
    2. **A**
    3. **A** and **B**
    4. **D**
    5. **C**
    (See Chapter 92 in *Nelson Textbook of Pediatrics,* 16th ed.)

27. 1. **C**
    2. **A**
    3. **D**
    4. **B**
    5. **E**
    (See Chapter 93 in *Nelson Textbook of Pediatrics,* 16th ed.)

28. **D.** Klumpke paralysis involves injury to the 7th and 8th cervical nerves and the 1st thoracic nerve. It is usually unilateral due to traction injury of the brachial plexus. (See Chapter 95 in *Nelson Textbook of Pediatrics,* 16th ed.)

29. **C.** Transition of the spinal cord may occur in vertex and breech positions and may be noted with normal vertebral body anatomy. It would manifest as in this

patient and with shock, hypothermia, and bowel and bladder dysfunction. With time, hypotonia resolves into hypertonia and hyperreflexia. (See Chapter 95 in *Nelson Textbook of Pediatrics,* 16th ed.)

30. **A.** Stage I hypoxic ischemic encephalopathy is the mildest stage, with an overall excellent prognosis for survival and for developmental outcome. (See Chapter 95 in *Nelson Textbook of Pediatrics,* 16th ed.)

31. **B and D.** A pneumothorax this early (in the delivery room) is unusual in the absence of high positive-pressure resuscitation. A PDA usually develops 2–4 days after therapy for RDS and is rarely symptomatic at birth. TTN does not require 100% O_2 or mechanical ventilation. RDS may have been prevented by antenatal glucocorticoids, whereas group B streptococcal sepsis may have been prevented by intrapartum penicillin. (See Chapter 97 in *Nelson Textbook of Pediatrics,* 16th ed.)

32. **B, C,** and **D** are fortunately true. However, and unexpectedly, the incidence of chronic lung disease (bronchopulmonary dysplasia) has not been reduced by surfactant therapy. (See Chapter 97 in *Nelson Textbook of Pediatrics,* 16th ed.)

33. **A, B.** Blood loss into the peritoneum (**A**) or cerebral ventricles (**B**) may produce this picture. IVH of this magnitude has a poor prognosis. (See Chapter 97 in *Nelson Textbook of Pediatrics,* 16th ed.)

34. **E.** **A → D** are appropriate laboratory tests in a pale neonate with significant hyperbilirubinemia. (See Chapter 98 in *Nelson Textbook of Pediatrics,* 16th ed.)

35. **C.** The patient has indirect hyperbilirubinemia that, if untreated, poses a risk for kernicterus. At this time and without evidence of neurologic signs of kernicterus and exchange, transfusion is not needed. (See Chapter 98 in *Nelson Textbook of Pediatrics,* 16th ed.)

36. **C.** The pattern on first presentation with hemologic jaundice, reticulocytosis, mild anemia (for a term infant), and a hemolytic smear plus the family history of anemia and jaundice helps provide clues to the diagnosis. The patient (and

family) has the autosomal dominant form of hereditary spherocytosis. Once the liver matures and can conjugate and excrete the bilirubin load from hemolysis, the hemolytic disease nonetheless continues. By the way, the same late-onset anemia may also be seen with Coombs-positive hemolytic anemia due to ABO blood group incompatibility. Therefore, always check serial hematocrits after discharge if hemolysis is suspected. (See Chapter 98 in *Nelson Textbook of Pediatrics,* 16th ed.)

37. **E.** Anemia due to fetal to maternal transfusion probably lowers the risk of jaundice due to decreased bilirubin production. (See Chapter 98 in *Nelson Textbook of Pediatrics,* 16th ed.)

38. **E.** Gilbert disease is due to polymorphisms of the bilirubin UDP glucuronyl transferase enzyme and manifests only as indirect hyperbilirubinemia. (See Chapter 98 in *Nelson Textbook of Pediatrics,* 16th ed.)

39. **A.** Physiologic jaundice never lasts this long. As noted by the remaining possible causes of prolonged or recurrent jaundice, many pose significant medical risks for the infant. Breast milk jaundice, although usually benign, has also been associated with kernicterus. (See Chapter 98 in *Nelson Textbook of Pediatrics,* 16th ed.)

40. **C.** Hypoglycemia is a potential early complication of erythroblastosis fetalis and is thought to be due to pancreatic islet cell hyperplasia. Graft-vs.-host disease is eliminated when using irradiated blood for intrauterine and neonatal exchange transfusions. Portal vein thrombosis is due to the use of umbilical venous catheters with the very late (years) development of portal hypertension. (See Chapter 99 in *Nelson Textbook of Pediatrics,* 16th ed.)

41. **A.** A higher than normal hematocrit is not always associated with hyperviscosity. Hematocrits > 65% may not produce hyperviscosity, whereas those < 65% may be hyperviscous. (See Chapter 99 in *Nelson Textbook of Pediatrics,* 16th ed.)

42. 1. **D**
    2. **E**
    3. **A**

4. **B**
5. **C**
(See Chapter 99 in *Nelson Textbook of Pediatrics*, 16th ed.)
43. **C.** IUGR occurs only with severe maternal vascular disease such as nephropathy or retinopathy. A class B diabetic mother with poor diabetic control would have a macrosomic (LGA) infant. (See Chapter 103 in *Nelson Textbook of Pediatrics*, 16th ed.)
44. **C.** All the others, as well as the new category of familial hyperinsulinemic hypoglycemias (nesidioblastosis is one form), are causes of hyperinsulinemic hypoglycemia. (See Chapter 103 in *Nelson Textbook of Pediatrics*, 16th ed.)
45. **D.** Total parenteral nutrition (not supplemented with trace minerals) and chronic diarrhea may produce a zinc deficiency state due to reduced intake and increased loss, respectively. Because alkaline phosphatase is a zinc-containing enzyme, its levels will be reduced. The clinical picture is similar to acrodermatitis enteropathica. (See Chapter 98 in *Nelson Textbook of Pediatrics*, 16th ed.)
46. **D.** Infants of diabetic mothers often experience hypocalcemia within 24–48 hours after birth due, in part, to an attenuated parathyroid gland response to reduced calcium levels. The IDM also develops hypomagnesemia which, if uncorrected, results in persistent hypocalcemia due to the dependency of parathyroid function on magnesium. (See Chapter 102 in *Nelson Textbook of Pediatrics*, 16th ed.)

12 *Special Health Problems During Adolescence*

1. **D.** Oral contraceptive agents in the available doses contain too little estrogen to close growth plates. In addition, most females use oral contraceptive agents after the adolescent growth spurt. Other complications of oral contraceptives are quite rare in adolescent patients, and thrombophlebitis or diabetes is very unusual. (See Chapter 117 in *Nelson Textbook of Pediatrics*, 16th ed.)
2. **F.** All of the conditions listed in the question produce a false-positive result in the VDRL or other nontreponemal test for syphilis. This patient actually had systemic lupus erythematosus (SLE). (See Chapter 119 in *Nelson Textbook of Pediatrics*, 16th ed.)
3. **D.** Bacterial vaginosis due to *G. vaginalis* or other pathogens typically is associated with these biochemical and microscopic features. Treatment in nonpregnant women is metronidazole. (See Chapter 119 in *Nelson Textbook of Pediatrics*, 16th ed.)
4. **D.** Narcan is indicated in this patient with intravenous drug misuse and a heroin overdose. Nonetheless, the patient will need the ABCs of resuscitation addressed if he is cyanotic, and so forth. Securing an airway while providing oxygen and artificial ventilation is the first priority—followed by Narcan, the antidote for opiates. (See Chapter 113 in *Nelson Textbook of Pediatrics*, 16th ed.)
5. **F.** Both acute and chronic effects of organic solvent misuse produce significant morbidity and mortality. (See Chapter 113 in *Nelson Textbook of Pediatrics*, 16th ed.)
6. **A.** School performance usually deteriorates as a result of mood changes and aggressive behavior. (See Chapter 113 in *Nelson Textbook of Pediatrics*, 16th ed.)
7. 1. **C**
   2. **D**
   3. **B**
   4. **A**
   5. **A**
   6. **B**
   7. **A**
   8. **C**
   9. **A**
   10. **A**
   11. **D**
   12. **C**
   (See Chapter 112 in *Nelson Textbook of Pediatrics*, 16th ed.)
8. **B.** Such severe wasting is compatible with anorexia nervosa. Bulimia does not produce such severe weight loss. Additional features of anorexia nervosa include bradycardia, hypothermia, amenorrhea, and hypokalemia. (See

Chapter 112 in *Nelson Textbook of Pediatrics,* 16th ed.)

9. **D.** Anemia is rare in adolescent males and common in females. Nonetheless, hospitalization is usually not warranted. (See Chapter 107 in *Nelson Textbook of Pediatrics,* 16th ed.)

10. **A. B → E** are all correct. (See Chapter 107 in *Nelson Textbook of Pediatrics,* 16th ed.)

11. **A.** Learning problems most likely were identified earlier than adolescence and are not part of the AAP guidelines. They are part of the AMA's annual screening, however. (See Chapter 108 in *Nelson Textbook of Pediatrics,* 16th ed.)

12. **B.** Late-maturing boys are at moderate risk. Low-risk categories are older age, stable relationships, and regular contraceptive use. (See Chapter 108 in *Nelson Textbook of Pediatrics,* 16th ed.)

13. **D.** Children who are less than 18 years old but who are no longer subject to parental control (married, military, economic self-sufficiency) are considered emancipated. (See Chapter 108 in *Nelson Textbook of Pediatrics,* 16th ed.)

14. **D.** Sexual activity is an absolute indication for a Pap smear. Two successive cervical scrapings increase the yield and avoid false-negative results. (See Chapter 108.2 in *Nelson Textbook of Pediatrics,* 16th ed.)

15. **B.** Depression is probably under-reported in the teenager. (See Chapter 109 in *Nelson Textbook of Pediatrics,* 16th ed.)

16. **C. A, B, D → F** are important considerations in the differential diagnosis. (See Chapter 109 in *Nelson Textbook of Pediatrics,* 16th ed.)

17. **B.** Depression requires a comprehensive treatment plan. Untreated, it may last 7–9 months; most patients become depressed again in the next 7 years. (See Chapter 109 in *Nelson Textbook of Pediatrics,* 16th ed.)

18. **D.** Males are more likely to complete suicide, whereas females are more likely to attempt suicide. (See Chapter 110 in *Nelson Textbook of Pediatrics,* 16th ed.)

19. **C.** Ideation is relatively common, but more serious cofactors such as an adverse event (breaking up with a loved one,

family discord) and a specific plan raise the level of concern. (See Chapter 110 in *Nelson Textbook of Pediatrics,* 16th ed.)

20. 1. **B**
    2. **C**
    3. **A**
    4. **A**
    5. **F**
    (See Chapter 111 in *Nelson Textbook of Pediatrics,* 16th ed.)

21. **A.** These are consequences of weight loss; others include postural hypotension, bone marrow hypoplasia, constipation, and dry lanugo-like skin. (See Chapter 112 in *Nelson Textbook of Pediatrics,* 16th ed.)

22. **A. B → E** are diagnostic of bulimia. (See Chapter 112 in *Nelson Textbook of Pediatrics,* 16th ed.)

23. 1. **B**
    2. **C**
    3. **A**
    4. **D**
    (See Chapter 113 in *Nelson Textbook of Pediatrics,* 16th ed.)

24. 1. **D**
    2. **A**
    3. **E**
    4. **B**
    5. **C**
    (See Chapter 113 in *Nelson Textbook of Pediatrics,* 16th ed.)

25. **A.** Athletes of both sexes use anabolic steroids to enhance athletic performance. This student was on the wrestling team and, like over 500,000 high school students, had used anabolic steroids. (See Chapter 113.9 in *Nelson Textbook of Pediatrics,* 16th ed.)

26. **B.** The patient had a prolactin-secreting pituitary adenoma detected by a CT scan. Other potential causes of galactorrhea include oral contraceptive pills, some antihypertensive medications, and some tranquilizers. (See Chapter 115 in *Nelson Textbook of Pediatrics,* 16th ed.)

27. **E.** All the rest plus at least a dozen other drugs may produce gynecomastia in males. (See Chapter 115 in *Nelson Textbook of Pediatrics,* 16th ed.)

28. 1. **E**
    2. **A**
    3. **D**

4. **C**
5. **B**
(See Chapter 116 in *Nelson Textbook of Pediatrics,* 16th ed.)
29. **A.** The patient has hypergonadotropic hypogonadism—primary ovarian failure. Her phenotype is compatible with Turner syndrome (45,X). (See Chapter 116 in *Nelson Textbook of Pediatrics,* 16th ed.)
30. **C.** The hematocrit is 27% (MCV 65), and her tachycardia responds to the administration of 1 L of normal saline (intravenous). (See Chapter 116.2 in *Nelson Textbook of Pediatrics,* 16th ed.)
31. **C.** Dysfunctional uterine bleeding occurs after anovulatory cycles and is due to lack of estrogen build-up of the endometrium. Some women also have von Willebrand disease. (See Chapter 116.2 in *Nelson Textbook of Pediatrics,* 16th ed.)
32. **A.** Estrogens such as Premarin or as part of a combination oral contraceptive pill are the treatment of choice. Don't forget to treat the iron-deficiency anemia with iron. (See Chapter 116.3 in *Nelson Textbook of Pediatrics,* 16th ed.)
33. **E.** A → D are correct, but fortunately quite rare, events and are even rarer in nonsmokers. (See Chapter 117 in *Nelson Textbook of Pediatrics,* 16th ed.)
34. **D.** The goal is at least 200 μg of ethinyl estradiol and 2 mg of norgestrel given twice 12 hours apart. Don't forget to provide advice about proper nonemergency contraception too. (See Chapter 117 in *Nelson Textbook of Pediatrics,* 16th ed.)
35. 1. **B**
    2. **C**
    3. **B**
    4. **A**
    5. **C**
    6. **D**
    7. **E**
    (See Chapter 119 in *Nelson Textbook of Pediatrics,* 16th ed.)
36. **D.** Norplant is a reasonable choice, but many adolescents have trouble with its side effects (weight gain, irregular periods) and often ask to have it removed. (See Chapter 117 in *Nelson Textbook of Pediatrics,* 16th ed.)

13 *The Immunologic System and Disorders*

1. **E.** Because of chronic or recurrent infections, most patients with CGD demonstrate hypergammaglobulinemia. (See Chapter 130.5 in *Nelson Textbook of Pediatrics,* 16th ed.)
2. **B.** Nitroblue tetrazolium (NBT) tests the neutrophils' ability to generate superoxide anion and thus kill ingested bacteria. (See Chapter 130.5 in *Nelson Textbook of Pediatrics,* 16th ed.)
3. **C.** CGD in the patient described in the question is X-linked (seen in 50–55%) and is associated with an absence of cytochrome b. NBT testing reveals failure to generate intracellular superoxide anion. (See Chapter 130.5 in *Nelson Textbook of Pediatrics,* 16th ed.)
4. **B.** Interferon-γ increases superoxide anion generation in vitro and reduces the incidence of new infections. Long-term use of trimethoprim-sulfamethoxazole may also be effective in reducing infections. (See Chapter 130.5 in *Nelson Textbook of Pediatrics,* 16th ed.)
5. **D.** Transient, benign neutropenia associated with various non–life-threatening viral infections is the most common cause of neutropenia in previously healthy children. Neonatal neutropenia due to alloimmune, autoimmune, or preeclamptic processes is often asymptomatic and transient. (See Chapter 131 in *Nelson Textbook of Pediatrics,* 16th ed.)
6. 1. **C**
   2. **A**
   3. **B**
   4. **E**
   5. **D**
   (See Chapter 134 in *Nelson Textbook of Pediatrics,* 16th ed.)
7. **E.** Because T-lymphocyte deficiency is present at birth, most patients with complete (severe) disease manifest serious infections before the age of 1 year. It should be noted that many patients have partial or incomplete DiGeorge syndrome and that these patients may have sufficient lymphocyte activity to avoid serious infections. (See Chapter 125 in *Nelson Textbook of Pediatrics,* 16th ed.)

8. 1. **B**
   2. **C**
   3. **E**
   4. **A**
   5. **F**
   6. **G**
   7. **D**
   8. **J**
   9. **I**
   10. **H**
   (See Chapter 122 in *Nelson Textbook of Pediatrics,* 16th ed.)

9. **D.** This infant has the clinical picture of sepsis plus persistence of the umbilical cord, extreme leukocytosis, and a family history of early childhood death. This pattern is consistent with a leukocyte adhesion deficiency. Absence of this molecule predisposes to sepsis and delayed neutrophil-induced separation of the umbilical cord. (See Chapter 122 in *Nelson Textbook of Pediatrics,* 16th ed.)

10. **D.** Immune evaluations should be initiated for children with unusual, chronic, or recurrent infections, such as two or more systemic bacterial infections, or infections at unusual sites or with unusual organisms. (See Chapter 122 in *Nelson Textbook of Pediatrics,* 16th ed.)

11. **E.** The nitroblue tetrazolium test is useful to exclude chronic granulomatous disease but is generally not part of the initial immunologic evaluation unless there is a family history of recurrent staphylococcal infections in males. The CBC, platelet count, and immunoglobulins are cost-effective screening tests. (See Chapter 122 in *Nelson Textbook of Pediatrics,* 16th ed.)

12. **D.** The *Candida* skin test is a cost-effective test of T-cell function. The absolute lymphocyte count and flow cytometry measure T-cell numbers and subsets but not function. (See Chapter 122 in *Nelson Textbook of Pediatrics,* 16th ed.)

13. **E.** X-linked agammaglobulinemia (XLA or Bruton agammaglobulinemia) is suggested by low concentrations of all Ig classes. These patients are also unable to respond to immunizations, unlike infants with transient agammaglobulinemia of infancy. (See Chapter 124.1 in *Nelson Textbook of Pediatrics,* 16th ed.)

14. **B.** Selective IgA deficiency is the most common well-defined immunodeficiency disorder, with a frequency of 1 in 333 persons. Most affected persons are healthy, but this is occasionally associated with illness. (See Chapter 124.3 in *Nelson Textbook of Pediatrics,* 16th ed.)

15. **A.** The genetic defect for X-linked lymphoproliferative (XLP) syndrome also predisposes to severe primary EBV infection, which is associated with 80% mortality in these patients. (See Chapter 124.7 in *Nelson Textbook of Pediatrics,* 16th ed.)

16. **D.** In persons with DiGeorge syndrome, the absolute lymphocyte count is usually only moderately low for age. Lymphocyte responses to mitogen stimulation are absent, reduced, or normal, depending on the degree of thymic deficiency. (See Chapter 125.1 in *Nelson Textbook of Pediatrics,* 16th ed.)

17. **D.** The combination of atopic dermatitis, thrombocytopenic purpura, and susceptibility to infection in males is the classic presentation of Wiskott-Aldrich syndrome. Leukopenia is not a feature. (See Chapter 126.11 in *Nelson Textbook of Pediatrics,* 16th ed.)

18. **E.** The hyper-IgE syndrome is inherited as an autosomal dominant trait with variable expressivity that is associated with recurrent pneumonias and pneumatoceles. Abnormalities in dentition, bones, and connective tissue are common. (See Chapter 126.14 in *Nelson Textbook of Pediatrics,* 16th ed.)

19. **D.** Neutrophils and monocytes share primary functions, including the ability to ingest organisms. Neutrophils persist for 6 hours in the circulation. Monocytes persist for 26–104 hours in the circulation and can persist in tissues as macrophages for months. (See Chapters 127 and 128 in *Nelson Textbook of Pediatrics,* 16th ed.)

20. **D.** Eosinophilia is associated with tissue-invasive helminthic parasites but not parasitic infections that are solely intraluminal such as giardiasis (*Giardia lamblia*) or pinworms (*Enterobius vermicularis*). (See Chapter 129 in *Nelson Textbook of Pediatrics,* 16th ed.)

21. **C.** Chronic granulomatous disease is

characterized by the ability of neutrophils and monocytes to ingest but not kill catalase-positive organisms. (See Chapter 130.5 in *Nelson Textbook of Pediatrics*, 16th ed.)

22. **D.** Children with phagocyte dysfunction may have a history of delayed separation of the umbilical cord, frequently also associated with infection of the cord stump. (See Chapter 130 in *Nelson Textbook of Pediatrics*, 16th ed.)

23. **B.** Schwachman-Diamond syndrome is an autosomal recessive disorder characterized by digestive abnormalities and leukopenia. (See Chapter 131 in *Nelson Textbook of Pediatrics*, 16th ed.)

24. **A.** Persons with leukocyte adhesion deficiency have impaired transendothelial migration. The circulating neutrophil count with infection is typically above 30,000/mm³ and can surpass 100,000/mm³, with a paucity of neutrophils in the infected tissues. (See Chapter 131 in *Nelson Textbook of Pediatrics*, 16th ed.)

25. **E.** Congenital deficiency of the terminal components of complement (especially C5, C6, C7, or C8) have been associated with repeated meningococcal and extragenital gonococcal infections. (See Chapter 134.2 in *Nelson Textbook of Pediatrics*, 16th ed.)

26. **D.** Although severe life-threatening sepsis may occur, it is extremely rare in patients with cyclic neutropenia. (See Chapter 131 in *Nelson Textbook of Pediatrics*, 16th ed.)

27. **C.** Kostmann disease, an autosomal recessive severe infantile form of agranulocytosis, manifests with persistently low absolute neutrophil counts (<200) and severe recurrent and at times lethal (by age 3 years) infection. (See Chapter 131 in *Nelson Textbook of Pediatrics*, 16th ed.)

28. **D.** Granulocyte colony-stimulating factor (G-CSF) is the treatment of choice and has dramatically improved the neutrophil count while reducing the incidence and severity of infection. (See Chapter 131 in *Nelson Textbook of Pediatrics*, 16th ed.)

29. **D.** AIDS has not been reported as a complication of the use of intravenous immunoglobulin (IVIG) prepared from human donors. Donors are screened for human immunodeficiency virus and hepatitis B seropositivity, and preparative methods would inactivate both of these viruses. The remaining choices are rare but reported complications of IVIG therapy. Nonetheless, IVIG has been a remarkable aid in the treatment of patients with congenital antibody deficiency states. (See Chapter 124 in *Nelson Textbook of Pediatrics*, 16th ed.)

14 *Allergic Disorders*

1. **A.** Although allergens have been implicated in the etiology of eczema, the precise role of allergen or of IgE is unknown. (See Chapter 146 in *Nelson Textbook of Pediatrics*, 16th ed.)

2. 1. **B**
   2. **A**
   3. **B**
   4. **B**
   5. **A**
   6. **A**
   7. **A**
   8. **C**
   9. **D**
   (See Chapter 146 in *Nelson Textbook of Pediatrics*, 16th ed.)

3. **A.** Epinephrine is the treatment of choice. It may be given subcutaneously, but intramuscularly is an ideal route. If the blood pressure does not respond, lactated Ringer's solution should be given. Benadryl, cimetidine, and prednisone are second-line therapies to be given after epinephrine and fluids. (See Chapter 148 in *Nelson Textbook of Pediatrics*, 16th ed.)

4. **D.** Anaphylaxis to penicillin usually occurs within 30–90 minutes of administration of this drug. Anaphylactic shock is often missed as a diagnosis unless there is a high index of suspicion *and* a complete history is taken. (See Chapter 148 in *Nelson Textbook of Pediatrics*, 16th ed.)

5. **A.** *Giardia* is not an "invasive" parasite and thus does not elicit eosinophilia. Allergic eosinophilia usually involves no greater than 15–20% of the leukocytes on peripheral smear. Higher levels suggest rheumatic, oncologic, parasitic, or toxic

causes. (See Chapter 141 in *Nelson Textbook of Pediatrics,* 16th ed.)

6. **D.** Smoking cigarettes or marijuana and eating charcoal-cooked meats, in addition to various drugs (rifampin, anticonvulsants) and diseases (hyperthyroidism, cystic fibrosis), increase theophylline clearance and thus decrease serum levels of theophylline. (See Chapter 143 in *Nelson Textbook of Pediatrics,* 16th ed.)

7. **E.** Allergic rhinitis is often seasonal and associated with allergic conjunctivitis. Eosinophils predominate in the nasal secretions. (See Chapter 144 in *Nelson Textbook of Pediatrics,* 16th ed.)

8. **A.** Sinusitis is a possible complication of allergic rhinitis. A change in the nature of the nasal discharge, facial pain, and fever may all herald the onset of sinusitis. (See Chapter 144 in *Nelson Textbook of Pediatrics,* 16th ed.)

9. **B.** Local reactions to Hymenoptera venom in children are not managed by immunotherapy. (See Chapter 151 in *Nelson Textbook of Pediatrics,* 16th ed.)

10. **A.** Immunotherapy in children is indicated only for systemic reactions. (See Chapter 151 in *Nelson Textbook of Pediatrics,* 16th ed.)

11. **B.** The urticarial reaction described in the question may develop into anaphylaxis; the latter requires emergency treatment. In addition, the penicillin should be stopped and a substitute nonpenicillin antibiotic chosen. (See Chapter 148 in *Nelson Textbook of Pediatrics,* 16th ed.)

12. **C.** The erythromycin component of Pediazole inhibits hepatic theophylline metabolism, thus potentially producing theophylline toxicity. (See Chapter 143 in *Nelson Textbook of Pediatrics,* 16th ed.)

13. **B.** Type II hypersensitivity (cytotoxic reaction) is characterized by antigen-antibody interaction on the cell surface, similar to type I hypersensitivity, but also includes the activation of complement with destruction of the involved cell. There is no type V hypersensitivity. (See Chapter 141 in *Nelson Textbook of Pediatrics,* 16th ed.)

14. **C.** Mast cells release histamine and eosinophil chemotactic factor. Other factors that participate in immediate-type hypersensitivity that are not derived from mast cells include eosinophil major basic protein and peroxidase, bradykinin, platelet-activating factor, and serotonin. (See Chapter 141 in *Nelson Textbook of Pediatrics,* 16th ed.)

15. **A.** Dennie lines (Dennie-Morgan folds) are wrinkles below the lower eyelids. Like allergic shiners and the allergic salute, they are signs of persistent rhinorrhea associated with allergic rhinitis. A "silent chest" in a patient with asthma (answer **E**) is a severe sign suggesting inspiratory and expiratory obstruction. Cyanosis is always present in such severe cases. (See Chapter 142 in *Nelson Textbook of Pediatrics,* 16th ed.)

16. **D.** The RAST (radioallergosorbent test) determines the serum IgE concentrations against specific antigens. The RAST correlates well with medical history and allergy skin testing but is somewhat less sensitive than skin testing. (See Chapter 142 in *Nelson Textbook of Pediatrics,* 16th ed.)

17. **C.** Positive skin test results obtained by the puncture technique correlate better than the more sensitive intradermal tests with measurements of specific IgE antibody and with the appearance of clinical symptoms on exposure to the allergen. (See Chapter 142 in *Nelson Textbook of Pediatrics,* 16th ed.)

18. **B.** Because skin tests are more sensitive than RAST, they are more reliable than RAST in confirming risk of life-threatening anaphylactic conditions. All the other responses are incorrect. (See Chapter 142 in *Nelson Textbook of Pediatrics,* 16th ed.)

19. **D.** Household humidity should be kept at < 50% to inhibit survival of mites. Use of vaporizers should be avoided. Dehumidifiers may be necessary in damp basements. Clothes and bedding should be washed in hot water to kill dust mites. Noncarpeted flooring is recommended. (See Chapter 143 in *Nelson Textbook of Pediatrics,* 16th ed.)

20. **E.** Agents with greater β_2-selective activity provide effective bronchodilation with less of the increase in heart rate

than may occur with agents with $\beta_1 + \beta_2$ activity. (See Chapter 143.1 in *Nelson Textbook of Pediatrics,* 16th ed.)

21. **E.** There is little reason to choose one antihistamine over another except for avoidance of adverse effects, such as sedation, impairment of function, and cost. The chemical classification of antihistamines (type 1 to type VI) does not have functional significance. Second-generation antihistamines have fewer sedative adverse effects. (See Chapter 143.1 in *Nelson Textbook of Pediatrics,* 16th ed.)

22. **E.** Cromolyn prevents bronchoconstriction caused by immunologic as well as nonimmunologic stimuli (e.g., frigid air, exercise). It has no bronchodilator properties and is useful only if given prophylactically. (See Chapter 143.1 in *Nelson Textbook of Pediatrics,* 16th ed.)

23. **C.** Topical nasal corticosteroids (beclomethasone, budesonide, flunisolide, or mometasone) should be used in children with allergic rhinitis that is resistant to antihistamine-decongestant therapy. (See Chapter 144 in *Nelson Textbook of Pediatrics,* 16th ed.)

24. **D.** For mild intermittent symptoms of asthma, recommended treatment is with a short-acting inhaled β_2-agonist as needed for symptoms. The intensity of treatment depends on the severity of exacerbations. The need for short-acting inhaled β_2-agonist use more than two times a week may indicate the need to initiate long-term-control therapy. (See Chapter 145 in *Nelson Textbook of Pediatrics,* 16th ed.)

25. **D.** For moderate persistent symptoms of asthma, recommended treatment is with a daily-inhaled corticosteroid and a long-acting inhaled β_2-agonist. Alternatives to the β_2-agonist are sustained-release theophylline or a long-acting β_2 agonist in tablet form. In addition, for moderate persistent symptoms of asthma, a short-acting β_2-agonist is also used as needed for quick relief of symptoms. (See Chapter 145 in *Nelson Textbook of Pediatrics,* 16th ed.)

26. **C.** Angioedema is similar to urticaria but has deeper tissue involvement. Urticaria

and angioedema are not characteristic features of atopic dermatitis. (See Chapter 146 in *Nelson Textbook of Pediatrics,* 16th ed.)

27. **C.** To minimize atopic dermatitis, garments should be of smooth-textured cotton. Wool garments and carpeting should be avoided. (See Chapter 146 in *Nelson Textbook of Pediatrics,* 16th ed.)

28. **D.** With control of trigger factors and appropriate local treatment, reasonable but not complete resolution of symptoms is usually possible. Improvement in childhood atopic dermatitis usually occurs over a period of several years. (See Chapter 146 in *Nelson Textbook of Pediatrics,* 16th ed.)

29. **E.** No laboratory test confirms or excludes the diagnosis of urticaria. In the absence of any specific clues, elimination diets and skin testing are generally not helpful. A skin biopsy is indicated only if urticarial vasculitis is suspected. (See Chapter 147 in *Nelson Textbook of Pediatrics,* 16th ed.)

30. **E.** A nonsedating antihistamine is the preferred therapy of urticaria. This is especially important for school-age children to minimize the effect on learning and school performance. (See Chapter 147 in *Nelson Textbook of Pediatrics,* 16th ed.)

31. **C.** Food-dependent, exercise-induced anaphylaxis occurs during exercise within 2 hours of ingestion of the food to which the patient has specific IgE. Exercise-induced anaphylaxis may also occur after ingestion of aspirin or nonsteroidal anti-inflammatory drugs. Exercise is typically tolerated 3 hours or more after ingestion. (See Chapter 148 in *Nelson Textbook of Pediatrics,* 16th ed.)

32. **D.** The treatment of choice of anaphylaxis is aqueous epinephrine, 1:1,000, 0.01 mL/kg (maximum 0.3 mL for a child or 0.5 mL for an adult) by intramuscular injection, which can achieve more rapid effective concentrations than occurs by subcutaneous injection. Fluids may also be needed for hypotension. Intravenous epinephrine may be added as a continuous drip for persistent shock. (See

Chapter 148 in *Nelson Textbook of Pediatrics,* 16th ed.)

33. **D.** With anaphylaxis due to injection of allergen extract or to a Hymenoptera sting on an extremity, one half of the dose of epinephrine may be diluted in 2 mL of normal saline and infiltrated subcutaneously at the site of the sting to slow absorption. A tourniquet above the site can also slow systemic distribution. The tourniquet can be loosened after improvement or briefly at intervals of 3 minutes. (See Chapter 148 in *Nelson Textbook of Pediatrics,* 16th ed.)

34. **E.** Serum sickness is a classic example of a type III hypersensitivity reaction, or immune complex disease. The symptoms develop as antibodies appear against the antigen at a time when the antigen is still present. Immune complexes may stimulate complement and deposit in joints, the skin, and the renal glomeruli. (See Chapter 149 in *Nelson Textbook of Pediatrics,* 16th ed.)

35. **D.** Risk factors for adverse reactions to drugs include the dose of the drug, route of administration, and duration and frequency of administration. (See Chapter 150 in *Nelson Textbook of Pediatrics,* 16th ed.)

36. **E.** Clinical findings in inhalant allergy caused by insects are similar to those occurring with usual inhalant allergens (e.g., rhinitis, conjunctivitis, and asthma). Biting insects may cause local reactions that do not involve IgE. Venom from stinging insects causes IgE-mediated sensitivity that may lead to anaphylaxis. (See Chapter 151 in *Nelson Textbook of Pediatrics,* 16th ed.)

37. **E.** There are patients with convincing histories of sting anaphylaxis with negative skin test results and RAST results. (See Chapter 151 in *Nelson Textbook of Pediatrics,* 16th ed.)

38. **E.** Allergic conjunctivitis in the patient with hay fever generally responds well to topical application of sympathomimetics (naphazoline or phenylephrine) or lodoxamide tromethamine (a mast cell stabilizer) eye drops. Topical corticosteroids should be used in the eyes, with caution, for severe cases of allergic conjunctivitis. (See Chapter 152 in *Nelson Textbook of Pediatrics,* 16th ed.)

39. **B.** Rashes and diarrhea after ingestion of fruits and juices are common during the first 3 years of life. There is no evidence of an immunologic basis for these reactions. (See Chapter 153 in *Nelson Textbook of Pediatrics,* 16th ed.)

15 *Rheumatic Diseases of Childhood*

1. **E.** Cancel the operation until the patient described in the question is further examined and the results of the urinalysis are considered. (See Chapter 167.1 in *Nelson Textbook of Pediatrics,* 16th ed.)

2. **B.** Henoch-Schönlein purpura is a common form of vasculitis in childhood and manifests with involvement of the skin (nonthrombocytopenic petechiae), joints (arthritis), kidneys (nephritis), and intestine (vasculitis, mucosal hemorrhage, intussusception). (See Chapter 167.1 in *Nelson Textbook of Pediatrics,* 16th ed.)

3. **D.** An echocardiogram reveals a moderate-sized pericardial effusion, the most probable cause of this boy's chest pain. An ESR is not diagnostic and occasionally shows low values in serious inflammatory, infectious, or oncologic diseases. A chest radiograph may reveal cardiomegaly due to pericardial effusion; nonetheless, an x-ray does not distinguish cardiomegaly from heart failure or effusion. A bone marrow aspirate may be of value if leukemia is a consideration. (See Chapter 156 in *Nelson Textbook of Pediatrics,* 16th ed.)

4. **D.** An oral anti-inflammatory agent or steroids would improve this boy's pericardial effusion. (See Chapter 156 in *Nelson Textbook of Pediatrics,* 16th ed.)

5. **A.** Systemic-onset JRA often manifests with prolonged fevers, a salmon-pink macular rash, asymptomatic pericarditis, leukocytosis, anemia of chronic inflammatory disease, hepatosplenomegaly, and lymphadenopathy. Arthralgia or myalgia may be present, but arthritis does not usually develop until later in the course of the illness. SLE and rheumatic fever may also produce rheumatologic symptoms

and pericardial effusion. (See Chapter 156 in *Nelson Textbook of Pediatrics*, 16th ed.)

6. 1. **C**
    2. **A**
    3. **B**
    4. **E**
    5. **D**

    (See Chapter 156 in *Nelson Textbook of Pediatrics*, 16th ed.)

7. **B.** CPK is 7500 IU/mL. (See Chapter 160 in *Nelson Textbook of Pediatrics*, 16th ed.)

8. **B.** Dermatomyositis classically affects preadolescent females with an insidious onset of muscle weakness. Vasculitic rashes may be present over knuckles, the malar area, or the eyelids (violet tinged). (See Chapter 160 in *Nelson Textbook of Pediatrics*, 16th ed.)

9. 1. **D**
    2. **E**
    3. **A**
    4. **B**
    5. **F**
    6. **C**
    7. **G**

    (See Chapter 154 in *Nelson Textbook of Pediatrics*, 16th ed.)

10. **B.** Erythema nodosum in itself is not a disease but is associated with other primary inflammatory or infectious disorders. (See Chapter 154 in *Nelson Textbook of Pediatrics*, 16th ed.)

11. **E.** A positive ANA is a nonspecific sign of increased lymphocyte activity and is noted in many infections (EBV) and inflammatory states (IBD, SLE, JRA, ITP). (See Chapter 154 in *Nelson Textbook of Pediatrics*, 16th ed.)

12. **A.** Nephrotic syndrome has normal levels of complement. Immune complex–mediated diseases reduce total hemolytic complement levels. (See Chapter 154 in *Nelson Textbook of Pediatrics*, 16th ed.)

13. **B.** Naproxen, more than other NSAIDs, can produce this skin lesion characterized by small hypopigmented flat scars after a blister formation. (See Chapter 155 in *Nelson Textbook of Pediatrics*, 16th ed.)

14. 1. **D**
    2. **B**
    3. **A**
    4. **C**
    5. **E**

(See Chapter 155 in *Nelson Textbook of Pediatrics*, 16th ed.)

15. 1. **B**
    2. **D**
    3. **A**
    4. **B**
    5. **C**
    6. **C**
    7. **E**
    8. **E**

    (See Chapter 156 in *Nelson Textbook of Pediatrics*, 16th ed.)

16. **D.** The ESR may be normal in patients with active JRA. The CRP may be elevated as well as the platelet count. Nonetheless, the ESR is not always elevated. (See Chapter 156 in *Nelson Textbook of Pediatrics*, 16th ed.)

17. **A.** All the others are associated with axial arthritis and nearly universally with HLA-B27. (See Chapter 157 in *Nelson Textbook of Pediatrics*, 16th ed.)

18. **E.** Agents may produce arthritis by immune complex deposition, cross-reactivity to shared antigenic epitopes between the synovium and the agent, or direct infection. (See Chapter 158 in *Nelson Textbook of Pediatrics*, 16th ed.)

19. **D.** Diagnosis of SLE requires 4 or more of the 11 criteria outlined in Table 159–4 of *Nelson's Textbook of Pediatrics*. (See Chapter 159 in *Nelson Textbook of Pediatrics*, 16th ed.)

20. **E.** SLE is defined by arthritis, mouth ulcers, photosensitivity, thrombocytopenia, hemolytic anemia, and hematuria. All manifestations need not be present at the same time. (See Chapter 159 in *Nelson Textbook of Pediatrics*, 16th ed.)

21. **D.** Prednisone is the treatment of choice for SLE exacerbations. (See Chapter 159 in *Nelson Textbook of Pediatrics*, 16th ed.)

22. **C.** In general, complement levels reflect the activity of the disease and return to normal levels when symptoms are in remission. Familial and thus congenital deficiency of complement components predisposes to the development of SLE in some, but not in all, family members. (See Chapter 159 in *Nelson Textbook of Pediatrics*, 16th ed.)

23. **B.** The CPK is 2000, approximately 40 times normal. An ANA is positive but is

not diagnostic. (See Chapter 160 in *Nelson Textbook of Pediatrics,* 16th ed.)

24. **A.** Striated muscle weakness of the oropharynx produces dysphagia and possible airway compromise. (See Chapter 160 in *Nelson Textbook of Pediatrics,* 16th ed.)

25. **C.** Dermatomyositis, an autoimmune inflammatory disease, is characterized by involvement of skeletal muscle and at times the cardiac muscle. Treatment with prednisone is usually efficacious. (See Chapter 160 in *Nelson Textbook of Pediatrics,* 16th ed.)

26. **C.** Although outbreaks are common, it is uncommon to catch Kawasaki disease from an affected patient. (See Chapter 166 in *Nelson Textbook of Pediatrics,* 16th ed.)

27. **B.** Splenic rupture has not been reported, nor has splenomegaly. (See Chapter 166 in *Nelson Textbook of Pediatrics,* 16th ed.)

28. **D.** In the early stage of disease, before aneurysm of the coronary arteries occurs, severe myocarditis may produce cardiogenic shock. (See Chapter 166 in *Nelson Textbook of Pediatrics,* 16th ed.)

29. **A.** The marked skeletal muscle involvement should make this too obvious. (See Chapter 166 in *Nelson Textbook of Pediatrics,* 16th ed.)

30. **C.** HSP is a common vasculitis among children and presents with the classic findings of abdominal pain with or without rectal bleeding, vasculitic rash, arthritis, and nephritis. The platelet count is normal, and the gastrointestinal involvement may progress to intussusception. (See Chapter 167 in *Nelson Textbook of Pediatrics,* 16th ed.)

31. **B.** This occurs most often in the other common childhood vasculitis—Kawasaki disease. (See Chapter 167.1 in *Nelson Textbook of Pediatrics,* 16th ed.)

32. **A.** End-stage renal disease is an uncommon sequela of HSP. Nonetheless, 1% of patients do have persistent renal abnormalities. (See Chapter 167.1 in *Nelson Textbook of Pediatrics,* 16th ed.)

33. 1. **E**
    2. **A**
    3. **B**
    4. **C**

5. **D**
   (See Chapter 169 in *Nelson Textbook of Pediatrics,* 16th ed.)

34. **B.** Antineutrophil cytoplasmic antibodies that are directed to protease-3 (PR3) of the neutrophil alpha-granule is the appropriate test and is markedly positive. (See Chapter 167.4 in *Nelson Textbook of Pediatrics,* 16th ed.)

35. **C.** This vascular pulmonary renal syndrome is not that rare and fortunately responds to therapy. (See Chapter 167.4 in *Nelson Textbook of Pediatrics,* 16th ed.)

36. **C and D** have both been valuable in improving the outcome. (See Chapter 167.4 in *Nelson Textbook of Pediatrics,* 16th ed.)

37. **D.** Nonsteroidal anti-inflammatory agents would be the appropriate medication for the patient with a Reiter-like syndrome after *Chlamydia* urethritis as described in the question. (See Chapter 119 in *Nelson Textbook of Pediatrics,* 16th ed.)

38. **E.** Polyarthritis with rheumatoid factor seropositivity, female sex, older age, hand/wrist joint involvement, erosions, nodules, and unremitting course are all associated with poor prognosis for JRA. (See Chapter 156 in *Nelson Textbook of Pediatrics,* 16th ed.)

39. **E.** Reactive arthritis may follow enteric infection (*Shigella, Salmonella, Yersinia enterocolitica, Campylobacter jejuni*) or genitourinary tract infection with *Chlamydia trachomatis.* (See Chapter 158 in *Nelson Textbook of Pediatrics,* 16th ed.)

40. **A.** Nonsteroidal anti-inflammatory drugs are the cornerstones of drug treatment of most rheumatic diseases in children. They are the only drugs needed for at least half of patients, and they provide significant relief for many of the remaining patients. (See Chapter 155 in *Nelson Textbook of Pediatrics,* 16th ed.)

41. **B.** The diagnosis for SLE is confirmed by the combination of 4 of 11 criteria, including neurologic disorders such as seizures and psychosis in the absence of other identified causes. Leukopenia, malar rash, false-positive serologic results for syphilis, and nonerosive arthritis are also components of the diagnostic criteria.

(See Chapter 159 in *Nelson Textbook of Pediatrics,* 16th ed.)

42. **D.** The onset of familial Mediterranean fever is usually before 5 years of age and is characterized by brief, acute, self-limited episodes of fever and polyserositis recurring at irregular intervals. (See Chapter 164 in *Nelson Textbook of Pediatrics,* 16th ed.)

43. 1. **F**
    2. **E**
    3. **B**
    4. **A**
    5. **D**
    6. **C**

16 *Infectious Diseases*

1. **D.** *Ascaris* is not a known cause of daycare-associated diarrheal epidemics, but choices **A–C** are. (See Chapter 303 in *Nelson Textbook of Pediatrics,* 16th ed.)

2. **D.** HHV-6 is the agent of roseola (erythema subitum), the childhood exanthem present in the infant described in the question. (See Chapter 249 in *Nelson Textbook of Pediatrics,* 16th ed.)

3. **E.** Pertussis is a "family" disease with various degrees of symptoms and colonization. (See Chapter 195 in *Nelson Textbook of Pediatrics,* 16th ed.)

4. **E.** The child has herpetic gingivostomatitis; he has autoinoculated his (sucking) thumb and herpetic whitlow has developed. (See Chapter 245 in *Nelson Textbook of Pediatrics,* 16th ed.)

5. **C.** The CSF profile and temporal lobe lesion are highly suggestive of HSV encephalitis. (See Chapter 245 in *Nelson Textbook of Pediatrics,* 16th ed.)

6. **C.** The infant described in the question requires a complete course of therapy for neurosyphilis. (See Chapter 215 in *Nelson Textbook of Pediatrics,* 16th ed.)

7. **A.** *Nocardia* infection is characterized by remissions and exacerbations. (See Chapter 190 in *Nelson Textbook of Pediatrics,* 16th ed.)

8. **D.** Pelvic actinomycosis is an unusual complication of IUD use. (See Chapter 189 in *Nelson Textbook of Pediatrics,* 16th ed.)

9. **A.** A patient who has only been in an urban area and has not participated in agricultural activities, has never traveled to areas endemic for hydatid transmission (e.g., in North America, areas where there are moose), and has not had contact with sheep or dogs is unlikely to acquire echinococcal infection. The sensitivity of an echinococcal serologic study varies from 60% to 90%. Healthy hydatid cysts may not stimulate much of an immune response. The other choices mentioned are not relevant to cystic liver disease. (See Chapter 300 in *Nelson Textbook of Pediatrics,* 16th ed.)

10. **E.** Hypoglycemia and seizures suggest a poor outcome for cholera. (See Chapter 199 in *Nelson Textbook of Pediatrics,* 16th ed.)

11. **D.** Typhoid fever may or may not be associated with diarrhea or constipation and is a prolonged, serious illness. (See Chapter 196.2 in *Nelson Textbook of Pediatrics,* 16th ed.)

12. **E.** There is no indication for antimotility agents in children with acute gastroenteritis. (See Chapter 176 in *Nelson Textbook of Pediatrics,* 16th ed.)

13. **B.** Ileus, coma with a risk of aspiration, shock, and peritonitis (e.g., pneumoperitoneum) are contraindications to oral therapy. (See Chapter 176 in *Nelson Textbook of Pediatrics,* 16th ed.)

14. **D.** *C. jejuni* is a commonly associated pathogen in Guillain-Barré syndrome (autoimmune polyneuropathy). (See Chapter 200 in *Nelson Textbook of Pediatrics,* 16th ed.)

15. **C.** *E. coli* 0157:H7 is an enterhemorrhagic pathogen and is responsible for most episodes of hemolytic-uremic syndrome. *Shigella dysenteriae* is occasionally responsible for the hemolytic-uremic syndrome. (See Chapter 197 in *Nelson Textbook of Pediatrics,* 16th ed.)

16. **C.** *Shigella* usually causes diarrhea and fever and sometimes, particularly in young infants, seizures. (See Chapter 197 in *Nelson Textbook of Pediatrics,* 16th ed.)

17. **B.** Adenovirus 11 or 21 probably is the cause. (See Chapter 254 in *Nelson Textbook of Pediatrics,* 16th ed.)

18. **G.** Congenital toxoplasmosis is associated with organ dysfunction, inflammation, growth retardation, thrombocytopenia, hepatitis, retinitis, and microcephaly, but not with true congenital anomalies. (See Chapter 280 in *Nelson Textbook of Pediatrics,* 16th ed.)

19. **B.** Severe combined immunodeficiency (SCID), with its T-lymphocyte deficiency, predisposes to *P. carinii* pneumonia (PCP). (See Chapter 281 in *Nelson Textbook of Pediatrics,* 16th ed.)

20. **C.** Amoxicillin is the treatment of choice for this early lesion of erythema migrans. (See Chapter 219 in *Nelson Textbook of Pediatrics,* 16th ed.)

21. **B.** The risk of Lyme disease is very small, and observing the patient for the development of a rash is reasonable. Most patients with Lyme disease experience erythema migrans even if a tick bite is not remembered. (See Chapter 219 in *Nelson Textbook of Pediatrics,* 16th ed.)

22. **B.** *Sporothrix* infection can come from sources other than rose thorns. (See Chapter 238 in *Nelson Textbook of Pediatrics,* 16th ed.)

23. **E.** Hyperinflation due to air trapping is not always noted with allergic bronchopulmonary aspergillosis, nor is hilar lymphadenopathy. The inflammatory response does not necessarily produce either of these lesions. (See Chapter 233 in *Nelson Textbook of Pediatrics,* 16th ed.)

24. **B.** Dogs do not carry oocysts. The other sources listed in the question are compatible with transmission of toxoplasmosis. (See Chapter 280 in *Nelson Textbook of Pediatrics,* 16th ed.)

25. **A.** In addition to gonococcal disease, Fitz-Hugh-Curtis syndrome may also be due to *Chlamydia.* (See Chapter 192 in *Nelson Textbook of Pediatrics,* 16th ed.)

26. **C.** Even with disseminated disease (bacteremia, arthritis, meningitis), ceftriaxone is the drug of choice because of the high rate of penicillin resistance.

(See Chapter 192 in *Nelson Textbook of Pediatrics,* 16th ed.)

27. **E.** The thick smear of peripheral blood should be diagnostic, especially if repeated. Laboratory manuals help identify the morphologic forms needed to distinguish the different malarial species. (See Chapter 278 in *Nelson Textbook of Pediatrics,* 16th ed.)

28. **C.** Malaria is the first diagnosis to be considered in this patient, who had the unfavorable prognostic features of hypoglycemia and coma. (See Chapter 278 in *Nelson Textbook of Pediatrics,* 16th ed.)

29. **C.** Psittacosis, a bird-borne chlamydial disease, produces severe pneumonia with systemic manifestations similar to *Mycoplasma pneumoniae* or Legionnaire's disease. (See Chapter 224 in *Nelson Textbook of Pediatrics,* 16th ed.)

30. **C.** Culture is of poor value, but serologic studies are the diagnostic tests of choice in the patient described in Question 29. (See Chapter 224 in *Nelson Textbook of Pediatrics,* 16th ed.)

31. **D.** The oculoglandular (conjunctivitis, lymph node) syndrome is the most frequent atypical manifestation of cat-scratch disease. (See Chapter 207.2 in *Nelson Textbook of Pediatrics,* 16th ed.)

32. **C.** Fever occurs in only 30% of cases of cat-scratch disease. (See Chapter 207.2 in *Nelson Textbook of Pediatrics,* 16th ed.)

33. **C.** The lag phase after a cat scratch may be 3–30 days, with an average incubation of 7–12 days. (See Chapter 207.2 in *Nelson Textbook of Pediatrics,* 16th ed.)

34. **E.** *Listeria monocytogenes* may contaminate dairy products (milk, cheese) and may survive, replicate, and spread in a family's refrigerator. (See Chapter 188 in *Nelson Textbook of Pediatrics,* 16th ed.)

35. **A.** Many patients affected by *Y. pseudotuberculosis* do not have diarrhea, and thus a stool culture is not considered. If the involvement is mesenteric adenitis, the stool culture results may be negative. (See Chapter 201.2 in *Nelson Textbook of Pediatrics,* 16th ed.)

36. **E.** *Y. enterocolitica* infection most often develops from contaminated food (animals, milk, water), from animals (dogs), or from human-to-human contact. Transfusion-related disease remains a risk but is uncommon. (See Chapter 201.1 in *Nelson Textbook of Pediatrics,* 16th ed.)

37. **E.** Tularemia, an important zoonotic infection, is most often acquired from a tick bite or directly from rabbits. Flies, fleas, mosquitos, lice, and many animals (squirrels, beavers, birds) are additional vectors. (See Chapter 204 in *Nelson Textbook of Pediatrics,* 16th ed.)

38. **B.** Sensorineural hearing loss is a risk after asymptomatic congenital CMV infection. The incidence of neonatal CMV-positive urine is much greater than the incidence of symptomatic neonatal CMV inclusion disease (e.g., microencephaly, retinitis, being small for gestational age, petechiae). (See Chapter 248 in *Nelson Textbook of Pediatrics,* 16th ed.)

39. **C.** Parvovirus B19, the agent of fifth disease (erythema infectiosum), produces congenital infection of the fetal erythrocyte precursor cells, producing transient fetal anemia. If the anemia is severe, it produces nonimmune hydrops with the possibility of intrauterine fetal demise. Intrauterine (umbilical venous) blood transfusion is curative but poses risk. (See Chapter 244 in *Nelson Textbook of Pediatrics,* 16th ed.)

40. **D.** Treatment of HIV-positive mothers can dramatically reduce the incidence of HIV infection in infants. Treatment reduces the overall risk of infection from approximately 25–30% to 8%. Treatment begins any time after 14 weeks of gestation and continues during labor and delivery and for another 6 weeks (in the infants). (See Chapter 268 in *Nelson Textbook of Pediatrics,* 16th ed.)

41. **D.** Guillain-Barré syndrome, or autoimmune peripheral neuropathy, is symmetric and involves sensory but more so motor nerves. Polio is an anterior horn cell disease and is purely motor. (See Chapter 243.1 in *Nelson Textbook of Pediatrics,* 16th ed.)

42. 1. **D**
    2. **A**
    3. **B**
    4. **C**
    5. **E**
    (See Section 14 in *Nelson Textbook of Pediatrics,* 16th ed.)

43. **D.** *Schistosoma haematobium* is not endemic to the areas visited. It also does not affect the portal circulation, preferring the ureteral and bladder veins. (See Chapter 296 in *Nelson Textbook of Pediatrics,* 16th ed.)

44. **A.** The treatment of choice of symptomatic nontuberculous mycobacterial lymphadenitis is complete excision. Fine-needle aspiration may help with the diagnosis, but excisional biopsy is the cure. (See Chapter 214 in *Nelson Textbook of Pediatrics,* 16th ed.)

45. **B.** The live measles virus is contraindicated in patients with T-cell immunodeficiency because disseminated disease may occur. Nonetheless, it is recommended that HIV-infected patients be given this vaccine because measles itself is a serious illness once AIDS develops. (See Chapter 240 in *Nelson Textbook of Pediatrics,* 16th ed.)

46. **D.** These are current recommendations of the World Health Organization *and* the American Academy of Pediatrics for the treatment of diarrhea. (See Chapter 176 in *Nelson Textbook of Pediatrics,* 16th ed.)

47. **A.** A careful history and physical examination help direct the evaluation of FUO and avoid unnecessary, invasive, risky, or expensive testing. (See Chapter 172 in *Nelson Textbook of Pediatrics,* 16th ed.)

48. **C.** Vancomycin is the current treatment of choice for penicillin/cephalosporin-resistant pneumococci. (See Chapter 183 in *Nelson Textbook of Pediatrics,* 16th ed.)

49. **E.** Other than low-risk, febrile, and stable children, patients with any of the manifestations in choices **A–D** require inpatient management for presumed bacterial sepsis. The combination of splenic hypofunction and a deficiency of the properdin system of complement activation places patients with sickle cell

anemia at even greater risk for bacteremia from encapsulated organisms. (See Chapter 172 in *Nelson Textbook of Pediatrics,* 16th ed.)

50. **D.** Ancestry rarely predisposes to urinary tract infections, whereas choices **A, B, C,** and **E** all are significant risk factors. (See Chapter 172 in *Nelson Textbook of Pediatrics,* 16th ed.)

51. **B.** Human ehrlichiosis is a rickettsia-like multisystem illness, with or without a rash. It is endemic and probably is more common than reported. (See Chapter 228 in *Nelson Textbook of Pediatrics,* 16th ed.)

52. **A.** *S. aureus* is the most common cause of osteomyelitis in all age groups. Group A *Streptococcus* is next in frequency but causes < 10% of cases. Group B *Streptococcus* is common in neonates. *P. aeruginosa* osteochondritis is usually associated with puncture wounds of the foot. *Salmonella* osteomyelitis is common in patients with sickle-cell anemia. (See Chapter 178 in *Nelson Textbook of Pediatrics,* 16th ed.)

53. **B.** In immunocompromised persons, fever is a sensitive and specific sign of infection. Almost any organism can cause severe and even life-threatening infection. Absolute neutrophil counts of ≤ 500 cells/mm³ are predictive of infection, with the risk directly proportional to the duration and depth of neutropenia. Multiple infections, either concomitant or sequential, are common. (See Chapter 179 in *Nelson Textbook of Pediatrics,* 16th ed.)

54. **D.** Many strains of *S. aureus* produce toxins. Exfoliatins A and B are associated with localized (e.g., bullous impetigo) or generalized (e.g., scalded skin syndrome) eruptions. Staphylococcal enterotoxins A, B, C_1, C_2, D, and E are associated with food poisoning. TSST-1 is the toxin of toxic shock syndrome. (See Chapter 182 in *Nelson Textbook of Pediatrics,* 16th ed.)

55. **D.** The diagnosis of toxic shock syndrome is based on the clinical manifestations. In severe cases, the hypotension may progress to shock. Kawasaki disease is uncommon after 5 years of age, is not as severe or as progressive, and is not associated with hypotension or diarrhea. (See Chapter 182.2 in *Nelson Textbook of Pediatrics,* 16th ed.)

56. **B.** Slime produced by coagulase-negative staphylococci surrounds the organism, resists phagocytosis, and enhances adhesion to foreign surfaces, including indwelling catheters and prostheses. (See Chapter 182.3 in *Nelson Textbook of Pediatrics,* 16th ed.)

57. **E.** Most coagulase-negative staphylococci are resistant to nafcillin. Vancomycin is the drug of choice. (See Chapter 182.3 in *Nelson Textbook of Pediatrics,* 16th ed.)

58. **C.** Scarlet fever is the result of infection with a strain of group A *Streptococcus* that produces one of three pyrogenic (erythrogenic) exotoxins (A, B, or C). (See Chapter 184 in *Nelson Textbook of Pediatrics,* 16th ed.)

59. **E.** The classic rash of scarlet fever has a texture of gooseflesh or coarse sandpaper. Pastia lines are areas of hyperpigmentation that do not blanch with pressure that may appear in creases, particularly in the antecubital fossae. White strawberry tongue is characteristic of the early illness; as the white coat desquamates, the red strawberry tongue persists. Skin desquamation begins toward the end of the first week of illness. Preauricular lymphadenopathy is not typical. (See Chapter 184 in *Nelson Textbook of Pediatrics,* 16th ed.)

60. **B.** The diagnosis of cat-scratch disease, caused by *B. henselae,* is usually confirmed by serologic testing but can also be confirmed by culture. (See Chapter 207.2 in *Nelson Textbook of Pediatrics,* 16th ed.)

61. **D.** Botulism immune globulin can be obtained from the California Department of Health Services. Use of BIG significantly reduces both mean hospital stay and hospital costs. In many centers, **E** is correct because BIG has not been universally available. (See Chapter 208 in *Nelson Textbook of Pediatrics,* 16th ed.)

62. **C.** "Swimming pool granuloma" or "fish

tank granuloma" is caused by *M. marinum* after inoculation of the organism at the site of a minor abrasion. (See Chapter 214 in *Nelson Textbook of Pediatrics*, 16th ed.)

63. **B.** Doxycycline (for 14–21 days) is the treatment of choice for Lyme borreliosis in children ≥ 8 years of age, but amoxicillin (for 14–21 days) is the treatment of choice in children < 8 years of age. Where effective alternatives are available, children younger than 8 years should not be treated with doxycycline because it may cause permanent discoloration of the teeth. Erythromycin is an alternative for persons who cannot take either doxycycline or amoxicillin. (See Chapter 219 in *Nelson Textbook of Pediatrics*, 16th ed.)

64. **C.** The new macrolide antibiotics clarithromycin and azithromycin are preferred because they are tolerated better than erythromycin. Doxycycline is an alternative for persons ≥ 8 years of age. (See Chapter 220 in *Nelson Textbook of Pediatrics*, 16th ed.)

65. **E.** Several features of measles suggest the possibility of global eradication, including the absence of an animal reservoir, vector, and transmissible latent virus and the presence of only one serotype. (See Chapter 240 in *Nelson Textbook of Pediatrics*, 16th ed.)

66. **C.** There is an apparent correlation between retinol concentration and measles severity. Treatment with vitamin A reduces morbidity and mortality in children with severe measles in developing countries and is recommended for selected children with measles in the United States. (See Chapter 240 in *Nelson Textbook of Pediatrics*, 16th ed.)

67. **A.** Congenital rubella affects virtually all organ systems. Snuffles is a sign of congenital syphilis. (See Chapter 241 in *Nelson Textbook of Pediatrics*, 16th ed.)

68. **E.** Antimicrobial prophylaxis for pertussis is always given to all household contacts and other close contacts, such as those in daycare, regardless of age, history of immunization, or symptoms. (See Chapter 195 in *Nelson Textbook of Pediatrics*, 16th ed.)

69. **C.** The more serious adverse events associated with DTP vaccine, such as high fever, persistent crying, and hyporesponsive episodes, occur significantly less frequently with DTaP vaccine and are not considered contraindications to further doses. (See Chapter 195 in *Nelson Textbook of Pediatrics*, 16th ed.)

70. **C.** DTaP is the preferred vaccine for diphtheria, tetanus, and pertussis. It is recommended for all children at 2, 4, 6, and 15–18 months, with a booster at 4–6 years. Children ≥ 7 years of age and adults should receive only DT or dT vaccine, as indicated. (See Chapter 301 in *Nelson Textbook of Pediatrics*, 16th ed.)

71. **D.** Hepatitis A virus is now classified as enterovirus 72 but is antigenically distinct from the other enteroviruses. (See Chapter 301 in *Nelson Textbook of Pediatrics*, 16th ed.)

72. **E.** Approximately 90–95% of poliovirus infections are inapparent, causing no paralytic disease and no sequelae. (See Chapter 243 in *Nelson Textbook of Pediatrics*, 16th ed.)

73. **B.** Paralytic polio is characterized by aseptic meningitis accompanied by asymmetric flaccid paralysis without sensory loss. In Guillain-Barré syndrome, the paralysis is characteristically symmetric, and sensory changes (paresthesias) are common. Pleocytosis is common in polio, whereas the cerebrospinal fluid in Guillain-Barré syndrome usually shows only elevated protein and occasionally a few cells. (See Chapter 243 in *Nelson Textbook of Pediatrics*, 16th ed.)

74. **B.** VAPP, which follows reversion of the OPV strain to a neurovirulent strain, has accounted for all cases of polio in the United States since 1979. The risk is higher in vaccinees than in contacts, after the first dose, and in immunocompromised persons. (See Chapter 243 in *Nelson Textbook of Pediatrics*, 16th ed.)

75. **D.** Enteroviruses have a wide spectrum

of clinical manifestations. Herpangina is usually caused by echovirus type 9. Hand, foot, and mouth disease is usually caused by coxsackievirus A16. Diarrhea is probably less common than is taught. (See Chapter 243 in *Nelson Textbook of Pediatrics,* 16th ed.)

76. **D.** The rash occurs in three stages, which are not always clinically distinguishable. After the initial "slapped-cheek" appearance, the rash spreads to become a lacy, reticulated rash over the trunk and proximal extremities. Arthritis and arthralgia are much more common in adults, especially in females, than in children. The transient arrest of erythropoiesis is usually clinically silent in previously healthy persons. (See Chapter 244 in *Nelson Textbook of Pediatrics,* 16th ed.)

77. **C.** Only 15–20% of mothers of newborns with perinatal HSV have a history of obvious HSV infection, and only about 25% have any relevant symptoms at birth. (See Chapter 245 in *Nelson Textbook of Pediatrics,* 16th ed.)

78. **D.** Both the American Academy of Pediatrics and the American College of Obstetrics and Gynecology recommend cesarean section if primary, first-episode, or recurrent HSV lesions are present at the onset of labor. Only 15–20% of mothers of newborns with perinatal HSV have a history of HSV infection. (See Chapter 245 in *Nelson Textbook of Pediatrics,* 16th ed.)

79. **C.** Acyclovir treatment of all persons with varicella is acceptable but is not recommended by the American Academy of Pediatrics. Antiviral treatment of zoster is associated with a less severe disease and greatly decreased risk for postherpetic neuralgia. (See Chapter 246 in *Nelson Textbook of Pediatrics,* 16th ed.)

80. **C.** The IgM-VCA is the best single test to identify acute EBV infection. Anti-EBNA antibodies appear 3–4 months after infection and can be used to distinguish recent from past infection. (See Chapter 247 in *Nelson Textbook of Pediatrics,* 16th ed.)

81. **E.** EBV is associated with several

malignancies, including nasopharyngeal carcinoma, Burkitt lymphoma, Hodgkin disease, and lymphoproliferative diseases and leiomyosarcomas in immunocompromised persons. Kaposi sarcoma is associated with HHV-8. (See Chapter 247 in *Nelson Textbook of Pediatrics,* 16th ed.)

82. **C.** Infectious mononucleosis-like illnesses may also be caused by primary infection with cytomegalovirus, *T. gondii,* adenovirus, viral hepatitis, HIV, and possibly rubella virus. (See Chapter 247 in *Nelson Textbook of Pediatrics,* 16th ed.)

83. **C.** Only 5% of infected newborns have severe disease, and another 5% have mild disease. Most infected newborns are asymptomatic. Treatment has not been shown to be beneficial and is considered experimental. (See Chapter 248 in *Nelson Textbook of Pediatrics,* 16th ed.)

84. **B.** Approximately 60–90% of children 12 months of age and 80–100% of children 3–5 years of age have antibodies to HHV-6. Most newborns are seropositive as a result of transplacental transfer of maternal antibodies. (See Chapter 249 in *Nelson Textbook of Pediatrics,* 16th ed.)

85. **E.** The generally benign nature of roseola precludes consideration of antiviral therapy. The clinical efficacy of antiviral therapy for roseola has not been evaluated. (See Chapter 249 in *Nelson Textbook of Pediatrics,* 16th ed.)

86. 1. **G**
    2. **K**
    3. **I**
    4. **B**
    5. **F**
    6. **H**
    7. **A**
    8. **E**
    9. **D**
    10. **J**
    11. **C**

87. **D.** Otitis media and pneumonia, either viral or bacterial, are common complications of influenza in children. Reye syndrome may follow influenza, usually if salicylates are given for antipyresis, which is why they are not

recommended for persons with influenza or flu-like illnesses. (See Chapter 251 in *Nelson Textbook of Pediatrics,* 16th ed.)

88. **D.** Annual influenza vaccine is recommended for children with chronic pulmonary (e.g., asthma), cardiac, renal, or metabolic disorders (e.g., diabetes mellitus); children with hemoglobinopathies; children with immunosuppression; receiving long-term aspirin therapy; children with a family member at risk; and women who will be in the second or third trimester of pregnancy during the influenza season. (See Chapter 251 in *Nelson Textbook of Pediatrics,* 16th ed.)

89. **B.** Parainfluenza viruses account for approximately half of cases of croup and, unlike influenza virus and RSV infections, are not usually associated with fever or lower respiratory tract symptoms. (See Chapter 252 in *Nelson Textbook of Pediatrics,* 16th ed.)

90. **C.** RSV is the most common cause of bronchiolitis, which has the highest incidence from 2–7 months of age and usually occurs in the winter months. (See Chapter 253 in *Nelson Textbook of Pediatrics,* 16th ed.)

91. **E.** *C. trachomatis* has insidious onset of persistent cough and tachypnea, with the notable absence of fever. Rales are common, but wheezes are uncommon, which helps distinguish *C. trachomatis* from RSV pneumonia. (See Chapter 223.3 in *Nelson Textbook of Pediatrics,* 16th ed.)

92. **A.** *C. trachomatis* pneumonia is not associated with fever. (See Chapter 223.3 in *Nelson Textbook of Pediatrics,* 16th ed.)

93. **C.** The recommended treatment for *C. trachomatis* conjunctivitis or pneumonia is erythromycin 50 mg/kg/24 hours in two or four divided doses orally for 14 days. Topical therapy of conjunctivitis doesn't reduce the high risk of subsequent pneumonia. (See Chapter 223.3 in *Nelson Textbook of Pediatrics,* 16th ed.)

94. **B.** The steeple sign is visible on an anteroposterior radiograph of the neck. It is the progressive narrowing of the subglottic region that has the appearance of a tall, tapering church steeple. It is a sign of subglottic edema that is typical of croup, which is most frequently caused by parainfluenza viruses. (See Chapter 253 in *Nelson Textbook of Pediatrics,* 16th ed.)

95. **A.** RSV-IVIG is contraindicated and palivizumab is not recommended for infants with cyanotic heart disease. In studies with RSV-IVIG, mortality is higher in treated patients with heart disease. (See Chapter 253 in *Nelson Textbook of Pediatrics,* 16th ed.)

96. **E.** Adenoviruses cause a wide array of clinical illnesses, including pharyngitis, pneumonia, a pertussis-like syndrome, pharyngoconjunctival fever, conjunctivitis, myocarditis, diarrhea, and hemorrhagic cystitis. Leukocytosis and a high ESR may also be present. (See Chapter 254 in *Nelson Textbook of Pediatrics,* 16th ed.)

97. **A.** ICAM-1 (intercellular adhesion molecule 1) is present on the epithelium covering the lymphoepithelium of the adenoids and other epithelial cells of the nose, and is the cell receptor for most rhinoviruses. (See Chapter 255 in *Nelson Textbook of Pediatrics,* 16th ed.)

98. **B.** Rotaviruses, astrovirus, adenoviruses, and caliciviruses (e.g., Norwalk virus) are the medically important pathogens of human viral gastroenteritis. (See Chapter 256 in *Nelson Textbook of Pediatrics,* 16th ed.)

99. **E.** Papillomaviruses cause a variety of proliferative cutaneous and mucosal lesions. Condylomata acuminata are genital warts. Laryngeal papillomatosis follows acquisition of papillomaviruses during passage through an infected birth canal. (See Chapter 257 in *Nelson Textbook of Pediatrics,* 16th ed.)

100. **A.** Untreated warts may spontaneously regress, remain unchanged, or increase in size and number. There are many effective treatments, some of which are patient-applied and some of which are physician-applied, and some are painful and some are painless. Treatment of cervical warts may not decrease the risk

of cervical cancer. (See Chapter 257 in *Nelson Textbook of Pediatrics,* 16th ed.)

101. **D.** Eastern equine encephalitis has a low incidence of a few cases each year along the Atlantic and Gulf States. The case:infection ratio is 1:8 in children and 1:29 in adults. Unlike the other arboviral encephalitides, it has a poor prognosis. The case fatality rate is 33–75%, with many survivors having residual neurologic deficits. No specific treatment is available. (See Chapter 258 in *Nelson Textbook of Pediatrics,* 16th ed.)

102. **D.** Dengue is characterized by high fever, headache, myalgias and arthralgias, a transient blanching rash for the first 1–2 days of fever, and a maculopapular rash, sometimes with desquamation, that appears after defervescence. (See Chapter 260 in *Nelson Textbook of Pediatrics,* 16th ed.)

103. **A.** Dengue hemorrhagic fever is associated with increased capillary permeability, which leads to increased hematocrit and hypoalbuminemia. Dengue shock syndrome is dengue hemorrhagic fever plus hypotension or a narrow pulse pressure. (See Chapter 260 in *Nelson Textbook of Pediatrics,* 16th ed.)

104. **C.** Sin nombre virus is shed from saliva, urine, and feces of the deer mouse *Peromyscus maniculatus.* (See Chapter 264 in *Nelson Textbook of Pediatrics,* 16th ed.)

105. **A.** Healthy dogs, cats, and ferrets should be held for a 10-day observation. Postexposure prophylaxis for rabies should be given to the bitten person at the first sign of rabies in the animal, which should be euthanized immediately and tested. (See Chapter 265 in *Nelson Textbook of Pediatrics,* 16th ed.)

106. **B.** As much as possible of the dose of HRIG (20 IU/kg) should be infiltrated into the wound and the area around the wound, with the remainder administered intramuscularly at another site. HRIG should always be given with vaccine for postexposure prophylaxis of unimmunized persons. (See Chapter 265 in *Nelson Textbook of Pediatrics,* 16th ed.)

107. **D.** Bats, skunks, raccoons, foxes, and most other carnivores should be regarded as rabid unless the animal is proven rabies-negative by laboratory testing. Bites of squirrels, hamsters, guinea pigs, gerbils, chipmunks, rats, mice, other small rodents, rabbits, and hares almost never require prophylaxis; local public health officials should be consulted. (See Chapter 265 in *Nelson Textbook of Pediatrics,* 16th ed.)

108. **B.** Prion proteins cause the transmissible spongiform encephalopathies. Their primary structure is encoded by the host. Prion proteins from several species are similar but not identical in structure. They are very resistant to chemical and physical treatments. (See Chapter 267 in *Nelson Textbook of Pediatrics,* 16th ed.)

109. **B.** Kuru once affected many children, adolescents, and adults of Papua New Guinea but is now recognized only in older adults. This indicates that ritual cannibalism was probably the only mechanism of spread. (See Chapter 267 in *Nelson Textbook of Pediatrics,* 16th ed.)

110. **A.** HIV gp120 has significant heterogeneity among HIV strains, which is one reason for the difficulty in developing an effective HIV vaccine. (See Chapter 268 in *Nelson Textbook of Pediatrics,* 16th ed.)

111. **D.** Most cases of vertical-transmitted HIV infection occur from intrapartum transmission, but HIV can also be vertically transmitted in utero or by breast-feeding. (See Chapter 268 in *Nelson Textbook of Pediatrics,* 16th ed.)

112. **C.** Serologic diagnosis of HIV infection by ELISA and Western immunoblot is reliable only after 18 months of age. Before this age, residual maternal antibodies acquired transplacentally may be responsible for the positive serologic test results. (See Chapter 268 in *Nelson Textbook of Pediatrics,* 16th ed.)

113. **A.** Sustainable suppression of HIV is best achieved by combination antiretroviral therapy to which the patient has not been exposed previously and that is not cross-resistant to drugs given to the patient previously. (See Chapter 268 in *Nelson Textbook of Pediatrics,* 16th ed.)

114. **B.** Protease inhibitors act by preventing packaging of infectious virions before they leave the infected cell. (See Chapter 268 in *Nelson Textbook of Pediatrics,* 16th ed.)

115. **E.** All infants between 6 weeks and 1 year of age should receive prophylaxis for *P. carinii* regardless of CD4 cell count and percentage. After 12 months of age, prophylaxis is prescribed according to the CD4 cell count and percentage. (See Chapter 268 in *Nelson Textbook of Pediatrics,* 16th ed.)

116. **D.** The regimen of prenatal oral zidovudine during the second and third trimesters, intravenous zidovudine during labor, and postnatal zidovudine given to the infant reduces vertical HIV transmission to as low as 3–4%. Regimens of only one or two of these components provide some reduction. Combination prophylaxis with drugs more potent than zidovudine and that may provide greater effectiveness is being studied. (See Chapter 268 in *Nelson Textbook of Pediatrics,* 16th ed.)

117. **C.** Monthly IVIG to prevent bacterial infections is recommended only for HIV-infected children who have had two or more serious bacterial infections within 1 year, have a documented inability to make antigen-specific immunoglobulin, or have hypogammaglobulinemia. (See Chapter 268 in *Nelson Textbook of Pediatrics,* 16th ed.)

118. **B.** HTLV-I is prevalent in Japan and the Caribbean, where breast-feeding is a major mode of transmission. Testing of all blood products for HTLV-I/II antibodies was implemented in the United States in 1997. (See Chapter 269 in *Nelson Textbook of Pediatrics,* 16th ed.)

119. **D.** *Naegleria* organisms are found in many freshwater sources, including ponds, lakes, and stagnant pools. Therapy is often difficult, and morbidity and mortality are high. (See Chapter 270 in *Nelson Textbook of Pediatrics,* 16th ed.)

120. **C.** Amebic colitis caused by *Entamoeba histolytica* has the highest incidence in children 1–5 years of age. *E. dispar* is associated only with an asymptomatic

carrier state. *Giardia lamblia* does not cause bloody colitis. Amebiasis is uncommon in temperate climates. (See Chapter 271 in *Nelson Textbook of Pediatrics,* 16th ed.)

121. **A.** All persons with *Entamoeba histolytica* trophozoites or cysts in their stools should be treated, whether they have symptoms or not. (See Chapter 271 in *Nelson Textbook of Pediatrics,* 16th ed.)

122. **E.** Contaminated water is the most common source of *Giardia* organisms, especially surface water treated by faulty or inadequate water purification systems. Other sources include contaminated swimming pools (*Giardia* is resistant to chlorination), mountain streams, and contaminated food. *Giardia* is very common in children in child-care centers and in male homosexuals. (See Chapter 272 in *Nelson Textbook of Pediatrics,* 16th ed.)

123. **E.** Symptomatic persons with *G. lamblia* should be treated. Asymptomatic persons usually do not need treatment except in specific instances such as outbreak control, prevention of household transmission to pregnant women, and patients with hypogammaglobulinemia or cystic fibrosis. (See Chapter 272 in *Nelson Textbook of Pediatrics,* 16th ed.)

124. **A.** *G. lamblia* is a flagellated protozoan. (See Chapter 273 in *Nelson Textbook of Pediatrics,* 16th ed.)

125. **B.** *Cryptosporidium* is prevalent in developing countries and in children < 2 years of age. It causes watery, nonbloody diarrhea that is usually self-limited but may persist for several weeks. Because illness is self-limited in immunocompetent persons, no specific therapy is required. Treatment of immunocompromised persons is with paromomycin, with or without azithromycin. (See Chapter 273 in *Nelson Textbook of Pediatrics,* 16th ed.)

126. **B.** Trichomoniasis is characterized by copious malodorous vaginal discharge, vulvovaginal irritation, dysuria, and dyspareunia. (See Chapter 274 in *Nelson Textbook of Pediatrics,* 16th ed.)

127. 1. **E**

2. **I**
3. **B**
4. **F**
5. **D**
6. **A**
7. **G**
8. **J**
9. **C**
10. **K**
11. **H**
128. **A.** *P. falciparum* malaria is the most severe form and carries fatality rates of 25–35% in untreated persons. (See Chapter 278 in *Nelson Textbook of Pediatrics*, 16th ed.)
129. **D.** The diagnosis of malaria is best established by identification of organisms on Giemsa-stained thick and thin blood smears. (See Chapter 278 in *Nelson Textbook of Pediatrics*, 16th ed.)
130. **B.** Most persons are infected with *P. carinii* before 4 years of age. In the immunocompetent host, most primary infections are asymptomatic. (See Chapter 281 in *Nelson Textbook of Pediatrics*, 16th ed.)
131. **C.** The recommended treatment regimen for enterobiasis is albendazole, 400 mg orally, with a repeat dose in 2 weeks. An alternative treatment is mebendazole, 100 mg orally, with a repeat dose in 2 weeks. (See Chapter 284 in *Nelson Textbook of Pediatrics*, 16th ed.)
132. **B.** In trichinosis, migrating larvae of *Trichinella spiralis* cause symptoms of fever and myalgias, and they elicit an eosinophilic response. (See Chapter 294 in *Nelson Textbook of Pediatrics*, 16th ed.)
133. **D.** The most useful diagnostic test for neurocysticercosis is either computed tomography (CT) or magnetic resonance imaging (MRI), which typically reveals a solitary cyst with or without contrast enhancement. (See Chapter 299 in *Nelson Textbook of Pediatrics*, 16th ed.)
134. 1. **F**
    2. **D**
    3. **A**
    4. **C**
    5. **B**
    6. **E**
    7. **G**

(See Chapter 301 in *Nelson Textbook of Pediatrics*, 16th ed.)
135. **D.** Vaccines made by different manufacturers but directed against the same infections are generally considered interchangeable, with the exception of DTaP vaccines. (See Chapter 301 in *Nelson Textbook of Pediatrics*, 16th ed.)
136. **B.** The National Childhood Vaccine Injury Act requires that, for vaccines mandated in childhood, health care providers document the date of administration, manufacturer, lot number, and name of the health care provider administering the vaccine. (See Chapter 301 in *Nelson Textbook of Pediatrics*, 16th ed.)
137. **C.** No cases of HIV transmission in out-of-home daycare have been reported. (See Chapter 303 in *Nelson Textbook of Pediatrics*, 16th ed.)
138. 1. **E**
    2. **A**
    3. **C**
    4. **B**
    5. **G**
    6. **F**
    7. **D**

(See Chapter 225 in *Nelson Textbook of Pediatrics*, 16th ed.)
139. **D.** The diagnosis of Rocky Mountain spotted fever should be suspected in persons with an acute febrile illness with headache and myalgias, especially during the spring through the fall with a history of tick exposure. The maculopapular rash progresses to petechia and purpura and classically involves the palms or soles. (See Chapter 225 in *Nelson Textbook of Pediatrics*, 16th ed.)
140. **C.** Early laboratory clues to Rocky Mountain spotted fever include normal to slightly low leukocyte count, a shift to the left (increased bands), thrombocytopenia, and low serum sodium. (See Chapter 225 in *Nelson Textbook of Pediatrics*, 16th ed.)
141. **C.** Chloramphenicol and tetracyclines have proven efficacy against Rocky Mountain spotted fever, but chloramphenicol may be associated with higher mortality. Dental staining is

unlikely with a single course of tetracyclines. Doxycycline is recommended because the risk of dental staining is less than with other tetracyclines. (See Chapter 225 in *Nelson Textbook of Pediatrics,* 16th ed.)

142. **C.** Unlike with *Rickettsia rickettsii,* the cause of Rocky Mountain spotted fever, chloramphenicol is not effective against *Ehrlichia* spp. Dental staining is unlikely with a single course of tetracyclines. Doxycycline is recommended because the risk of dental staining is less than with other tetracyclines. (See Chapter 225 in *Nelson Textbook of Pediatrics,* 16th ed.)

143. **C.** *H. capsulatum* is found in the soil throughout the midwestern United States. *Blastomyces* is found in the same areas but is less common except in the northern midwestern states (Wisconsin). (See Chapter 234 in *Nelson Textbook of Pediatrics,* 16th ed.)

144. **C.** Bats are infected with *H. capsulatum,* which can be transmitted to humans after exposure to bat guano. (See Chapter 234 in *Nelson Textbook of Pediatrics,* 16th ed.)

145. **E.** *C. immitis* is found in arid areas of California's San Joaquin Valley (Valley fever), central and southern Arizona, and southwestern Texas. (See Chapter 236 in *Nelson Textbook of Pediatrics,* 16th ed.)

146. **C.** Sunken eyes are a sign of severe dehydration; hypotension, tachypnea, and tachycardia are also present in severe dehydration. (See Chapter 55 in *Nelson Textbook of Pediatrics,* 16th ed.)

147. **B.** The optimal solution for oral rehydration is WHO solution or commercial preparations based on WHO recommendations. (See Chapter 55 in *Nelson Textbook of Pediatrics,* 16th ed.)

148. **D.** Fecal leukocytes and blood or mucus in the stool suggest bacterial enteritis. (See Chapter 176 in *Nelson Textbook of Pediatrics,* 16th ed.)

149. **B.** *Shigella* usually responds to treatment, although the infection is usually self-limited. (See Chapter 176 in *Nelson Textbook of Pediatrics,* 16th ed.)

150. **B.** *Listeria* isolates are usually sensitive to penicillin, ampicillin, erythromycin, and tetracycline but are not susceptible to the cephalosporins, including the third-generation cephalosporins. The addition of an aminoglycoside (e.g., gentamicin) lowers the minimum bacteriocidal concentration. (See Chapter 188 in *Nelson Textbook of Pediatrics,* 16th ed.)

151. **B.** Meningococcus group B polysaccharide is poorly immunogenic. There is no vaccine available for this serogroup. (See Chapter 188 in *Nelson Textbook of Pediatrics,* 16th ed.)

152. **D.** Occult bacteremia (bacteremia without an obvious focus of infection) due to *Streptococcus pneumoniae, H. influenzae* type b, *N. meningitidis,* and *Salmonella* species occurs in approximately 4% of relatively well-appearing children between 3 and 36 months of age with fever (rectal temperature ≥ 38.0° C). *S. pneumoniae* accounts for 85% of cases of occult bacteremia. (See Chapter 172 in *Nelson Textbook of Pediatrics,* 16th ed.)

153. **A.** Poor prognostic signs for meningococcal disease include hypotension and shock, purpura fulminans, seizures, leukopenia, thrombocytopenia, and high circulating levels of endotoxin and tumor necrosis factor. The presence of petechiae for less than 12 hours before admission, hyperpyrexia, and the absence of meningitis reflect rapid clinical progression and poorer prognosis. (See Chapter 191 in *Nelson Textbook of Pediatrics,* 16th ed.)

154. **B.** Gonococcal infections range from asymptomatic carriage to localized urogenital infections, culture-negative tenosynovitis, suppurative arthritis, and disseminated gonococcal infection with bacteremia. Most genital tract infections in children are symptomatic, but as many as 80% of sexually active mature females with urogenital gonorrhea infections are asymptomatic. Conjunctivitis occurs in neonates born to mothers with genital tract gonorrhea. (See Chapter 192 in *Nelson Textbook of Pediatrics,* 16th ed.)

155. **E.** Chemoprophylaxis for contacts of a person with proven or suspected *N. meningitidis* infection is indicated for all household, daycare, and nursery care contacts. The index patient should also receive rifampin prophylaxis if penicillin was used for treatment. (See Chapter 191 in *Nelson Textbook of Pediatrics,* 16th ed.)

156. **C.** Chemoprophylaxis for contacts of a person with proven *H. influenzae* type b infection is indicated if the close contact group includes one or more children younger than 48 months of age who are not fully immunized; under these circumstances, rifampin prophylaxis is indicated for all members of the close contact group, including the index patient. (See Chapter 193 in *Nelson Textbook of Pediatrics,* 16th ed.)

157. **C.** The unusual lymph node tenderness, especially in the presence of systemic toxicity, distinguishes bubonic plague caused by *Y. pestis* from the typical lymphadenopathy associated with cat-scratch disease or tularemia. (See Chapter 201.3 in *Nelson Textbook of Pediatrics,* 16th ed.)

158. **E.** Mucoid strains of *P. aeruginosa* are common in persons with cystic fibrosis, causing insidious but progressive respiratory deterioration, but are rarely encountered in other persons. *B. cepacia* is an opportunist that rarely infects immunocompetent persons but is especially common in persons with cystic fibrosis and causes acute respiratory syndrome with fever, leukocytosis, and progressive respiratory failure. (See Chapters 203.1 and 203.2 in *Nelson Textbook of Pediatrics,* 16th ed.)

159. **E.** *F. tularensis*, the cause of tularemia, can be transmitted by many different modes, but person-to-person transmission has not occurred. (See Chapter 204 in *Nelson Textbook of Pediatrics,* 16th ed.)

160. **A.** Gentamicin or streptomycin is the treatment of choice for tularemia. Chloramphenicol and third-generation cephalosporins are associated with a high clinical failure rate. (See Chapter 204 in *Nelson Textbook of Pediatrics,* 16th ed.)

161. **C.** Because of the difficulty in culture techniques and the inconsistency of seroconversion, the urinary antigen test for *Legionella* is a useful method in the prompt diagnosis of *Legionella* infection. (See Chapter 206 in *Nelson Textbook of Pediatrics,* 16th ed.)

162. **D.** Erythromycin, with or without rifampin, has been established empirically as effective therapy for legionellosis. The newer macrolides (azithromycin and clarithromycin) and the quinolones also have excellent activity in vitro. (See Chapter 206 in *Nelson Textbook of Pediatrics,* 16th ed.)

163. **C.** Group B *Streptococcus* organisms are the major cause of severe systemic and focal infections in the newborn. Coagulase-negative *Staphylococcus* spp. are the most common nosocomial infection in the neonatal intensive care unit. (See Chapter 185 in *Nelson Textbook of Pediatrics,* 16th ed.)

164. **B.** Group B *Streptococcus* colonization rates are increased in women under 20 years of age, blacks, and lower socioeconomic groups. (See Chapter 185 in *Nelson Textbook of Pediatrics,* 16th ed.)

165. **D.** Using the risk factor–only-based approach, mothers should receive intrapartum prophylaxis for group B *Streptococcus* if one or more of the following is present: (1) previous infant with invasive group B *Streptococcus* disease, (2) maternal group B *Streptococcus* bacteriuria during pregnancy, (3) delivery at < 37 weeks' gestation, (4) maternal age < 21 years, and (5) intrapartum temperature ≥ 38°C (100.4°F).

166. **B.** For group B *Streptococcus* prophylaxis, the AAP and CDC recommend penicillin G, 5,000,000 units at the onset of labor, followed by 2,500,000 units every 4 hours until delivery. Ampicillin is an alternative. For penicillin-allergic patients, clindamycin or erythromycin may be used. (See Chapter 185 in *Nelson Textbook of Pediatrics,* 16th ed.)

167. **A.** Tuberculosis *infection* typically occurs after inhalation of *M. tuberculosis*. A

reactive skin test and the absence of clinical and radiographic manifestations of *disease* are the hallmark of this stage. (See Chapter 212 in *Nelson Textbook of Pediatrics,* 16th ed.)

168. **B.** If left untreated, 5–10% of asymptomatic persons with *M. tuberculosis* infection will experience disease in the future. (See Chapter 212 in *Nelson Textbook of Pediatrics,* 16th ed.)

169. **D.** Almost all transmission of *M. tuberculosis* is from person-to-person spread by airborne mucus droplet nuclei, usually from an actively infected person with cavitary TB and coughing. (See Chapter 212 in *Nelson Textbook of Pediatrics,* 16th ed.)

170. **C.** The 5-TU PPD skin test is administered by intradermal injection and is read by measuring the amount of induration (not erythema) 48–72 hours after administration. Corticosteroids may decrease the reaction, but this is variable. Up to 50% of persons with tuberculous meningitis or disseminated disease do not react initially to PPD; most become reactive after several months of therapy. (See Chapter 212 in *Nelson Textbook of Pediatrics,* 16th ed.)

171. **C.** Pulmonary tuberculosis is best confirmed by culture and isolation of *M. tuberculosis.* The best culture specimen in young children is three consecutive early-morning gastric aspirates obtained before the child has arisen and before peristalsis has emptied the stomach contents. The yield is approximately 50%, but the yield from bronchoscopy is even lower. Negative cultures never exclude the diagnosis of tuberculosis. (See Chapter 212 in *Nelson Textbook of Pediatrics,* 16th ed.)

172. **C.** *M. tuberculosis* drug resistance is chromosomally mediated and is not transferable. The estimated frequency of naturally drug-resistant organisms varies from 10^{-5} to $10^{-8.}$ Drug resistance to any one drug is independent of resistance to other drugs. (See Chapter 212 in *Nelson Textbook of Pediatrics,* 16th ed.)

173. **C.** Rapid acetylation of isoniazid is more frequent in African-Americans and Asians than among whites. There is no correlation between acetylation rate and either efficacy or adverse reactions in children. (See Chapter 212 in *Nelson Textbook of Pediatrics,* 16th ed.)

174. **D.** The American Academy of Pediatrics and the Centers for Disease Control recommend that children with pulmonary tuberculosis be treated with 6 months of isoniazid and rifampin supplemented with pyrazinamide for the first 2 months. (See Chapter 212 in *Nelson Textbook of Pediatrics,* 16th ed.)

175. **E.** Isoniazid therapy for newborns has been so effective that separation of the mother and infant is no longer mandatory unless the mother is ill enough to require hospitalization or is expected to not adhere to her treatment. (See Chapter 212 in *Nelson Textbook of Pediatrics,* 16th ed.)

176. **E.** *C. difficile* produces two toxins, A and B, that, in the appropriate clinical setting, are markers for the disease. It is not known whether the toxins are responsible, alone or together, for causing *Clostridium difficile*–associated diarrhea in humans. (See Chapter 210 in *Nelson Textbook of Pediatrics,* 16th ed.)

177. **D.** Antibiotics that impair growth of normal gut flora but not *C. difficile* are the most common risk factor for *C. difficile*–associated diarrhea. (See Chapter 210 in *Nelson Textbook of Pediatrics,* 16th ed.)

178. **E.** *C. difficile* is frequently isolated from the stool of infants. The interpretation of a positive stool culture or toxin requires clinical correlation. No treatment would be indicated for an asymptomatic infant. (See Chapter 210 in *Nelson Textbook of Pediatrics,* 16th ed.)

179. **C.** Anaerobic infections should be suspected with foul-smelling pus, which is present in half of anaerobic infections. In addition, the culture may be negative if not handled properly under anaerobic conditions. (See Chapter 211 in *Nelson Textbook of Pediatrics,* 16th ed.)

180. **A.** Tuberculoid and lepromatous leprosy forms the ends of the spectrum of leprosy. Tuberculoid leprosy responds well to treatment, but complete

resolution may take 8–12 months. Response of lepromatous leprosy to therapy may take 2–5 years. (See Chapter 213 in *Nelson Textbook of Pediatrics,* 16th ed.)

181. **B.** Lymphadenitis of the superior or anterior cervical or submandibular areas is the most frequent manifestation of atypical mycobacterial infections in children. (See Chapter 214 in *Nelson Textbook of Pediatrics,* 16th ed.)

182. **E.** Complete surgical excision is the preferred treatment of lymphadenitis caused by atypical mycobacteria. Antimycobacterial therapy is necessary only if there is concern for *M. tuberculosis* or if chronic drainage develops. (See Chapter 214 in *Nelson Textbook of Pediatrics,* 16th ed.)

183. **D.** Nontreponemal tests (VDRL, RPR) can be quantified and usually become nonreactive with 1 year of adequate therapy for primary syphilis and within 2 years of adequate therapy for secondary syphilis. Treponemal tests (MHA-TP, FTA-ABS) are not quantified and usually remain positive for life, even with adequate therapy. (See Chapter 215 in *Nelson Textbook of Pediatrics,* 16th ed.)

184. **D.** There is limited cross-reactivity of the treponemal tests (MHA-TP, FTA-ABS) with other spirochetes. Only *T. pallidum* and *Borrellia burgdorferi,* the causative organism of Lyme disease, are endemic in the United States. (See Chapter 215 in *Nelson Textbook of Pediatrics,* 16th ed.)

185. **B.** A biphasic course is characteristic of icteric leptospirosis (Weil syndrome). Hepatorenal dysfunction follows anicteric leptospirosis in < 10% of cases. (See Chapter 217 in *Nelson Textbook of Pediatrics,* 16th ed.)

186. **E.** Most immunologically normal children who acquire *T. gondii* have no clinically recognizable disease. (See Chapter 280 in *Nelson Textbook of Pediatrics,* 16th ed.)

187. **A.** The PPD test usually does not yield positive results initially in children with congenital tuberculosis, but results become positive in 1–3 months. The most important clue for diagnosis is a family history of tuberculosis. (See Chapter 212 in *Nelson Textbook of Pediatrics,* 16th ed.)

188. **D.** Risk factors for congenital syphilis are maternal treatment that was inadequate, unknown, or undocumented; treatment ≤ 30 days before delivery; treatment with a nonpenicillin regimen; or serial maternal VDRL titers that do not decrease sufficiently (at least fourfold) to demonstrate a cure. (See Chapter 215 in *Nelson Textbook of Pediatrics,* 16th ed.)

189. **C.** Bone abnormalities are common in congenital syphilis. Periostitis, occurring in the long bones, is most typical of congenital syphilis. Osteochondritis is a common finding of congenital cytomegalovirus, rubella, and syphilis infections. (See Chapter 215 in *Nelson Textbook of Pediatrics,* 16th ed.)

190. **D.** Chorioretinitis occurs in only approximately 22% of newborns with congenital toxoplasmosis, but almost all untreated persons will have chorioretinal lesions by adulthood and about half will have severe visual impairment. (See Chapter 280 in *Nelson Textbook of Pediatrics,* 16th ed.)

191. **C.** Cats ingest *Toxoplasma* oocysts in infected meat or from the feces of other infected cats. Cats that are strictly kept indoors, maintained on prepared diets, and not fed fresh, uncooked meat should not contact encysted *T. gondii* or shed oocysts. Pregnant women who are seronegative for *T. gondii* should avoid contact with cat feces. (See Chapter 280 in *Nelson Textbook of Pediatrics,* 16th ed.)

192. **B.** The six hepatotropic viruses (designated A, B, C, D, E, and G) are a heterogeneous group of viruses that cause similar acute clinical illness except for the most recently discovered virus, hepatitis G, which appears to cause a mild or no disease. (See Chapter 177 in *Nelson Textbook of Pediatrics,* 16th ed.)

193. **E.** Contact with infected persons, daycare attendance including household contacts of daycare attendees, contaminated food and water, homosexuality, and travel to endemic

areas are all associated with increased risk of hepatitis A infection. (See Chapter 177 in *Nelson Textbook of Pediatrics,* 16th ed.)

194. **D.** Hepatitis A vaccine is preferred for pre-exposure prophylaxis, and with IG for children ≥ 2 years of age for postexposure prophylaxis if future exposure is likely. The hepatitis A vaccine is licensed only for children ≥ 2 years of age. For children < 2 years of age who require postexposure prophylaxis, IG alone is used. (See Chapter 177 in *Nelson Textbook of Pediatrics,* 16th ed.)

17 *The Digestive System*

1. **C.** If an avulsed tooth is clean and the risk of aspiration is not too high, the tooth should be reimplanted in its socket and held in place on the way to the dentist. If this is not possible, the tooth should be placed in milk or water. (See Chapter 314 in *Nelson Textbook of Pediatrics,* 16th ed.)

2. **A.** The therapeutic window for fluoride and mild mottling of teeth is narrow. (See Chapter 312 in *Nelson Textbook of Pediatrics,* 16th ed.)

3. **E.** Appendicitis may produce infectious (wound, right lower quadrant, hepatic abscesses) and noninfectious (e.g., systemic inflammatory response syndrome—acute respiratory distress syndrome, disseminated intravascular coagulation) complications. Chronic complications include infertility in females and intestinal obstruction from adhesions. (See Chapter 343 in *Nelson Textbook of Pediatrics, 16th ed.)*

4. **B.** Inflammatory bowel disease is one of the most common causes of significant chronic or recurrent abdominal pain in adolescents. Functional abdominal pain (irritable bowel) is in the differential diagnosis but is precluded by the presence of anemia and weight loss. (See Chapter 337 in *Nelson Textbook of Pediatrics,* 16th ed.)

5. 1. **E**
   2. **D**
   3. **F**
   4. **A**
   5. **B**
   6. **C**
   (See Chapter 345 in *Nelson Textbook of Pediatrics,* 16th ed.)

6. **B.** Choices **A, B,** and **C** must be considered because each may produce similar hepatic and extrahepatic manifestations. Chronic active hepatitis of the autoimmune (lupoid hepatitis) type is often associated with other autoimmune diseases (the patient described in the question had Hashimoto thyroiditis) and is more prevalent in adolescent females. High titers of liver-kidney microsomal antibodies are present. The antinuclear antibody response is also positive in many patients. (See Chapter 361 in *Nelson Textbook of Pediatrics,* 16th ed.)

7. **C.** In the patient described in the question, the hepatic abscess developed as a complication of a partially treated ruptured appendix after acute appendicitis. The over-the-counter medication was an oral antibiotic that suppressed some of the signs of appendicitis. The right lower quadrant fullness is a walled-off appendiceal abscess. This is treated with antibiotics and resected at a later date.

   The hepatic abscess developed after septic embolization into the portal vein (during the acute appendicitis) and subsequently the liver. The organisms are usually enteric anaerobes in this form of liver abscess. Treatment includes antibiotics (including metronidazole or clindamycin) and percutaneous drainage under ultrasonographic or computed tomographic guidance. (See Chapter 358 in *Nelson Textbook of Pediatrics,* 16th ed.)

8. **D.** Vitamin E deficiency has a long latency before it eventually produces ataxia, posterior (spinal cord) column signs, and peripheral neuropathy. Early treatment with water-soluble vitamin E may reverse these neurologic processes. (See Chapter 340.3 in *Nelson Textbook of Pediatrics,* 16th ed.)

9. 1. **A**
   2. **A**
   3. **B**
   4. **C**

5. **C**
6. **A**
7. **B**
8. **B**
9. **A**
10. **B**
11. **B**
12. **A**

(See Chapter 355 in *Nelson Textbook of Pediatrics,* 16th ed.)

10. **B.** Pancreatitis may develop in patients with total body casts. Associated features may also include hypercalcemia and hypertension. (See Chapter 351 in *Nelson Textbook of Pediatrics,* 16th ed.) An alternative diagnosis is superior mesenteric artery syndrome with compression of the artery over the duodenum. (See Chapter 332.2 in *Nelson Textbook of Pediatrics,* 16th ed.)

11. 1. **E**
    2. **D**
    3. **C**
    4. **B**
    5. **A**
    6. **F**
    7. **G**

(See Chapter 340 in *Nelson Textbook of Pediatrics,* 16th ed.)

12. **D.** All of the choices in the question must be included in the differential diagnosis. Pelvic inflammatory disease often presents with lower abdominal suprapubic pain, a vaginal discharge, and signs of peritoneal irritation. A ruptured ectopic pregnancy would be unlikely but not unheard of in a Tanner stage 2 girl. Mesenteric adenitis may present in a similar manner as appendicitis (pseudoappendicitis) and can be detected by abdominal ultrasonography or CT scan. This patient has the characteristic appendicitis sequence of periumbilical pain, followed more often by nausea and less often by emesis and then followed by right lower quadrant pain. The 2-day history is typical of appendicitis, as is the apprehension about the examiner's hand during the abdominal palpation. (See Chapter 343 in *Nelson Textbook of Pediatrics,* 16th ed.)

13. **D.** Intussusception should be suspected in any toddler or young child with an acute illness characterized by intermittent episodes of abdominal pain (colic) and blood in the stool. A physical examination, abdominal kidney-ureter-bladder (KUB) radiograph, or most likely ultrasonography may show that the bowel is being pulled into the next segment of the bowel. Nonetheless, the diagnostic test of choice and treatment of choice is a barium or air enema. Hydrostatic pressure during the enema reduces the intussusception in approximately 80–90% of patients. (See Chapter 333.3 in *Nelson Textbook of Pediatrics,* 16th ed.)

14. **E.** Pyloric stenosis is most often encountered in a first-born boy after the second or third week of life. Recurrent emesis of gastric contents results in dehydration plus loss of H^+, K^+, and Cl^-, resulting in hypokalemic metabolic alkalosis. On physical examination immediately after feeding the patient described in the question, an olive-shaped mass was felt in the epigastrium. Surgical pyloromyotomy cured the patient, who was taking oral feeding 12 hours later. (See Chapter 329 in *Nelson Textbook of Pediatrics,* 16th ed.)

15. **C.** Scrubbing an avulsed tooth, especially the root, can cause permanent damage and prevent reimplantation. The remaining choices, including plugging the sink drain to avoid losing the tooth, are all correct. (See Chapter 314 in *Nelson Textbook of Pediatrics,* 16th ed.)

16. **C.** Pancreatitis is rarely associated with the other conditions listed in the question despite elevations of serum amylase levels. (See Chapter 351 in *Nelson Textbook of Pediatrics,* 16th ed.)

17. **C.** Remember that a mass in the labium of a female may be a gonad (testis, ovum-testis, ovary). (See Chapter 346 in *Nelson Textbook of Pediatrics,* 16th ed.)

18. **E.** Hearing aid batteries are highly corrosive and must be removed if swallowed. The location in the boy described in the question also suggests that it will not pass into his stomach. (See Chapter 334 in *Nelson Textbook of Pediatrics,* 16th ed.)

19. **C.** The pneumococcus is a common

pathogen producing peritonitis (primary) in any condition causing ascites (nephrosis, cirrhosis). Next in frequency is *Escherichia coli.* (See Chapter 370.1 in *Nelson Textbook of Pediatrics,* 16th ed.)

20. **B.** Despite the initial success of the Kasai operation, patients with biliary atresia either go directly to transplantation or undergo transplantation later in life after the Kasai procedure fails. (See Chapter 367 in *Nelson Textbook of Pediatrics,* 16th ed.)

21. **C.** With current immunosuppressive therapy, most patients experience mild graft rejection; causes of mortality include opportunistic infections and lymphoproliferative disease. (See Chapter 367 in *Nelson Textbook of Pediatrics,* 16th ed.)

22. **D.** All live virus vaccines place an immunosuppressed patient at increased risk for adverse vaccine-related complications. (See Chapter 367 in *Nelson Textbook of Pediatrics,* 16th ed.)

23. **A.** EBV produces a lymphoproliferative disease and lymphoma that may respond to a reduction of immunosuppression and EBV-specific chemotherapy or immune modulation. (See Chapter 367 in *Nelson Textbook of Pediatrics,* 16th ed.)

24. **A.** B–F must be considered as well as increased intracranial pressure. Be wary of emesis in the absence of diarrhea when you consider a diagnosis of gastroenteritis. (See Chapter 306 in *Nelson Textbook of Pediatrics,* 16th ed.)

25. **D.** Dysphagia is a sensation that swallowing is difficult because of "something stuck." Odynophagia is pain on swallowing. (See Chapter 306 in *Nelson Textbook of Pediatrics,* 16th ed.)

26. **E.** A–D are all correct. Nystagmus should suggest serious central nervous system disease or vestibular disease. (See Chapter 306 in *Nelson Textbook of Pediatrics,* 16th ed.)

27. 1. **D**
    2. **A**
    3. **B**
    4. **E**
    5. **C**
    6. **F**

(See Chapter 306 in *Nelson Textbook of Pediatrics,* 16th ed.)

28. **D.** Indeed, this drug may cause abdominal pain and loose stools. (See Chapter 306 in *Nelson Textbook of Pediatrics,* 16th ed.)

29. **B.** A is normal; any other misalignment with the upper and lower molars is abnormal. (See Chapter 309 in *Nelson Textbook of Pediatrics,* 16th ed.)

30. **D.** This is quite false. Indeed, palatopharyngeal incompetence may first become evident or exacerbated after adenoid removal. (See Chapter 310 in *Nelson Textbook of Pediatrics,* 16th ed.)

31. **C.** Intrusion up into the maxillary bone may be a common problem in children with the appearance of an avulsed tooth. (See Chapter 314 in *Nelson Textbook of Pediatrics,* 16th ed.)

32. **B.** A barium esophagram demonstrated marked dilatation of the proximal esophagus with extreme narrowing of the esophageal sphincter. (See Chapter 321 in *Nelson Textbook of Pediatrics,* 16th ed.)

33. **D.** Pylorospasm is uncommon in GERD. If present, it should suggest another cause of regurgitation such as pyloric stenosis, peptic ulcer disease, or inflammatory bowel disease. (See Chapter 323 in *Nelson Textbook of Pediatrics,* 16th ed.)

34. **D.** The event occurred while the patient was eating gumdrops. One hour after admission, all symptoms resolved, probably as the gumdrop passed to the stomach. If symptoms had persisted, endoscopic removal would have been indicated. (See Chapter 327 in *Nelson Textbook of Pediatrics,* 16th ed.)

35. **D.** Feeding initiates the pylorospasm, which may be visualized in a thin infant or palpated in the right upper or mid upper quadrants. (See Chapter 329 in *Nelson Textbook of Pediatrics,* 16th ed.)

36. **A.** B–E are all correct. (See Chapter 329 in *Nelson Textbook of Pediatrics,* 16th ed.)

37. **C.** Malrotation, and with this patient volvulus (a bowel and life-threatening complication), usually presents with bowel obstruction before 1 year of age. The oldest reported patient, however, was over 80 years old. Most cases present before age 3 years. Superior mesenteric

artery obstruction of the intestines may also produce bile-stained emesis; however, intestinal infarction is not observed. (See Chapters 330 and 332 in *Nelson Textbook of Pediatrics,* 16th ed.)

38. **E.** A Meckel scan is positive. The hemoglobin is 12 g/dL, and the vital signs are normal. (See Chapter 331 in *Nelson Textbook of Pediatrics,* 16th ed.)

39. **C.** Surgery is the treatment of choice for symptomatic Meckel diverticulum. (See Chapter 331 in *Nelson Textbook of Pediatrics,* 16th ed.)

40. **E.** Cystic fibrosis is not associated with malrotation. (See Chapter 332 in *Nelson Textbook of Pediatrics,* 16th ed.)

41. **D.** Pseudo-obstruction, a chronic group of disorders, may be due to abnormalities of the intestinal innervation or to its muscle layers. Most are sporadic cases. (See Chapter 332 in *Nelson Textbook of Pediatrics,* 16th ed.)

42. **C.** Imperforate anus is associated with VATER syndrome. Hirschsprung disease is the most common anatomic cause of lower intestinal obstruction in neonates. (See Chapter 332 in *Nelson Textbook of Pediatrics,* 16th ed.)

43. **B.** Intussusception may present with lethargy out of proportion to the intestinal signs and symptoms. (See Chapter 333 in *Nelson Textbook of Pediatrics,* 16th ed.)

44. **B.** Air or barium hydrostatic reduction is indicated unless there are signs of perforation or peritonitis; at that point surgical reduction is indicated. (See Chapter 333 in *Nelson Textbook of Pediatrics,* 16th ed.)

45. **B, E.** Both are correct. The child has a TEF and abnormal vertebra compatible with VATER syndrome. (The patient also had a VSD.) The TEF is the most urgent and requires surgery as soon as the patient's condition is stabilized. (See Chapter 319 in *Nelson Textbook of Pediatrics,* 16th ed.)

46. **D.** Peptic ulcer disease in children over 6 years of age presents similarly to that in adults. Infants may only manifest acute bleeding of perforation. *Giardia* does not cause intestinal bleeding. (See Chapter 336 in *Nelson Textbook of Pediatrics,* 16th ed.)

47. **A.** Gastroduodenal endoscopy picks up all significant ulcers and is more sensitive than upper tract barium studies. (See Chapter 336 in *Nelson Textbook of Pediatrics,* 16th ed.)

48. **D.** Although therapy is still being defined, an H$_2$-blocker or hydrogen pump inhibitor plus at least two antibiotics effective against *H. pylori* are needed to treat the acute episode of ulceration and to prevent recurrences. (See Chapter 336 in *Nelson Textbook of Pediatrics,* 16th ed.)

49. **B.** The risk of colonic cancer is higher than the general population in both diseases but much higher in patients with ulcerative colitis. (See Chapter 337 in *Nelson Textbook of Pediatrics,* 16th ed.)

50. 1. **A**
    2. **B**
    3. **A**
    4. **A**
    5. **B**
    6. **B**
    7. **D**
    8. **B**
    9. **B**
    10. **C**
    (See Chapter 337 in *Nelson Textbook of Pediatrics,* 16th ed.)

51. **B.** Celiac disease or gluten-sensitive enteropathy occurs only after the introduction of gluten-containing foods (wheat, rye, barley). Small bowel mucosal biopsy reveals flattened villi and mucosal atrophy. (See Chapter 340 in *Nelson Textbook of Pediatrics,* 16th ed.)

52. **E.** SLE is not a predisposing condition for celiac disease. (See Chapter 340 in *Nelson Textbook of Pediatrics,* 16th ed.)

53. **B.** This is the serum diagnostic test of choice and is almost 100% sensitive and specific except in IgA-deficient patients. (See Chapter 340 in *Nelson Textbook of Pediatrics,* 16th ed.)

54. 1. **B**
    2. **D**
    3. **A**
    4. **C**

5. **F**

6. **E**

(See Chapter 340 in *Nelson Textbook of Pediatrics,* 16th ed.)

55. **A.** Female tubo-ovarian inflammation produces scarring and reduced fertility after appendicitis; no such effect has been observed in males. (See Chapter 343 in *Nelson Textbook of Pediatrics,* 16th ed.)

56. 1. **C**

2. **A**

3. **D**

4. **B**

5. **F**

6. **E**

(See Chapter 356 in *Nelson Textbook of Pediatrics,* 16th ed.)

57. **A.** B–F represent the hepatic, neurologic, and renal (plus hematologic) findings. Ocular disease is detected by Kayser-Fleischer corneal rings, which may be absent in younger patients, who usually manifest hepatic disease. (See Chapter 357 in *Nelson Textbook of Pediatrics,* 16th ed.)

58. **D.** Chronic fatigue syndrome would not be associated with jaundice. (See Chapter 717 in *Nelson Textbook of Pediatrics,* 16th ed.)

59. **B.** Chronic active or autoimmune hepatitis is associated with these auto-antibodies. (See Chapter 361 in *Nelson Textbook of Pediatrics,* 16th ed.)

60. **E.** Prednisone is the treatment of choice for autoimmune hepatitis. (See Chapter 361 in *Nelson Textbook of Pediatrics,* 16th ed.)

61. **B.** A facial space inflammatory response to a tooth abscess is the cause of such facial swelling until proved otherwise. (See Chapter 312 in *Nelson Textbook of Pediatrics,* 16th ed.)

62. **C.** Direct tenderness, particularly localized to the right lower quadrant, is a valuable sign in appendicitis. This may be absent in an appendix located in the retrocecum or pelvis or early in the progression of the disease. (See Chapter 343 in *Nelson Textbook of Pediatrics,* 16th ed.)

63. **B.** Administration of milk helps calm a child and helps dilute the alkali in the esophagus and stomach. (See Chapter

324 in *Nelson Textbook of Pediatrics,* 16th ed.

64. **D.** Endoscopy is indicated to assess the severity of inflammation and necrosis. Even without oral lesions, significant esophageal involvement is possible. Prednisone is of no value in preventing strictures. (See Chapter 324 in *Nelson Textbook of Pediatrics,* 16th ed.)

65. 1. **A**

2. **A**

3. **B**

4. **B**

5. **A**

(See Chapter 332 in *Nelson Textbook of Pediatrics,* 16th ed.)

66. **E.** Vitamin E deficiency is a major cause of morbidity in patients with prolonged cholestasis. (It is also responsible for symptoms in abetalipoproteinemia.) Previously, the management of this deficiency was difficult, and parenteral therapy occasionally was necessary. Awareness of this problem is mandatory for physicians who are caring for patients with cholestasis. (See Chapter 356 in *Nelson Textbook of Pediatrics,* 16th ed.)

67. **D.** ERCP is an endoscopic-radiographic technique for visualization of the ducts of the pancreas and biliary tree. Ductal disorders such as strictures, choledochal cyst, and intraductal stones are common causes of recurrent pancreatitis. Serum amylase determination confirms the diagnosis of pancreatitis. A CT scan or ultrasonography can confirm the diagnosis of pancreatitis and diagnose complications such as pseudocyst but cannot determine the underlying causes of pancreatitis. Undiagnosed cystic fibrosis is an unlikely cause of recurrent pancreatitis. (See Chapter 351 in *Nelson Textbook of Pediatrics,* 16th ed.)

68. **E.** Choices **A–D** must be considered in the differential diagnosis but are usually discernible by the history and the findings on physical examination. (See Chapter 346 in *Nelson Textbook of Pediatrics,* 16th ed.)

69. **B.** Many patients with a rectourethral fistula may pass meconium through the fistula. (See Chapter 335 in *Nelson Textbook of Pediatrics,* 16th ed.)

18 *The Respiratory System*

1. **D.** Choanal atresia is complete obstruction of the nasal passages, usually due to bony obliteration of the nasal airway. Mouth breathing during crying bypasses the obstruction, but in quiet states, an affected newborn may become an obligate nasal breather. Treatment requires an oral airway and eventual nasal surgery. (See Chapter 378 in *Nelson Textbook of Pediatrics,* 16th ed.)

2. 1. **A**
   2. **C**
   3. **A**
   4. **B**
   5. **C**
   6. **B**
   7. **B**
   8. **A**
   9. **A**
   10. **B**
   (See Chapter 381 in *Nelson Textbook of Pediatrics,* 16th ed.)

3. **D.** Foreign body aspiration into the trachea or bronchi is often heralded by the abrupt onset of cough, choking, and wheezing. The age group at highest risk is small children younger than 3 years. Either bronchus may contain a foreign body. (See Chapter 386 in *Nelson Textbook of Pediatrics,* 16th ed.)

4. **D.** Pulmonary embolism must be considered with the sudden onset of chest pain, dyspnea, and cyanosis. A normal-appearing chest radiograph with significant hypoxia is classic for pulmonary embolism. A spiral CT is a useful test to determine the presence of a pulmonary embolism. (See Chapter 409 in *Nelson Textbook of Pediatrics,* 16th ed.)

5. **D.** Other intestinal obstruction is possible and includes neonatal meconium ileus, congenital ileal atresia, neonatal mucus plus syndrome, meconium ileus equivalent (from insufficient use of pancreatic enzyme replacement), intussusception, inguinal hernias, and appendiceal obstruction. (See Chapter 416 in *Nelson Textbook of Pediatrics,* 16th ed.)

6. **D.** Peritonsillar abscess often follows or complicates pharyngitis. As the tonsillar abscess develops, trismus, deviation of the uvula away from the abscess, drooling, and intense pain ensue. Treatment is with penicillin and aspiration of the abscess cavity. (See Chapter 381.7 in *Nelson Textbook of Pediatrics,* 16th ed.)

7. **C.** Empyema and chylothorax are not sudden in onset, and staphylococcal pneumonia is not likely in adolescents. (See Chapter 419 in *Nelson Textbook of Pediatrics,* 16th ed.)

8. **B.** Bronchoscopy is the approach of choice to visualize and remove a bronchial foreign body. (See Chapter 386 in *Nelson Textbook of Pediatrics,* 16th ed.)

9. 1. **B**
   2. **A**
   3. **A**
   4. **D**
   5. **A**
   (See Chapter 375 in *Nelson Textbook of Pediatrics,* 16th ed.)

10. 1. **A**
    2. **B**
    3. **C**
    4. **D**
    5. **D**
    (See Chapter 375 in *Nelson Textbook of Pediatrics,* 16th ed.)

11. 1. **B**
    2. **C**
    3. **B**
    4. **D**
    5. **D**
    (See Chapter 375 in *Nelson Textbook of Pediatrics,* 16th ed.)

12. **C.** The onset of CCHS is in early infancy, usually a few hours after birth. With sleep, the P_{CO_2} rapidly rises to over 80 mm Hg, but with awake infants, the P_{CO_2} rapidly returns to normal. (See Chapter 375 in *Nelson Textbook of Pediatrics,* 16th ed.)

13. **E.** High-resolution CT is the method of choice to help guide the surgeon's plan. (See Chapter 378 in *Nelson Textbook of Pediatrics,* 16th ed.)

14. **D.** Such things as food, crayons, toys, erasers, paper, and beads all wind up in young children's noses. (See Chapter 379 in *Nelson Textbook of Pediatrics,* 16th ed.)

15. **D.** Topical anesthesia followed by forceps or suction removal of the foreign body is all that is usually needed. Phenylephrine may be helpful to reduce swelling.

Antibiotics are not needed. (See Chapter 379 in *Nelson Textbook of Pediatrics*, 16th ed.)

16. **E.** HSP usually doesn't just present with recurrent epistaxis without other manifestations of HSP (renal, cutaneous, abdominal, joint). Thrombocytopenia is not part of HSP. (See Chapter 379 in *Nelson Textbook of Pediatrics*, 16th ed.)

17. **C.** The presence of a mass and epistaxis in a pubertal male is a classic presentation for a juvenile nasopharyngeal angiofibroma. (See Chapter 379 in *Nelson Textbook of Pediatrics*, 16th ed.)

18. **E.** Up to 25% of children with cystic fibrosis experience nasal polyps. (See Chapter 380 in *Nelson Textbook of Pediatrics*, 16th ed.)

19. **B.** Reovirus infection is common, but it is only an occasional cause of colds. (See Chapter 381 in *Nelson Textbook of Pediatrics*, 16th ed.)

20. **F.** None is of any proven efficacy in children. Fever is best controlled by acetaminophen or ibuprofen. Chicken soup may help as a way to keep hydrated, although my grandmother remains convinced that it is more effective than combination cold remedies. (See Chapter 381 in *Nelson Textbook of Pediatrics*, 16th ed.)

21. **B.** QD amoxicillin has been proven effective for the treatment of streptococcal pharyngitis. Its ability to prevent rheumatic fever is untested. (See Chapter 381 in *Nelson Textbook of Pediatrics*, 16th ed.)

22. **E.** Adenoid hypertrophy may be confused with a rhabdomyosarcoma; chronic sinusitis is another possible presentation of this tumor. (See Chapter 382 in *Nelson Textbook of Pediatrics*, 16th ed.)

23. **E.** Any disorder that causes relaxation of the oropharyngeal muscles or narrowing of the upper airway, including the nose, may produce OSA/H. (See Chapter 383 in *Nelson Textbook of Pediatrics*, 16th ed.)

24. **D.** Children don't consistently manifest daytime hypersomnolence. (See Chapter 383 in *Nelson Textbook of Pediatrics*, 16th ed.)

25. **C.** This is a classic manifestation for laryngomalacia. (See 384 in *Nelson Textbook of Pediatrics*, 16th ed.)

26. **E.** Choanal atresia is exacerbated when the mouth is closed and relieved during crying. There is no stridor. (See Chapter 384 in *Nelson Textbook of Pediatrics*, 16th ed.)

27. 1. **C**
    2. **A**
    3. **B**
    4. **C**
    5. **A**
    6. **B**
    (See Chapter 384 in *Nelson Textbook of Pediatrics*, 16th ed.)

28. **A.** Croup (LTB) is common in this age group and is frequently a benign disorder. However, because of the small diameter of the child's airway, acute obstruction is always a serious possibility. (See Chapter 385 in *Nelson Textbook of Pediatrics*, 16th ed.)

29. **D.** Croup may also be caused by RSV, which more often causes bronchiolitis. (See Chapter 385 in *Nelson Textbook of Pediatrics*, 16th ed.)

30. **A.** Racemic epinephrine and oral or intramuscular long-acting steroids are indicated in patients with croup who have significant distress and stridor at rest. Oxygen is appropriate for all cyanotic infants. (See Chapter 385 in *Nelson Textbook of Pediatrics*, 16th ed.)

31. **E.** Bacterial tracheitis is a serious, uncommon, but well-recognized complication of viral croup. Because of the small airway, the tracheal mucosal inflammation creates a significant risk of acute airway obstruction and respiratory arrest. (See Chapter 385 in *Nelson Textbook of Pediatrics*, 16th ed.)

32. **A.** HIB is not a common cause of trachitis. It was the most common cause of bacteremic epiglottitis and remains the cause of epiglottitis in children who have not received the very effective HIB vaccine. (See Chapter 385 in *Nelson Textbook of Pediatrics*, 16th ed.)

33. **D.** The marked hyperinflation of one lung (obstructive emphysema) is a classic finding of an aspirated radiolucent foreign body, particularly on an expiratory film.

(See Chapter 386 in *Nelson Textbook of Pediatrics,* 16th ed.)

34. **D.** This facilitates visualization and removal of the aspirated object. (See Chapter 386 in *Nelson Textbook of Pediatrics,* 16th ed.)

35. **E.** Oxygen plus supporting and protecting his airway are the first priorities. Inducing emesis with ipecac or possibly provoking emesis with a nasogastric tube are not needed and are potentially dangerous. Routine use of antibiotics is not recommended, and steroids may increase the risk of infection. (See Chapter 393 in *Nelson Textbook of Pediatrics,* 16th ed.)

36. **C.** Clubbing is not universally present, and fever is quite unusual. (See Chapter 400 in *Nelson Textbook of Pediatrics,* 16th ed.)

37. **E.** Cardiac lesions that increase pulmonary venous pressure may result in pulmonary hemorrhage; mitral stenosis is a classic lesion, not aortic stenosis. (See Chapter 402 in *Nelson Textbook of Pediatrics,* 16th ed.)

38. **C.** The mediastinum is shifted to the right, and the left lung is hyperinflated (either because of asthma or secondary to compensation for the right-sided atelectasis). (See Chapter 406 in *Nelson Textbook of Pediatrics,* 16th ed.)

39. **D.** Intractable hiccups may be due to CNS lesions and peripheral causes that irritate the vagus nerve or that act locally on the diaphragm. Folk remedies (sugar, hyperventilating, breath holding) usually don't work; mediates (haloperidol, metoclopramide) sometimes are needed for chronic hiccups. (See Chapter 414 in *Nelson Textbook of Pediatrics,* 16th ed.)

40. **B.** Chronic cough that is present during wakefulness and disappears with sleep (not necessarily at night) suggests a habit. (See Chapter 415 in *Nelson Textbook of Pediatrics,* 16th ed.)

41. 1. **C**
    2. **A** or **D**
    3. **B** or **A**
    4. **D**
    5. **D**
    (See Chapter 415 in *Nelson Textbook of Pediatrics,* 16th ed.)

42. **A.** The incidence of cystic fibrosis is highest in northern European whites (1 in 3500) and lowest in Asian infants in Hawaii (1 in 90,000). (See Chapter 416 in *Nelson Textbook of Pediatrics,* 16th ed.)

43. **C.** The cough begins as dry and nonproductive but progresses to loose and productive of purulent sputum. (See Chapter 416 in *Nelson Textbook of Pediatrics,* 16th ed.)

44. **E.** Enteric manifestations affect the small and large bowel, the liver and bile ducts, and the pancreas. Cystic fibrosis may protect patients from certain bacterial causes of diarrhea. (See Chapter 416 in *Nelson Textbook of Pediatrics,* 16th ed.)

45. 1. **D**
    2. **A**
    3. **B**
    4. **D**
    5. **C**
    6. **E**
    (See Chapter 416 in *Nelson Textbook of Pediatrics,* 16th ed.)

46. **D.** Although immune deficiency is an important consideration, the combination of situs inversus, chronic sinusitis and otitis, and pneumonia leading to bronchiectasis suggests the diagnosis of primary client dyskinesia (immobile cilia syndrome). Otitis is not common in cystic fibrosis but is common in ciliary dyskinesia. (See Chapter 417 in *Nelson Textbook of Pediatrics,* 16th ed.)

47. **E.** Although *Mycoplasma* occasionally is associated with a pleural effusion, it is usually a parapneumonic effusion and not an empyema. (See Chapter 418 in *Nelson Textbook of Pediatrics,* 16th ed.)

19 *The Cardiovascular System*

1. **C.** The murmur may represent a patent ductus arteriosus (PDA). If the PDA closes, marked cyanosis would supervene and result in acidosis, shock, and death. Prostaglandin E_1 (PGE_1) maintains patency of the ductus arterious between the pulmonary artery and the aorta. (See Chapter 436 in *Nelson Textbook of Pediatrics,* 16th ed.)

2. **D.** Pulmonary atresia is manifested by a small right ventricle, decreased

pulmonary vascular markings, early and marked cyanosis without heart failure, and ductal dependence to maintain some pulmonary blood flow. (See Chapter 437.3 in *Nelson Textbook of Pediatrics,* 16th ed.)

3. **C.** The child described in the question has tetralogy of Fallot with exercise-induced cyanosis. The more serious episode is a cyanotic, blue, or "tet" spell and may be due to decreased systemic vascular resistance, increased pulmonary artery pressure, or right ventricular outflow tract obstruction. The murmur of tetralogy (the pulmonary stenosis) often disappears or lessens during a spell. (See Chapter 437.1 in *Nelson Textbook of Pediatrics,* 16th ed.)

4. **A.** Epinephrine is potentially dangerous because it may exacerbate inotropy and contractile forces, which may obstruct the right ventricular infundibulum. Indeed, propranolol has been used to treat "tet" spells. (See Chapter 437.1 in *Nelson Textbook of Pediatrics,* 16th ed.)

5. **B.** Poor pulses, reduced left ventricular forces on ECG, cardiogenic shock, and severe cyanosis are typical of hypoplastic left heart syndrome. (See Chapter 438.10 in *Nelson Textbook of Pediatrics,* 16th ed.)

6. **C.** Supraventricular tachycardia is a frequent cause of heart failure in this age group with a structurally normal heart. (See Chapter 442.2 in *Nelson Textbook of Pediatrics,* 16th ed.)

7. **B.** Placing an iced saline bag over a neonate's face is the vagal maneuver of choice to break supraventricular tachycardia (SVT). Verapamil may decrease contractility and is dangerous in this age group. (See Chapter 442.2 in *Nelson Textbook of Pediatrics,* 16th ed.)

8. 1. **C**
   2. **D**
   3. **A**
   4. **E**
   5. **B**
   6. **G**
   7. **F**
   (See Chapter 431 in *Nelson Textbook of Pediatrics,* 16th ed.)

9. 1. **C**
   2. **A**

3. **B**
4. **E**
5. **F**
6. **D**
7. **H**
8. **G**
9. **I**
(See Chapter 429 in *Nelson Textbook of Pediatrics,* 16th ed.)

10. **C.** A large VSD with a large left-to-right shunt produces significant heart failure. The age of onset usually corresponds to the time when the normally high fetal pulmonary vascular resistance declines in the first 1–3 months of life. With decreasing pulmonary artery pressure, the left-to-right shunt increases. (See Chapter 433.6 in *Nelson Textbook of Pediatrics,* 16th ed.)

11. **C.** Balloon valvuloplasty has greatly improved the management of stenotic lesions of the pulmonic and aortic valves. (See Chapter 434.1 in *Nelson Textbook of Pediatrics,* 16th ed.)

12. **A.** Paradoxic pulse is also noted in asthma. (See Chapter 446 in *Nelson Textbook of Pediatrics,* 16th ed.)

13. **C.** Rib notching is caused by increased collateral arteries trying to supply the lower trunk and extremities and bypass the aortic coarctation. (See Chapter 434.6 in *Nelson Textbook of Pediatrics,* 16th ed.)

14. 1. **D**
    2. **B**
    3. **A**
    4. **C**
    (See Chapter 429 in *Nelson Textbook of Pediatrics,* 16th ed.)

15. 1. **B**
    2. **A**
    3. **D**
    4. **C**
    (See Chapter 429 in *Nelson Textbook of Pediatrics,* 16th ed.)

16. **B.** Most pediatric patients with an ASD are asymptomatic. Heart failure is rare in childhood. (See Chapter 433 in *Nelson Textbook of Pediatrics,* 16th ed.)

17. **D.** The atrial and/or the atrial-ventricular defects both have a higher tendency for an earlier and more rapid onset of pulmonary hypertension. The ECG of an A-V septal defect is characteristic because

of the superior left deviation of the QRS axis. (See Chapter 433 in *Nelson Textbook of Pediatrics*, 16th ed.)

18. **A.** A small VSD (<0.5 cm²) produces a loud murmur, perhaps with a thrill but no other abnormalities due to the limited left-to-right shunt. Many of these will close spontaneously. (See Chapter 435 in *Nelson Textbook of Pediatrics*, 16th ed.)

19. **C.** There is an increased risk of bacterial endocarditis with a small VSD. In addition, adult patients who have had a small but unclosed VSD may have symptoms (arrhythmias, exercise intolerance). (See Chapter 433 in *Nelson Textbook of Pediatrics*, 16th ed.)

20. **D.** A PDA often presents like a large VSD except that there is a continuous murmur and the diastolic run-off, which produces the wide pulse pressure and bounding pulses. (See Chapter 433 in *Nelson Textbook of Pediatrics*, 16th ed.)

21. **E.** Aortic stenosis without significant aortic regurgitation (insufficiency) produces an inactive precordium, normal or weak pulses, and pressure overload of the left ventricle. (See Chapter 433 in *Nelson Textbook of Pediatrics*, 16th ed.)

22. **B** and **C.** A PDA manifesting in any patient other than a premature infant does not close spontaneously. Surgery carries low morbidity and even lower mortality. However, transcatheter closure with coils or umbrellas has reduced the need for surgery in many patients. (See Chapter 433 in *Nelson Textbook of Pediatrics*, 16th ed.)

23. **E.** Echocardiology has replaced most methods of visualizing the anatomy of congenital and other heart lesions. In many circumstances, the echo diagnosis is all that is needed before surgery or other therapies. (See Chapter 434 in *Nelson Textbook of Pediatrics*, 16th ed.)

24. **C.** Critical pulmonic stenosis often presents in the neonate. Cyanosis is due to elevated right-sided pressures and right-to-left shunting at the patent former orale. (See Chapter 434 in *Nelson Textbook of Pediatrics*, 16th ed.)

25. **D.** Balloon pulmonary valvuloplasty is a remarkable nonsurgical method to dilate the valve and partially relieve the obstruction to right ventricular outflow. (See Chapter 434 in *Nelson Textbook of Pediatrics*, 16th ed.)

26. **D.** Echocardiography is essential to identify valve disease, estimate gradients, and detect signs of endocardial fibroelastosis. (See Chapter 434 in *Nelson Textbook of Pediatrics*, 16th ed.)

27. **C.** Severe aortic stenosis may develop gradually, progressing over 5–10 years. (See Chapter 434 in *Nelson Textbook of Pediatrics*, 16th ed.)

28. **E.** Rheumatic fever is acquired, whereas most cases of aortic stenosis in children in the United States are congenital. Rheumatic fever can produce aortic stenosis if there are repeated episodes that are poorly treated. (See Chapter 434 in *Nelson Textbook of Pediatrics*, 16th ed.)

29. **E.** Balloon dilatation valvotomy or surgically splitting the valve are treatments of choice. (See Chapter 434 in *Nelson Textbook of Pediatrics*, 16th ed.)

30. **D.** Splenomegaly, if present, may suggest hemolysis and anemia, which would be determined by the CBC. Splenomegaly is rare in congenital or acquired heart disease in neonates. In older children, it may suggest endocarditis. (See Chapter 434 in *Nelson Textbook of Pediatrics*, 16th ed.)

31. **E.** Coarctation in neonates is also associated with a VSD. Immediately after birth, the patent ductus provides flow to the lower extremity, bypassing the aortic obstruction. When the PDA closes, the coarctation becomes more prominent and obstructs flow. (See Chapter 434 in *Nelson Textbook of Pediatrics*, 16th ed.)

32. **D.** Hypertension may develop immediately after repair (the post-coarctotomy syndrome), or it may be delayed many years and appear as essential hypertension. (See Chapter 434 in *Nelson Textbook of Pediatrics*, 16th ed.)

33. **B.** TOF includes a VSD, pulmonary stenosis, right ventricular hypertrophy, and an overriding aorta between the two ventricles and above the VSD. In addition, 25% of patients have a right-sided aortic arch. (See Chapter 437 in *Nelson Textbook of Pediatrics*, 16th ed.)

34. **A.** Chronic hypoxia produces both the

clubbing and the polycythemia. High hematocrits (usually > 65% on a central blood sample) usually produce hyperviscosity, which impairs tissue perfusion. Therefore, up to a point, the raised hematocrit improves oxygen delivery; once hyperviscosity develops, the tissue microcirculation is compromised. (See Chapter 437 in *Nelson Textbook of Pediatrics,* 16th ed.)

35. **C.** Cerebrovascular accidents are a compilation of polycythemia and the right-to-left shunting in patients with TOF. Strokes are more common in children under 2 years of age and those with iron-deficiency anemia. Cerebral abscess formations are more common in children over 2 years of age. (See Chapter 437 in *Nelson Textbook of Pediatrics,* 16th ed.)

36. **B.** SVT in infants commonly presents with heart failure. The higher the rate and the longer the duration of SVT, the greater the risk of heart failure. (See Chapter 442 in *Nelson Textbook of Pediatrics,* 16th ed.)

37. **A.** Adenosine is the treatment of choice for all SVTs at most ages. Given by rapid intravenous infusion, it may be repeated and given with multiple doses. (See Chapter 442 in *Nelson Textbook of Pediatrics,* 16th ed.)

38. **E.** Synchronized cardioversion (0.5–2 watt sec/kg) is the treatment of choice for a patient with SVT who has poor cardiac output. It is used in urgent situations. Verapamil is dangerous in infants because its negative inotropic effects have caused cardiac arrest. (See Chapter 442 in *Nelson Textbook of Pediatrics,* 16th ed.)

39. **A.** This unusual event places the heart in asystole, which is unfortunately refractory to almost all resuscitative efforts. (See Chapter 442 in *Nelson Textbook of Pediatrics,* 16th ed.)

40. **A.** After repair of a simple ASD (secundum) or a PDA, there is no increased risk of endocarditis. (See Chapter 443 in *Nelson Textbook of Pediatrics,* 16th ed.)

41. **A.** These occur with dermatomyositis. Osler nodes occur in endocarditis. (See Chapter 443 in *Nelson Textbook of Pediatrics,* 16th ed.)

42. **D.** Pericarditis, in this child due to coxsackievirus, often presents with chest pain, tachycardia, narrow pulse pressure, and a pulsus paradoxus. The chest x-ray demonstrates cardiomegaly, which can be enlargement due to myocardial dilatation or expansion of the pericardial space from fluid. (See Chapter 446 in *Nelson Textbook of Pediatrics,* 16th ed.)

43. **E.** Immune complex and other immune mechanisms may produce a pericardial effusion, pericarditis, and rarely cardiac tamponade. (See Chapter 446 in *Nelson Textbook of Pediatrics,* 16th ed.)

20 *Diseases of the Blood*

1. **A.** A complete blood count (CBC) reveals a hemoglobin value of 12 g/dL, a white blood cell (WBC) count of 11,000, and a platelet count of 5000. (See Chapter 489 in *Nelson Textbook of Pediatrics,* 16th ed.)

2. **D.** Idiopathic thrombocytopenia (ITP) or autoimmune thrombocytopenia is an acute process that often follows an upper respiratory tract infection. Leukemia is always a worrisome possibility but is extremely unusual in the absence of anemia, leukopenia or blasts, lymphadenopathy, or hepatosplenomegaly. (See Chapter 489.4 in *Nelson Textbook of Pediatrics,* 16th ed.)

3. **B.** The boy described in the question has hemophilia A. His factor VIII level was 4%, which is in the moderate severity category. (See Chapter 482 in *Nelson Textbook of Pediatrics,* 16th ed.)

4. **D.** (See Chapter 482 in *Nelson Textbook of Pediatrics,* 16th ed.)

5. **B.** Factor VIII antibodies (IgG) develop in 10–15% of patients with hemophilia and are not related to the number of replacement therapies. (See Chapter 482 in *Nelson Textbook of Pediatrics,* 16th ed.)

6. **D.** Methemoglobinemia presents with intense cyanosis, desaturated hemoglobin, chocolate-colored blood, but a normal Pao_2. Treatment for significant methemoglobinemia includes methylene blue. Methemoglobinemia can be measured in the blood sample;

subsequent studies are needed to determine if this is a defect in the hemoglobin (hemoglobin M) or more likely in the NADH cytochrome b5 reductase system. (See Chapter 468 in *Nelson Textbook of Pediatrics,* 16th ed.)

7. 1. **D**
   2. **E**
   3. **F**
   4. **A**
   5. **G**
   6. **B**
   7. **C**
   (See Section 3, Part 20 in *Nelson Textbook of Pediatrics,* 16th ed.)

8. 1. **A**
   2. **B**
   3. **A**
   4. **B**
   5. **C**
   6. **A**
   7. **C**
   8. **B**
   (See Chapter 453 in *Nelson Textbook of Pediatrics,* 16th ed.)

9. 1. **A**
   2. **D**
   3. **B**
   4. **A**
   5. **B**
   (See Chapters 454 and 455 in *Nelson Textbook of Pediatrics,* 16th ed.)

10. **A.** This is a classic case of iron-deficiency anemia, undoubtedly nutritional in origin. Pica is a common symptom and makes lead poisoning a possible diagnosis but not the most likely diagnosis. (See Chapter 461 in *Nelson Textbook of Pediatrics,* 16th ed.)

11. **B.** Reticulocytosis peaks at 5–7 days. (See Chapter 461 in *Nelson Textbook of Pediatrics,* 16th ed.)

12. **C.** Stores of iron need to be repleted, and 4–8 weeks is required. (See Chapter 461 in *Nelson Textbook of Pediatrics,* 16th ed.)

13. **A, B,** and **E.** Sickle cell anemia is not usually seen in Caucasians, and urinary tract infection is highly unlikely in an otherwise healthy boy. (See Chapter 461 in *Nelson Textbook of Pediatrics,* 16th ed.)

14. 1. **B.** Purpura, but with normal counts
    2. **B.** Adhesiveness is impaired

3. **A.** Idiopathic thrombocytopenic purpura, obviously
4. **A.** Also, eczema and immune deficiency are present
5. **C.** Thrombocytosis is common
6. **A.** Platelets are consumed along with the coagulation factors
7. **A.** The name *thrombotic thrombocytopenic purpura* gives the answer again
8. **A.** On the basis of trapping of the platelets in the cavernous hemangioma
(See Chapter 489 in *Nelson Textbook of Pediatrics,* 16th ed.)

15. **E.** The risk of infection with pneumococci is greatly increased and may last for the life of the patient. Prophylaxis with penicillin is recommended. (See Chapter 493 in *Nelson Textbook of Pediatrics,* 16th ed.)

16. **D.** Oxidant drug-induced hemolysis with anemia and hemoglobinuria is common in G-6-PD–deficient patients. (See Chapter 469.3 in *Nelson Textbook of Pediatrics,* 16th ed.)

17. **B.** The enzyme assay is of value, but results may be falsely normal immediately after a hemolytic episode because younger cells may have normal G-6-PD levels. (See Chapter 469.3 in *Nelson Textbook of Pediatrics,* 16th ed.)

18. **B.** No treatment is required unless the anemia worsens and a transfusion is then needed. Forced diuresis is needed to prevent hemoglobinuric renal failure. (See Chapter 469.3 in *Nelson Textbook of Pediatrics,* 16th ed.)

19. **E.** Immune-mediated hemolysis often produces spherocytes. (See Chapter 470 in *Nelson Textbook of Pediatrics,* 16th ed.)

20. **D.** The Coombs tests detect antibody directed against RBCs. Further analysis determines the IgM or IgG nature of the autoantibodies. (See Chapter 470 in *Nelson Textbook of Pediatrics,* 16th ed.)

21. **D.** Many would begin prednisone as the initial treatment of choice for autoimmune hemolytic anemia, and some would use IVIG. (See Chapter 470 in *Nelson Textbook of Pediatrics,* 16th ed.)

22. **A.** The risk of pneumococcal sepsis and meningitis is much higher in patients

with sickle cell anemia. Prophylactic antibiotics begun as soon as possible significantly reduce this risk, even in this era of resistant pneumococci. (See Chapter 468.1 in *Nelson Textbook of Pediatrics,* 16th ed.)

23. **D.** Factor VII is an important coagulation factor of the extrinsic or tissue coagulation pathway. This factor is called *stable factor.* (See Chapter 483 in *Nelson Textbook of Pediatrics,* 16th ed.)

24. **C.** The bleeding time tests the platelet vascular endothelium interaction, and results are abnormal in conditions with thrombocytopenia, platelet dysfunction, or abnormal endothelium. (See Chapter 489 in *Nelson Textbook of Pediatrics,* 16th ed.)

25. **C.** Idiopathic thrombocytopenia purpura is an autoimmune process due to production of IgG antibodies against antigens on all platelets. Although splenectomy may improve the mother's platelet count, the autoimmune production of antiplatelet antibodies persists. Because IgG actively crossed the placenta, fetal and neonatal thrombocytopenia develops because of the presence of antiplatelet antibodies. (See Chapter 489.4 in *Nelson Textbook of Pediatrics,* 16th ed.)

26. **A.** TFR (serum transferrin receptor) levels are elevated in ineffective erythropoiesis and in iron deficiency but are reduced in bone marrow failure. (See Chapter 453 in *Nelson Textbook of Pediatrics,* 16th ed.)

27. **E.** Mutations of the EPO gene have not been identified after extensive investigation. (See Chapter 454 in *Nelson Textbook of Pediatrics,* 16th ed.)

28. **B.** Despite an association of poor nutrient balance, obesity is not commonly associated with iron deficiency. (See Chapter 461 in *Nelson Textbook of Pediatrics,* 16th ed.)

29. **B.** Chromosome breaks are common and can be induced in the laboratory. (See Chapter 474 in *Nelson Textbook of Pediatrics,* 16th ed.)

30. **D.** Immune-mediated thrombocytopenia (idiopathic thrombocytopenic purpura—ITP) rarely requires platelet

transfusion, especially in the absence of clinical bleeding or an invasive procedure. Intravenous immunoglobulin, oral prednisone, or no therapy is usually effective. Remember to avoid drugs that interfere with platelet function such as the various NSAIDs. (See Chapter 477 in *Nelson Textbook of Pediatrics,* 16th ed.)

31. **E.** The reptilase time is similar to the thrombin time except, in contrast with the thrombin time, the reptilase time is not influenced by the presence of heparin. (See Chapter 481 in *Nelson Textbook of Pediatrics,* 16th ed.)

32. **D.** This, plus a prothrombin mutation (G20210A), is the most common genetic cause of thrombophilia identified to date. (See Chapter 484 in *Nelson Textbook of Pediatrics,* 16th ed.)

33. **E.** TB is an uncommon cause of these hematologic problems. A Coombs test result will be positive in SLE and Evans syndrome (hemolytic anemia and immune thrombocytopenia). In some patients, Evans syndrome evolves into SLE. (See Chapter 490 in *Nelson Textbook of Pediatrics,* 16th ed.)

34. **D.** Wiskott-Aldrich syndrome, an immune deficiency syndrome, shares the gene for simple X-linked thrombocytopenia. (See Chapter 490 in *Nelson Textbook of Pediatrics,* 16th ed.)

35. 1. **B**
    2. **C**
    3. **A**
    4. **D**
    (See Chapter 496 in *Nelson Textbook of Pediatrics,* 16th ed.)

21 *Neoplastic Diseases and Tumors*

1. **C.** Chest radiography is important for two reasons, first to document mediastinal involvement and second to determine whether these lymph nodes threaten the patency of the airway. (See Chapter 503 in *Nelson Textbook of Pediatrics,* 16th ed.)

2. **D.** At this time, a lymph node biopsy can confirm suspicion of Hodgkin disease. Thereafter, CT scans and bone marrow biopsy are useful in staging the extent of

the lymph node and extranodal involvement. (See Chapter 503 in *Nelson Textbook of Pediatrics*, 16th ed.)

3. 1. **C**
    2. **A**
    3. **B**
    4. **A**
    5. **A**
    6. **A**
    7. **D**
    8. **B**
    9. **B**
    10. **A**
    11. **B**

(See Chapter 505 in *Nelson Textbook of Pediatrics*, 16th ed.)

4. **D.** Orbital rhabdomyosarcoma is a common site for rhabdomyosarcoma, which produces local signs as it grows and displaces normal tissues. (See Chapter 506 in *Nelson Textbook of Pediatrics*, 16th ed.)

5. 1. **A**
    2. **C**
    3. **B**
    4. **C**
    5. **A**
    6. **B**
    7. **D**
    8. **A**
    9. **C**
    10. **B**

(See Chapter 507 in *Nelson Textbook of Pediatrics*, 16th ed.)

6. **E.** Cases such as the one described in the question raise a suspicion of retinoblastoma and warrant immediate attention and visualization. A CT examination may also identify this ocular tumor. (See Chapter 508 in *Nelson Textbook of Pediatrics*, 16th ed.)

7. 1. **D**
    2. **A**
    3. **B**
    4. **C**
    5. **F**
    6. **D**
    7. **E**

(See Chapter 497 in *Nelson Textbook of Pediatrics*, 16th ed.)

8. **A.** Only about 1% of new cases of cancer in the United States occur in children, yet malignancy remains the major cause of

death due to disease between the ages of 1 and 15 years. (See Chapter 497 in *Nelson Textbook of Pediatrics*, 16th ed.)

9. 1. **F**
    2. **E**
    3. **B**
    4. **D**
    5. **A**
    6. **C**

(See Chapter 498 in *Nelson Textbook of Pediatrics*, 16th ed.)

10. 1. **C**
    2. **A**
    3. **F**
    4. **B**
    5. **E**
    6. **D**

(See Chapter 498 in *Nelson Textbook of Pediatrics*, 16th ed.)

11. **E.** Epstein-Barr virus is associated with Hodgkin disease, African (endemic) Burkitt lymphoma, nasopharyngeal carcinoma, post-transplantation lymphoma, lymphoma in persons with congenital immunodeficiencies (e.g., X-linked lymphoproliferative syndrome), and leiomyosarcomas in immunocompromised persons. (See Chapter 489 in *Nelson Textbook of Pediatrics*, 16th ed.)

12. **E.** Anticancer therapy can result in substantial breakdown of tumor cells (tumor lysis syndrome) with release of large quantities of phosphates and potassium into the circulation. Hypocalcemia can result in the setting of inadequate renal function. (See Chapter 501.1 in *Nelson Textbook of Pediatrics*, 16th ed.)

13. **C.** Many sequelae of radiation do not become apparent until the child is fully grown. Irradiation can result in infertility, second cancers, scoliosis, pulmonary fibrosis, leukoencephalopathy, impaired cognition and intelligence, hypothyroidism, isolated growth hormone deficiency, and panhypopituitarism. Cardiomyopathy is classically associated with the anthracyclines (doxorubicin and daunomycin). (See Chapter 501.3 in *Nelson Textbook of Pediatrics*, 16th ed.)

14. **D.** Cells for autologous transplantation (after removal of cancer cells) are

obtained from the patient. Cells for syngeneic transplantation are obtained from an identical twin. Cells for allogeneic transplantation are obtained from a nonidentical person. (See Chapter 501.4 in *Nelson Textbook of Pediatrics,* 16th ed.)

15. **E.** The clinical features of the childhood leukemias are similar, because all involve severe disruption of bone marrow function. There is marked variability in responses to therapy and prognosis. (See Chapter 502 in *Nelson Textbook of Pediatrics,* 16th ed.)

16. **B.** The French-American-British (FAB) system distinguishes three morphologic subtypes (L1, L2, and L3). Only the L3 subtype appears to be clinically meaningful. Because most patients present with disseminated disease that involves the bone marrow, spleen, liver, and lymph nodes, there is no anatomic staging system. (See Chapter 502 in *Nelson Textbook of Pediatrics,* 16th ed.)

17. **E.** Most children with leukemia present with less than 4 weeks of symptoms. Most children with ALL have pallor, 50% have petechiae or mucous membrane bleeding, 60% have lymphadenopathy, 25% have fever, and about 25% have bone pain and arthralgias caused by leukemic infiltration of the perichondral bone or joint or by leukemic expansion of the marrow cavity. (See Chapter 502 in *Nelson Textbook of Pediatrics,* 16th ed.)

18. **D.** The T-cell immunophenotype is associated with higher risk of relapse with childhood ALL than the more common B-cell immunophenotype. (See Chapter 502 in *Nelson Textbook of Pediatrics,* 16th ed.)

19. **E.** The most important extramedullary sites of relapse of ALL are the central nervous system and the testes. (See Chapter 502.1 in *Nelson Textbook of Pediatrics,* 16th ed.)

20. **C.** Neonates and infants with Down syndrome may experience transient myeloproliferative syndrome, which mimics congenital leukemia. These children have a higher incidence of subsequent acute leukemia, especially the acute megakaryocytic subtype of myeloid leukemia. (See Chapter 502.4 in *Nelson Textbook of Pediatrics,* 16th ed.)

21. **C.** The Philadelphia chromosome is associated with chronic myelogenous leukemia. (See Chapter 502.5 in *Nelson Textbook of Pediatrics,* 16th ed.)

22. **C.** The Philadelphia chromosome is associated with chronic myelogenous leukemia. (See Chapter 502.5 in *Nelson Textbook of Pediatrics,* 16th ed.)

23. **D.** Most neuroblastomas arise in the abdomen, either in the adrenal gland or in retroperitoneal sympathetic ganglia. Catecholamine production may cause hypertension, whereas other vasoactive substances may produce a secretory diarrhea. (See Chapter 504 in *Nelson Textbook of Pediatrics,* 16th ed.)

24. **A.** Children with neuroblastoma with early-stage disease without *mycn* or chromosome 1p deletion can usually be cured with surgery alone. Children < 1 year of age have a 95% 3-year survival rate, compared with 25–50% for children 1–5 years of age. (See Chapter 504 in *Nelson Textbook of Pediatrics,* 16th ed.)

25. **C.** Wilms tumor accounts for most renal neoplasms in children. (See Chapter 505 in *Nelson Textbook of Pediatrics,* 16th ed.)

26. **D.** The highest risk period for development of osteosarcoma is during the adolescent growth spurt. (See Chapter 507 in *Nelson Textbook of Pediatrics,* 16th ed.)

27. **B.** Pain and swelling are the most common presenting symptoms of osteosarcoma and Ewing sarcoma. Osteosarcoma has a characteristic sunburst pattern on x-ray. Ewing sarcoma is associated with periosteal elevation, or "onion-skinning," on x-ray. (See Chapter 507 in *Nelson Textbook of Pediatrics,* 16th ed.)

28. **A.** Retinoblastoma occurs in 1 of 18,000 live births in the United States. (See Chapter 508 in *Nelson Textbook of Pediatrics,* 16th ed.)

29. **B.** Hepatic tumors are rare in children, accounting for 1% of malignancies in childhood. Approximately two thirds of hepatic tumors in children are hepatoblastomas. (See Chapter 510 in *Nelson Textbook of Pediatrics,* 16th ed.)

30. **D.** Osteochondroma (exostosis) is one of the most common benign bone tumors in children. Many are asymptomatic or are detected when the child or parent notes a bony, nonpainful mass. Most arise in the metaphyses of long bones. (See Chapter 514 in *Nelson Textbook of Pediatrics,* 16th ed.)

31. **C.** Kasabach-Merritt syndrome is trapping of platelet and red blood cells within a hemangioma with activation of the clotting system within the vasculature of the hemangioma. (See Chapter 514.2 in *Nelson Textbook of Pediatrics,* 16th ed.)

32. **D.** For hemangiomas that are life threatening or that threaten vital functions such as eyesight, a trial of oral corticosteroids is warranted. Approximately 30% respond dramatically and begin to regress within a week, 40% stabilize or show minimal response, and the remainder do not respond. Other possible treatments for hemangiomas that do not respond to corticosteroids include interferon, laser therapy, or surgery. (See Chapter 514.2 in *Nelson Textbook of Pediatrics,* 16th ed.)

33. **C.** Leukocoria (white pupillary reflex) and strabismus are often the presenting signs of retinoblastoma.

22 *Nephrology*

1. **C.** The name gives the answer away. (See Chapter 526 in *Nelson Textbook of Pediatrics,* 16th ed.)

2. **D.** The abdominal mass in the patient described in the question is likely to be hydronephrosis. (See Chapter 546 in *Nelson Textbook of Pediatrics,* 16th ed.)

3. 1. **A**
   2. **B**
   3. **C**
   4. **A**
   5. **D**
   (See Chapters 519–525 in *Nelson Textbook of Pediatrics,* 16th ed.)

4. **C.** Hypoalbuminemia, proteinuria, edema, and hyperlipidemia constitute the nephrotic syndrome. Hypertension, azotemia, edema, or hematuria would suggest nephritis but may also be encountered in minimal lesion nephrotic syndrome. This patient has nephrotic syndrome, not nephritis. (See Chapter 535 in *Nelson Textbook of Pediatrics,* 16th ed.)

5. **E.** What is most remarkable is the pressure of hemoglobinuria but only 0–3 RBCs. (See Chapter 517 in *Nelson Textbook of Pediatrics,* 16th ed.)

6. **A.** Influenza-induced myositis presents with myalgia (often the calf muscles), fever, and red urine due to myoglobinuria. The last is a positive sign of hemoglobin on urine biochemical testing. Myoglobinuria may produce tubular injury and acute renal failure. Other causes of red urine include porphyrias beets, rifampin, deferoxamine, and blackberries. (See Chapter 517 in *Nelson Textbook of Pediatrics,* 16th ed.)

7. **C.** This form of nephritis rarely results with asymptomatic hematuria but in 50% of cases may manifest initially as acute renal failure. (See Chapter 517 in *Nelson Textbook of Pediatrics,* 16th ed.)

8. **A.** The onset is rapid if preceded by a URI. Poststreptococcal glomerulonephritis has a latent period of 7–12 days after the streptococcal infection. (See Chapter 518 in *Nelson Textbook of Pediatrics,* 16th ed.)

9. **C.** In contrast with poststreptococcal nephritis and lupus, IgA nephropathy has normal serum complement levels. (See Chapter 518 in *Nelson Textbook of Pediatrics,* 16th ed.)

10. **A.** This X-linked-dominant disorder produces end-stage renal disease in the 2nd to 3rd decade of life. Females usually have a normal life span. Any patient with renal failure or hematuria and hearing loss should be suspected of Alport syndrome. Renal biopsy confirms this diagnosis. (See Chapter 518 in *Nelson Textbook of Pediatrics,* 16th ed.)

11. **A.** Hypercalcemia must make one consider hyperparathyroidism or vitamin D intoxication. (See Chapter 518 in *Nelson Textbook of Pediatrics,* 16th ed.)

12. **E.** Poststrept GN is the most common cause of hypocomplementemic nephritis. Other causes include SLE, serum sickness, membranoproliferative

glomerulonephritis, bacterial endocarditis, and other postinfectious glomerulonephritides. (See Chapter 519 in *Nelson Textbook of Pediatrics,* 16th ed.)

13. **A.** Penicillin therapy does not prevent poststreptococcal glomerulonephritis but does stop the spread of the organism to others. This is true whether the streptococcal infection is impetigo or pharyngitis. (See Chapter 519 in *Nelson Textbook of Pediatrics,* 16th ed.)

14. **B.** DIC is rare, whereas local (toxin-mediated) endothelial cell injury and intrarenal thrombosis with thrombocytopenia are the general rule. (See Chapter 526 in *Nelson Textbook of Pediatrics,* 16th ed.)

15. **A.** Fomites are a rare cause of spread of *E. coli* and HUS. Nonetheless, hand-to-mouth, person-to-person spread may occur as evidenced by outbreaks in nursing homes. (See Chapter 526 in *Nelson Textbook of Pediatrics,* 16th ed.)

16. **E.** HUS with its associated renal failure, hypertension, hematuria, and normal albumin level is easily distinguished from nephrotic syndrome. (See Chapter 526 in *Nelson Textbook of Pediatrics,* 16th ed.)

17. **C.** Because of renal protein loss and hypoalbuminemia, there is reduced intravascular volume. This stimulates the renin-angiotensin system, resulting in enhanced renal sodium reabsorption. Eventually, the sodium partially contributes to the edema. (See Chapter 535 in *Nelson Textbook of Pediatrics,* 16th ed.)

18. **D.** Unfortunately, only 15–20% of cases respond to steroid therapy. This disease is progressive and often leads to end-stage renal disease. (See Chapter 535 in *Nelson Textbook of Pediatrics,* 16th ed.)

19. **D.** In the second half of the first year of life, one would expect to start to see minimal change idiopathic nephrotic syndrome. Drash syndrome is nephropathy, Wilms tumor, and genital anomalies. (See Chapter 535 in *Nelson Textbook of Pediatrics,* 16th ed.)

20.   1. **E**
    2. **A**
    3. **B**
    4. **A**

    5. **C**
    6. **D**
    7. **A**
    8. **B**
    9. **A**
  10. **C**
  11. **B**
  12. **A**
(See Chapter 537 in *Nelson Textbook of Pediatrics,* 16th ed.)

21. **G.** Diseases that interfere with ADH action (**A, B, C, E, F**) or ADH production (destruction of hypothalamic-pituitary region) produce diabetes insipidus. Nephrogenic diabetes insipidus is an X-linked disorder presenting in infancy with recurrent episodes of hypernatremic dehydration, polyuria, and very dilute urine (specific gravity of 1.001). (See Chapter 538 in *Nelson Textbook of Pediatrics,* 16th ed.)

22.   1. **C**
    2. **C**
    3. **C**
    4. **B**
    5. **B**
    6. **D**
(See Chapter 539 in *Nelson Textbook of Pediatrics,* 16th ed.)

23.   1. **C**
    2. **B**
    3. **A**
    4. **B**
    5. **B**
    6. **A**
    7. **A**
    8. **D**
(See Chapter 543 in *Nelson Textbook of Pediatrics,* 16th ed.)

24. **D.** Anemia is not a cause of seizures and is unusual in acute renal failure in the absence of hemolyte uremic syndrome, blood loss, or SLE. (See Chapter 543 in *Nelson Textbook of Pediatrics,* 16th ed.)

25. **E.** Indeed, clotting of vascular access sites has been reported. (See Chapter 543 in *Nelson Textbook of Pediatrics,* 16th ed.)

23 *Urologic Disorders in Infants and Children*

1. **F.** Primarily encountered in renal agenesis or dysplasia, the Potter

phenotype (flattened face, broad nose, low-set ears, receding chin, clubfoot) is also due to severe oligohydramnios. (See Chapter 545 in *Nelson Textbook of Pediatrics,* 16th ed.)

2. **E.** Chronic use of antibiotics is not a risk factor for urinary tract infection. All the other choices listed in the question are significant risks. (See Chapter 546 in *Nelson Textbook of Pediatrics,* 16th ed.)

3. **A.** A DMSA radionuclide scan helps to define photopenic images, which are accurate representations of chronic renal scarring. (See Chapter 546 in *Nelson Textbook of Pediatrics,* 16th ed.)

4. **A.** Renal masses are the most common lesions in neonates with an abdominal mass. Hydronephrosis and multicystic-dysplastic lesions are the most common renal masses. (See Chapter 545 in *Nelson Textbook of Pediatrics,* 16th ed.)

5. **B.** Renal agenesis results in no fetal urine output, resulting in oligohydramnios. The reduced amniotic fluid produces fetal constraint and compression, resulting in the abnormal physical features (**C, D, E**). (See Chapter 545 in *Nelson Textbook of Pediatrics,* 16th ed.)

6. **C.** Multicystic dysplastic kidneys are not inherited. In contrast, polycystic kidneys are bilateral and are either autosomal dominant (adult) or autosomal recessive (child) traits. (See Chapter 545 in *Nelson Textbook of Pediatrics,* 16th ed.)

7. **B.** Renal ultrasonography demonstrates a small left kidney with a deep groove in the lateral convexity of the kidney. The Doppler scan of blood flow in the renal arteries appears normal. (See Chapter 545 in *Nelson Textbook of Pediatrics,* 16th ed.)

8. **C.** Segmental hypoplasia, or Ask-Upmark kidney, produces severe hypertension, usually beginning at age 10 years when identified on routine examination. Nephrectomy is the treatment of choice. (See Chapter 545 in *Nelson Textbook of Pediatrics,* 16th ed.)

9. **E.** *E. coli* and other gram-negative enteric pathogens (e.g., *Proteus, Klebsiella*) are the most common pathogens for UTIs at all ages. (See Chapter 546 in *Nelson Textbook of Pediatrics,* 16th ed.)

10. **C.** Cystitis is not usually associated with fever. If there is fever, chills, or rigors, suspect pyelonephritis with or without urosepsis. (See Chapter 546 in *Nelson Textbook of Pediatrics,* 16th ed.)

11. **E.** HSP is not a risk factor for UTI. Other risks include bubble bath, wiping from back to front, reflux, instrumentation, tight underwear, and those listed in Question 9. (See Chapter 546 in *Nelson Textbook of Pediatrics,* 16th ed.)

12. **D** and **E,** possibly **C.** Renal ultrasonography demonstrates renal anomalies, obstruction, renal enlargement (pyelonephritis), or renal abscess. Unfortunately, it misses many renal scars. A VCUG is needed because vesicoureteral reflux is a common cause of UTI in children less than 6 years of age. A DMSA scan identifies acute pyelonephritis (if pyelonephritis is evident clinically, the role for DMSA is less important). A DMSA scan also shows scarring and is valuable to follow the progression of scarring and the possible need for further intervention. (See Chapter 546 in *Nelson Textbook of Pediatrics,* 16th ed.)

13. **E.** All the rest are important risk factors for reflux. Of note, approximately 35% of siblings of a child with reflux have reflux; 50% of the children of a mother with reflux have reflux. Reflux (primary) is uncommon in African-American children. (See Chapter 547 in *Nelson Textbook of Pediatrics,* 16th ed.)

14. **D.** Posterior urethral values may be detected by in utero ultrasound examinations or after birth if there is a big bladder, poor stream, UTI, or failure to thrive. Every parent of every boy should be questioned about the baby's urinary stream. (See Chapter 548 in *Nelson Textbook of Pediatrics,* 16th ed.)

15. **A.** This is a classic presentation of the pediatric unstable bladder. The bladder is smaller than normal and exhibits strong uninhibited contractions. Constipation and UTI may complicate the disorder. Treatment is with frequent, timed voiding and anticholinergic drugs. (See Chapter 551 in *Nelson Textbook of Pediatrics,* 16th ed.)

16. **C.** This child has testicular torsion until proven otherwise. If not relieved, testicular infarction may result in a necrotic organ in a sexually active male. Gonorrhea or chlamydia epididymitis must also be considered. (See Chapter 553 in *Nelson Textbook of Pediatrics*, 16th ed.)

24 *Gynecologic Problems in Childhood*

1. **C.** Patients with spontaneous galactorrhea should be screened by determining their prolactin level. (See Chapter 559 in *Nelson Textbook of Pediatrics*, 16th ed.)
2. **A.** Magnetic resonance imaging (MRI) or computed tomography (CT) of the cranium demonstrates a pituitary prolactinoma. Hypothyroidism also produces hyperprolactinemia and galactorrhea. The treatment of some small prolactinomas includes bromocriptine (Parlodel). Larger or persistently symptomatic lesions require surgery. (See Chapter 559 in *Nelson Textbook of Pediatrics*, 16th ed.)
3. 1. **B**
   2. **C**
   3. **D**
   4. **E**
   5. **A**
   (See Chapter 557 in *Nelson Textbook of Pediatrics*, 16th ed.)
4. **A.** Nonspecific vaginitis most often occurs in prepubertal girls who wear tight-fitting clothing (leotards) or are exposed to vaginal irritants (soaps) or have poor hygiene. It is often due to coliform bacteria or group A *Streptococcus.* (See Chapter 557 in *Nelson Textbook of Pediatrics*, 16th ed.)
5. **E.** Metronidazole is not indicated for this form of nonspecific vaginitis. If the process is recurrent, amoxicillin may be of value in addition to the suggestions in choices **A–D.** (See Chapter 557 in *Nelson Textbook of Pediatrics*, 16th ed.)
6. **A.** This type of vaginitis usually improves at puberty as the vaginal mucosa changes and the pH becomes more acidic. (See Chapter 557 in *Nelson Textbook of Pediatrics*, 16th ed.)
7. **E.** This is a disease that responds to supportive hygienic care and does not require antibiotics. In addition, because it occurs in young girls, tetracycline should not be given. (See Chapter 557 in *Nelson Textbook of Pediatrics*, 16th ed.)
8. **D.** Topical estrogen cream each evening for 1 week is effective in over 90% of cases. Further cleaning followed by petroleum ointment for 1–2 months helps prevent recurrences. (See Chapter 557 in *Nelson Textbook of Pediatrics*, 16th ed.)
9. **F.** This is very unlikely in the absence of any physical secondary sexual characterization of puberty (pubic hair, breast development). (See Chapter 558 in *Nelson Textbook of Pediatrics*, 16th ed.)
10. **B.** Breast pain occurs in cyclical patterns at the time of each menstrual cycle. (See Chapter 559 in *Nelson Textbook of Pediatrics*, 16th ed.)
11. **C.** Prolactin levels were markedly elevated. (See Chapter 559 in *Nelson Textbook of Pediatrics*, 16th ed.)
12. **C.** The head CT demonstrates a prolactinoma. (See Chapter 559 in *Nelson Textbook of Pediatrics*, 16th ed.)
13. **B.** Parlodel inhibits prolactin secretion and markedly reduces the size of the tumor. Surgery is rarely needed. (See Chapter 559 in *Nelson Textbook of Pediatrics*, 16th ed.)
14. **B.** Teratomas are usually benign but rarely are malignant. Calcification suggests the lesion is benign. (See Chapter 561 in *Nelson Textbook of Pediatrics*, 16th ed.)
15. **B.** X-Y gonadal dysgenesis carries a very high risk for this cancer, and this requires elective removal of the gonad. (See Chapter 561 in *Nelson Textbook of Pediatrics*, 16th ed.)
16. **B.** DES is an in utero carcinogen. (See Chapter 561 in *Nelson Textbook of Pediatrics*, 16th ed.)

25 *The Endocrine System*

1. 1. **C**
   2. **D**
   3. **A**
   4. **B**

5. **E**
(See Chapter 585 in *Nelson Textbook of Pediatrics,* 16th ed.)

2. **D.** Type I autoimmune polyendocrinopathy—also known as autoimmune polyendocrinopathy candidiasis, ectodermal dystrophy (APECED)—is associated with hypoparathyroidism, hypothyroidism, and Addison disease. (See Chapter 585 in *Nelson Textbook of Pediatrics,* 16th ed.)

3. 1. **D**
   2. **D**
   3. **C**
   4. **D**
   5. **A**
   6. **B**
   7. **B**
   8. **D**
(See Chapter 588 in *Nelson Textbook of Pediatrics,* 16th ed.)

4. **B.** Hypergonadotropic hypogonadism may result from testicular damage any time after the end of the first trimester. Absent or small testes and low serum testosterone levels are additional findings. (See Chapter 593 in *Nelson Textbook of Pediatrics,* 16th ed.)

5. **A.** The problem described in the question is transient and compatible with the physiology of puberty in normal males. Indeed, as many as 60% of boys have some degree of pubertal gynecomastia. Some cases are familial. (See Chapter 595 in *Nelson Textbook of Pediatrics,* 16th ed.)

6. 1. **A**
   2. **B**
   3. **B**
   4. **A**
   5. **B**
   6. **A**
   7. **C**
   8. **A**
   9. **C**
   10. **D**
(See Chapter 599 in *Nelson Textbook of Pediatrics,* 16th ed.)

7. **B.** For the patient described in the question, the serum total calcium is 6.0 mg/dL, the phosphorus level is 8.5 mg/dL, and the albumin is normal. (See Chapter 581 in *Nelson Textbook of Pediatrics,* 16th ed.)

8. **C.** Hyperparathyroidism is not an associated risk for acquired hypothyroidism. (See Chapter 575 in *Nelson Textbook of Pediatrics,* 16th ed.)

9. **B.** Patients with hyperthyroidism have heat intolerance because of their hypermetabolism. (See Chapter 578 in *Nelson Textbook of Pediatrics,* 16th ed.)

10. **C.** In patients with McCune-Albright syndrome, the insulin stimulation pathway is unaffected. However, because of a mis-sense mutation in the gene for the α-subunit of the G protein, which stimulates cyclic AMP, there is activation of these ACTH, TSH, LH, and FSH receptors. (See Chapter 572 in *Nelson Textbook of Pediatrics,* 16th ed.)

11. **F.** *Mycobacterium tuberculosis* may produce diabetes insipidus; atypical mycobacteria do not. (See Chapter 568 in *Nelson Textbook of Pediatrics,* 16th ed.)

12. **E.** Choices **A–D** in the question are true, but the mechanism of this growth delay is not known. Constitutional growth delay is not genetic short stature because these children may attain normal adult stature. (See Chapter 567 in *Nelson Textbook of Pediatrics,* 16th ed.)

13. **A.** Reassurance about lack of menarche is appropriate at age 14. Workup should be begun after 16 years of age. (See Chapter 571 in *Nelson Textbook of Pediatrics,* 16th ed.)

14. **A.** (See Chapter 585 in *Nelson Textbook of Pediatrics,* 16th ed.)

15. **A** and **B.** This is a case of Addison disease, and replacement therapy with both DOCA and hydrocortisone is necessary. (See Chapter 585 in *Nelson Textbook of Pediatrics,* 16th ed.)

16. **D.** Toxoplasmosis does not produce congenital anomalies. Holoprosencephaly, however, is a marker for pituitary hormone deficiencies. (See Chapter 567 in *Nelson Textbook of Pediatrics,* 16th ed.)

17. **E.** This is another syndrome that should suggest pituitary hormone deficiency. (See Chapter 567 in *Nelson Textbook of Pediatrics,* 16th ed.)

18. **E.** Again facial anomalies, especially if

short stature is present, suggest pituitary and thus growth hormone deficiency. (See Chapter 567 in *Nelson Textbook of Pediatrics*, 16th ed.)

19. **A.** Most children with isolated GH deficiency are of normal length and weight at birth. Those with multiple pituitary hormone deficiencies may demonstrate a shorter length. By 1 year of age, the children appear short but are not thin or wasted, as occurs in severe caloric deprivation. (See Chapter 567 in *Nelson Textbook of Pediatrics*, 16th ed.)

20. **E.** This is incorrect because calcium homeostasis and parathyroid hormone metabolism are not affected by GH. Nonetheless, whenever GH deficiency is suspected, other hormone levels should be determined (thyroid, cortisol, TSH) to look for panhypopituitarism. (See Chapter 567 in *Nelson Textbook of Pediatrics*, 16th ed.)

21. **E.** Wolfram syndrome (autosomal recessive or mitochondrial disorder on chromosome 4), destructive tumors, and mutations of the vasopressin, neurophysin gene on chromosome 20 are associated causes of central DI. (See Chapter 568 in *Nelson Textbook of Pediatrics*, 16th ed.)

22. **E.** Long-standing polyuria can produce these urologic findings. If the patient has access to large quantities of free water, hypernatremia as well as dehydration can be prevented. (See Chapter 568 in *Nelson Textbook of Pediatrics*, 16th ed.)

23. **E.** Most patients have some degree of mental retardation. Perceptual deficits are also common. (See Chapter 570 in *Nelson Textbook of Pediatrics*, 16th ed.)

24. **E.** Although theoretically feasible, this is not a reported cause of precocious puberty. (See Chapter 572 in *Nelson Textbook of Pediatrics*, 16th ed.)

25. **E.** Central precocious puberty involves idiopathic release of LH and a normal, albeit early, progression of puberty. (See Chapter 572 in *Nelson Textbook of Pediatrics*, 16th ed.)

26. **C** or **B.** In the absence of neurologic or visual signs, a pituitary or hypothalamic lesion is highly unlikely. In girls, the risk

of such a lesion is low; in boys, the risk of identifying a CNS lesion is 25–75%. In addition, the lesions are seldom malignant and rarely require neurosurgical intervention. (See Chapter 572 in *Nelson Textbook of Pediatrics*, 16th ed.)

27. **A.** Long-acting GnRH analogs in depot form help prevent gonadotropic cell release of their hormones, thus abating the early onset of puberty. (See Chapter 572 in *Nelson Textbook of Pediatrics*, 16th ed.)

28. **D.** TBG deficiency is an X-linked dominant disorder. The serum-free T_4 is normal. TBG deficiency occurs in 1 in 2400 males and is confused with congenital hypothyroidism because the total T_4 is low (not the free or active T_4). (See Chapter 574 in *Nelson Textbook of Pediatrics*, 16th ed.)

29. **D.** These autoantibodies have a minor role, if any, in the etiology of this disorder. However, thyroid growth blocking and cytotoxic antibodies may have a role in the etiology of congenital hypothyroidism. (See Chapter 575 in *Nelson Textbook of Pediatrics*, 16th ed.)

30. **E.** Congenital hypothyroidism may also demonstrate large fontanelles, feeding intolerance, distended abdomen, constipation, prolonged sleep, and a poor cry. (See Chapter 575 in *Nelson Textbook of Pediatrics*, 16th ed.)

31. **B.** The serum T_4 is markedly depressed. Most cases of congenital hypothyroidism are due to dysgenesis of the thyroid gland, and therefore the TSH is elevated and a thyroid scan shows no uptake or ectopic tissue. Nonetheless, the serum T_4 is the best of these tests. Central hypothalamic pituitary causes have a low TSH. Therapy with T_4 should be initiated immediately. Fortunately, state screening for congenital hypothyroidism has prevented this type of late presentation with the inherent risks of mental retardation. (See Chapter 575 in *Nelson Textbook of Pediatrics*, 16th ed.)

32. **A.** Hypothyroidism that is acquired is insidious in onset and primarily affects growth. Schoolwork is not as severely

affected, as one would expect. (See Chapter 575 in *Nelson Textbook of Pediatrics*, 16th ed.)

33. **B.** TPOAbs are present in 90% of children with Hashimoto autoimmune thyroiditis. (See Chapter 576 in *Nelson Textbook of Pediatrics*, 16th ed.)

34. **A.** The female:male sex ratio is actually 5:1. (See Chapter 578 in *Nelson Textbook of Pediatrics*, 16th ed.)

35. **D.** PTU and methimazole (Tapazole) inhibit incorporation of trapped inorganic iodine into organ iodine and are the drugs and treatment of choice for Graves disease. (See Chapter 578 in *Nelson Textbook of Pediatrics*, 16th ed.)

36. **E.** Early rickets is characterized by an elevated serum alkaline phosphatase and a low phosphate but maintenance of normal calcium levels. (See Chapter 581 in *Nelson Textbook of Pediatrics*, 16th ed.)

37. **D.** Muscle weakness, hypotension, anorexia, and hypoglycemia all suggest adrenal insufficiency. (See Chapter 585 in *Nelson Textbook of Pediatrics*, 16th ed.)

38. **A.** Also called autoimmune polyendocrinopathy—candidiasis—ectodermal dystrophy, this disorder causes severe mucocutaneous candidiasis, hypoparathyroidism, and adrenal insufficiency. Type II is Addison disease and thyroid disease or type I diabetes. (See Chapter 585 in *Nelson Textbook of Pediatrics*, 16th ed.)

39. 1. **B**
    2. **A**
    3. **D**
    4. **C**
    (See Chapter 586 in *Nelson Textbook of Pediatrics*, 16th ed.)

40. **B.** There is no chromosome duplication. A possible association to the type I neurofibromatosis loci on chromosome 17q has been reported. (See Chapter 593 in *Nelson Textbook of Pediatrics*, 16th ed.)

41. **C.** Patients are uniformly tall, and hypogonadism is present. (See Chapter 593 in *Nelson Textbook of Pediatrics*, 16th ed.)

42. **C.** Anti-GAD antibodies, also known as anti-islet antibodies, are present in at least 90% of children with insulin-dependent diabetes. (See Chapter 599 in *Nelson Textbook of Pediatrics*, 16th ed.)

43. **C.** Hyponatremia may be due to measurement artifacts of serum glucose levels. Failure of the serum sodium level to rise during therapy places the patient at risk for cerebral edema, as the serum osmolarity drops below that in the brain, resulting in fluid shifting to the CNS. (See Chapter 599 in *Nelson Textbook of Pediatrics*, 16th ed.)

44. **E.** Transcellular shifts of H+ into the cell with K+ leaving the cell during acidosis produce transient hyperkalemia, which is usually reversed with improvement in metabolism by insulin and improved tissue perfusion from isotonic fluids. Hypokalemia may develop during therapy with insulin; placing potassium salts in the intravenous solution given to the patient may reduce this risk. (See Chapter 599 in *Nelson Textbook of Pediatrics*, 16th ed.)

26 *The Nervous System*

1. **B.** Metachromatic leukodystrophy is a familial degenerative disease affecting both the central nervous system (CNS) and peripheral nervous system white matter, hence the loss of deep tendon reflexes with CNS symptoms. (See Chapter 608 in *Nelson Textbook of Pediatrics*, 16th ed.)

2. **E.** The young girl described in the question has tetralogy of Fallot and a brain abscess partly resulting from the right-to-left cardiac shunt. Predisposing factors for brain abscesses in other patients include chronic otic and sinus infections. (See Chapter 610 in *Nelson Textbook of Pediatrics*, 16th ed.)

3. 1. **B**
   2. **C**
   3. **B**
   4. **A**
   5. **B**
   6. **D**
   (See Chapter 601 in *Nelson Textbook of Pediatrics*, 16th ed.)

4. **E.** Congenital cytomegalovirus (CMV) usually causes microcephalus, not macrocephalus. Expansion of the bone

marrow (hemolytic anemias), storage diseases (lysosomal, leukodystrophies), excessive cerebrospinal fluid (CSF) (hydrocephalus) and blood (subdurals), and familial factors contribute to megalocephaly. (See Chapter 601 in *Nelson Textbook of Pediatrics*, 16th ed.)

5. **E.** Spina bifida with or without hydrocephalus but without other CNS lesions does not usually produce seizures. All the other diagnoses listed in the question are associated with neonatal seizures. (See Chapter 602 in *Nelson Textbook of Pediatrics*, 16th ed.)

6. 1. **E**
   2. **C**
   3. **A**
   4. **B**
   5. **A**
   6. **B**
   7. **C**
   8. **D**
   9. **A**
   10. **A**
   (See Chapter 605 in *Nelson Textbook of Pediatrics*, 16th ed.)

7. **B.** MRI is most useful in confirming the diagnosis of a possible demyelinating disease such as multiple sclerosis. MRI demonstrates small 3- to 4-mm plaques compatible with the disease. (See Chapter 608 in *Nelson Textbook of Pediatrics*, 16th ed.)

8. 1. **B**
   2. **D**
   3. **A**
   4. **E**
   5. **F**
   6. **B**
   7. **F**
   8. **C**
   9. **F**
   10. **C**
   11. **D**
   12. **A**
   (See Chapter 608 in *Nelson Textbook of Pediatrics*, 16th ed.)

9. **C.** A CT or MRI scan would reveal a cystic cerebellar astrocytoma. Positional and progressive headache, with or without head tilt, is a significant manifestation of a brain tumor. The poor visualization of the retina is probably due

to marked papilledema obscuring the optic disc. (See Chapter 611 in *Nelson Textbook of Pediatrics*, 16th ed.)

10. **D.** The patient described in the question underwent CT that revealed a frontal brain abscess due to anaerobic mouth flora from chronic tooth decay. As an aside, a patient with a history suspicious of chronic CNS infection (e.g., more than 2–3 days) should undergo head CT before a lumbar puncture. If a lumbar puncture is performed with a brain abscess, ICP may be increased (as in this patient) and cerebral herniation and death may ensue. If infection is suspected but a CT scan is indicated, the patient should be empirically treated for meningitis after a blood culture is obtained but before a lumbar puncture is performed. (See Chapter 610 in *Nelson Textbook of Pediatrics*, 16th ed.)

11. **D.** Arteriovenous malformation, like an aneurysm, may rupture, producing hemiplegia or coma. Blood in the subarachnoid space produces nuchal rigidity and may be detected by CT or a carefully performed lumbar puncture. (See Chapter 609 in *Nelson Textbook of Pediatrics*, 16th ed.)

12. 1. **B**
    2. **D**
    3. **A**
    4. **C**
    5. **E**
    (See Chapter 600 in *Nelson Textbook of Pediatrics*, 16th ed.)

13. **D.** Eighteen months with a range of 9–12 months. The usual size is 2×2 cm. (See Chapter 600 in *Nelson Textbook of Pediatrics*, 16th ed.)

14. **B.** The posterior fontanel closes first and is usually nonpalpable by 6–8 weeks of life. (See Chapter 600 in *Nelson Textbook of Pediatrics*, 16th ed.)

15. **A.** Acutely, the visual activity is usually not reduced in papilledema. This is in contrast with papillitis noted during optic neuritis; these patients have poor visual activity. (See Chapter 600 in *Nelson Textbook of Pediatrics*, 16th ed.)

16. **D.** Motor weakness, especially of the thighs, requires the child to stand from a supine position by using the arms to

"climb" up the legs to stand erect. (See Chapter 600 in *Nelson Textbook of Pediatrics*, 16th ed.)

17. **B.** AFP testing at 16–18 weeks' gestation is a helpful screening tool. High levels occur in open neural tube defects and other lesions such as omphalocele; therefore, follow-up fetal ultrasonography is needed as a next stage. (See Chapter 601 in *Nelson Textbook of Pediatrics*, 16th ed.)

18. **B.** Supplementation with folate is the most successful strategy to reduce the incidence of neural tube defects and possibly other non-neural congenital anomalies. (See Chapter 601 in *Nelson Textbook of Pediatrics*, 16th ed.)

19. 1. **D**
    2. **A**
    3. **B**
    4. **C**
    (See Chapter 601 in *Nelson Textbook of Pediatrics*, 16th ed.)

20. 1. **B**
    2. **A**
    3. **D**
    4. **C**
    5. **E**
    (See Chapter 601 in *Nelson Textbook of Pediatrics*, 16th ed.)

21. **A.** There is never a loss of consciousness in simple partial seizures. Actually, some patients may talk to you during the event. (See Chapter 602 in *Nelson Textbook of Pediatrics*, 16th ed.)

22. **C.** Sequelae may include hemiplegia, hemianopia, or aphasia. (See Chapter 602 in *Nelson Textbook of Pediatrics*, 16th ed.)

23. **B.** The disorder is more common in boys. The etiology is unknown, and the treatment of choice is valproic acid. (See Chapter 602 in *Nelson Textbook of Pediatrics*, 16th ed.)

24. **D.** HIE is usually easy to identify by a need for resuscitation and abnormalities of tone. By the way, febrile seizures never occur in newborns. Be careful to take a good history to identify benign familial seizures that do not recur after the neonatal period. (See Chapter 602 in *Nelson Textbook of Pediatrics*, 16th ed.)

25. 1. **A**
    2. **C**

3. **B**
4. **E**
5. **D**
6. **F**
(See Chapter 603 in *Nelson Textbook of Pediatrics*, 16th ed.)

26. **E.** A family history, particularly on the mother's side, is present in 90% of children with common migraine. The gene for familial hemiplegic migraine has also been localized; it is an autosomal dominant disorder. (See Chapter 604 in *Nelson Textbook of Pediatrics*, 16th ed.)

27. **A.** These constitute a separate classification of headaches that are unusual in children. (See Chapter 604 in *Nelson Textbook of Pediatrics*, 16th ed.)

28. **A.** Most children with mild migraine headaches respond well to acetaminophen or ibuprofen, bed rest, and elimination of initiating stimuli. Control of emesis and more severe pain may require additional medications. Aspirin increases the risk of Reye syndrome and is contraindicated in children. (See Chapter 604 in *Nelson Textbook of Pediatrics*, 16th ed.)

29. **D.** The ash leaf–shaped hypopigmented macule is most typical of tuberous sclerosis (being present in over 90% of affected children), another autosomal dominant disorder. (See Chapter 605 in *Nelson Textbook of Pediatrics*, 16th ed.)

30. **A.** NF-2 accounts for 10% of all NF cases, has distinctive chromosomal sites, and is characterized by bilateral acoustic neuromas. *Café-au-lait* macules may not be present. (See Chapter 605 in *Nelson Textbook of Pediatrics*, 16th ed.)

31. **C.** Postviral ataxia is probably an autoimmune response and typically follows varicella but may also follow enterovirus infection. (See Chapter 606 in *Nelson Textbook of Pediatrics*, 16th ed.)

32. **A.** Hypotonia is the rule. (See Chapter 606 in *Nelson Textbook of Pediatrics*, 16th ed.)

33. 1. **A**
    2. **D**
    3. **C**
    4. **A**
    5. **B**
    6. **B**

7. **B**
8. **C**
9. **C and D**
10. **C**
(See Chapter 608 in *Nelson Textbook of Pediatrics,* 16th ed.)

27 *Neuromuscular Disorders*

1. **B.** Guillain-Barré syndrome is an ascending peripheral polyneuropathy that is predominantly motor but may have mild sensory symptoms (paresthesias). An upper respiratory tract infection or diarrhea (often due to *Campylobacter*) often precedes the onset of paralysis. (See Chapter 623 in *Nelson Textbook of Pediatrics,* 16th ed.)

2. **E.** Pulmonary function tests, such as measurement of negative inspiratory force, are helpful in detecting impending respiratory failure due to intercostal or phrenic nerve involvement. Reductions in inspiratory force often precede abnormalities of the arterial blood gases (hypercarbia, hypoxia) and should be monitored frequently in any patient with acute progressive muscle weakness. (See Chapter 623 in *Nelson Textbook of Pediatrics,* 16th ed.)

3. **E.** Ticks (wood or dog) may produce a motor-sensory neuropathy indistinguishable from Guillain-Barré syndrome. On removal of the tick (often on the scalp), the paralysis rapidly resolves. (See Chapter 621 in *Nelson Textbook of Pediatrics,* 16th ed.)

4. 1. **A**
   2. **B**
   3. **D**
   4. **C**
   5. **A**
   (See Chapter 614 in *Nelson Textbook of Pediatrics,* 16th ed.)

5. 1. **D**
   2. **F**
   3. **A**
   4. **B**
   5. **C**
   6. **G**
   7. **E**
   (See Chapter 618 in *Nelson Textbook of Pediatrics,* 16th ed.)

6. **E.** Myasthenia gravis is characterized by progressive muscle weakness that is exacerbated by repetitive muscle use. The facial and extraocular muscles are classically involved. (See Chapter 619 in *Nelson Textbook of Pediatrics,* 16th ed.)

7. **C.** Duchenne muscular dystrophy is also called pseudohypertrophic muscular dystrophy. (See Chapter 616 in *Nelson Textbook of Pediatrics,* 16th ed.)

8. **D.** Creatine phosphokinase (CK) is one of several lysosomal enzymes released by damaged or degenerating muscle fibers and is the most useful in laboratory measurement of these enzymes in serum. CK is found in only three organs and may be separated into corresponding isozymes: MM for skeletal muscle, MB for cardiac muscle, and BB for brain. (See Chapter 614 in *Nelson Textbook of Pediatrics,* 16th ed.)

9. **C.** The definitive diagnosis of congenital neuromuscular disorders is best determined by histopathologic findings in the muscle biopsy sample. Most of the congenital myopathies are hereditary; some are sporadic. In a few conditions for which the defective gene has been identified, the diagnosis may be established using the specific molecular probe on lymphocytes. (See Chapter 615 in *Nelson Textbook of Pediatrics,* 16th ed.)

10. **E.** The muscular dystrophies are a group of unrelated disorders, each transmitted by a different gene and each differing in its clinical course and expression. The muscular dystrophies are distinguished from other neurogenic disorders by the four obligatory criteria listed in the question. (See Chapter 616 in *Nelson Textbook of Pediatrics,* 16th ed.)

11. **B.** Duchenne muscular dystrophy, the most common hereditary neuromuscular disorder, is inherited as an X-linked recessive trait. The gene is on the X chromosome at the Xp21 locus. (See Chapter 616 in *Nelson Textbook of Pediatrics,* 16th ed.)

12. **E.** Cardiomyopathy is a constant feature of Duchenne muscular dystrophy, although the severity of cardiac involvement does not necessarily correlate with the degree of skeletal

muscle weakness. Intellectual impairment occurs in all patients, although only 20–30% have an intelligence quotient (IQ) of less than 70. Scoliosis is common. (See Chapter 616.1 in *Nelson Textbook of Pediatrics,* 16th ed.)

13. **D.** Thyrotoxicosis causes proximal muscle weakness and wasting accompanied by electromyogram (EMG) changes. Hypothyroidism, whether congenital or acquired, consistently produces proximal muscle weakness and hypotonia. Hyperparathyroidism causes weakness and reversible muscle wasting. Both natural Cushing disease and exogenous corticosteroid administration may cause proximal muscle weakness. Hyperaldosteronism is accompanied by episodic and reversible muscle weakness. (See Chapter 614 in *Nelson Textbook of Pediatrics,* 16th ed.)

14. **B.** Acute episodes of malignant hyperthermia are precipitated by exposure to general anesthetics and occasionally to local anesthetic drugs. Acute attacks may be prevented by administration of dantrolene sodium before an anesthetic is administered. (See Chapter 618.2 in *Nelson Textbook of Pediatrics,* 16th ed.)

15. **D.** Myasthenia gravis is an autoimmune disorder. A rare familial form is probably an autosomal recessive trait but is not associated with plasma anti-ACh antibodies. (See Chapter 619 in *Nelson Textbook of Pediatrics,* 16th ed.)

16. **C.** Ptosis and some degree of extraocular muscle weakness are the earliest and most constant signs in myasthenia gravis. Older children may complain of diplopia. (See Chapter 619.1 in *Nelson Textbook of Pediatrics,* 16th ed.)

17. **C.** Myasthenia gravis is one of the few neuromuscular diseases in which an electromyogram (EMG) is more diagnostic than muscle biopsy. A decremental response occurs in response to repetitive nerve stimulation; the muscle potentials diminish rapidly in amplitude until the muscle becomes refractory to further stimulation. Motor nerve conduction velocity remains normal. Plasma anti-ACh antibodies

should be assayed but are inconsistently found in only one third of adolescents. (See Chapter 619.1 in *Nelson Textbook of Pediatrics,* 16th ed.)

18. **C.** If untreated, myasthenia gravis is usually progressive and may become life threatening because of respiratory muscle weakness. Cardiomyopathy is not a feature of myasthenia gravis, and electrocardiogram (ECG) findings remain normal. (See Chapter 619.1 in *Nelson Textbook of Pediatrics,* 16th ed.)

19. **C.** After the abnormal (maternally derived) antibodies disappear, offspring born to myasthenic mothers have normal muscle strength and are not at increased risk for myasthenia gravis in later life. (See Chapter 619.1 in *Nelson Textbook of Pediatrics,* 16th ed.)

20. **D.** Familial dysautonomia (Riley-Day syndrome) is usually expressed in infancy as poor sucking and feeding. Autonomic crises usually begin after 3 years of age. (See Chapter 622.1 in *Nelson Textbook of Pediatrics,* 16th ed.)

21. **D.** Guillain-Barré syndrome is a postinfectious polyneuropathy that causes demyelination, primarily in the motor nerves. The onset is typically gradual, with symmetric involvement that begins in the lower extremities and progressively involves the trunk and upper limbs. Bulbar involvement occurs in about half of cases. Spontaneous recovery usually occurs in 2–3 weeks. (See Chapter 624 in *Nelson Textbook of Pediatrics,* 16th ed.)

22. **D.** Bell palsy is an acute unilateral facial nerve palsy that is not associated with other cranial neuropathies of brainstem dysfunction. It is a common disorder at all ages and typically develops about 2 weeks after a systemic infection, especially herpes simplex virus and Lyme disease. (See Chapter 624 in *Nelson Textbook of Pediatrics,* 16th ed.)

28 *Disorders of the Eye*

1. 1. **B**
   2. **C**
   3. **A**
   4. **E** (congenital miosis)
   5. **D**

(See Chapter 629 in *Nelson Textbook of Pediatrics,* 16th ed.)

2. **F.** Coats disease is a rare problem in childhood; it does not produce leukokoria. (See Chapter 628 in *Nelson Textbook of Pediatrics,* 16th ed.)

3. **A.** Amblyopia is a vision loss that is not due to a specific organic lesion but rather to deprivation or disuse of the retina. Even after delayed removal of a cataract or correction of strabismus, the previously unused retina tunes out the image. (See Chapter 635 in *Nelson Textbook of Pediatrics,* 16th ed.)

4. 1. **C**
   2. **A**
   3. **D**
   4. **B**
   5. **F**
   6. **E**
   (See Chapter 630 in *Nelson Textbook of Pediatrics,* 16th ed.)

5. 1. **A**
   2. **B**
   3. **D**
   4. **A**
   5. **A**
   6. **B**
   7. **A**
   8. **B**
   9. **B**
   10. **C**
   (See Chapter 638 in *Nelson Textbook of Pediatrics,* 16th ed.)

6. **G.** Hyperoxia in preterm neonates usually causes retinopathy of prematurity, which occasionally is associated with cataracts. Oxygen does not directly cause cataracts. (See Chapter 635 in *Nelson Textbook of Pediatrics,* 16th ed.)

7. **E.** The acquired triad of nystagmus, head nodding, and torticollis, in its classic form, is self-limited and benign. Nonetheless, children with brain tumors may have signs resembling components of spasmus nutans. (See Chapter 630 in *Nelson Textbook of Pediatrics,* 16th ed.)

8. **D.** Rhabdomyosarcoma of the face, orbit, and sinus often presents early because of the space-occupying and displacement effects of tumor growth. (See Chapter 640 in *Nelson Textbook of Pediatrics,* 16th ed.)

9. **D.** The visual acuity of the newborn is estimated to be approximately 20/400 but improves with age and may reach 20/30–20/20 by 2–3 years of age. The cornea is normally clear in full-term newborns but may have a transient opalescent haze in premature newborns. Superficial retinal hemorrhages and subconjunctival hemorrhages may be visible after birth in normal newborns. The iris is light gray or blue at birth and undergoes progressive change of color as the pigmentation of the stroma increases in the first 6 months of life. Tears often are not present with crying until 1–3 months of age. (See Chapter 625 in *Nelson Textbook of Pediatrics,* 16th ed.)

10. **C.** Amblyopia occurs in visually immature children, and only before the cortex has become visually mature. Younger children are more susceptible to amblyopia but also show more rapid reversal than older children. Amblyopia is frequently asymptomatic. (See Chapter 628 in *Nelson Textbook of Pediatrics,* 16th ed.)

11. **D.** Approximately two thirds of cases of aniridia result from transmission of an autosomal dominant gene on the 11p13 region, with a high degree of penetrance. Most of the remainder of cases are sporadic and are considered to be new mutations. (See Chapter 629 in *Nelson Textbook of Pediatrics,* 16th ed.)

12. **E.** Aniridia should not be considered an isolated iris defect. Associated defects include macular and optic nerve hypoplasia, poor visual acuity (20/200 in most patients), and lens and corneal abnormalities. Wilms tumor may develop in one fifth of patients with aniridia, usually (but not always) in patients with sporadic aniridia. (See Chapter 629 in *Nelson Textbook of Pediatrics,* 16th ed.)

13. **D.** Dacryostenosis, or congenital nasolacrimal duct obstruction, presents with increased tearing after normal tear production develops. The primary treatment of uncomplicated nasolacrimal duct obstruction is a regimen of nasolacrimal massage, usually two to three times each day, accompanied by cleansing of the lids with warm water.

Topical antibiotics are used for significant mucopurulent discharge. (See Chapter 632 in *Nelson Textbook of Pediatrics,* 16th ed.)

14. **D.** The recommended treatment of chlamydial neonatal conjunctivitis is oral erythromycin (50 mg/kg/24 hours in four divided doses). Although chlamydial conjunctivitis is a self-limited disease that has no sequelae, approximately 10–20% of infants exposed to *Chlamydia trachomatis* do experience afebrile pneumonia. This may be prevented by oral erythromycin therapy. (See Chapter 633 in *Nelson Textbook of Pediatrics,* 16th ed.)

15. **C.** The clinical manifestations of retinoblastoma vary, but the initial sign in the majority of cases is leukocoria (white pupillary reflex, also known as "cat eye") instead of the normal red pupillary reflex. (See Chapter 637 in *Nelson Textbook of Pediatrics,* 16th ed.)

16. **D.** Papilledema is a neurologic emergency. Neuroimaging should be performed, and if no intracranial masses are found, a lumbar puncture for determination of cerebrospinal fluid pressure should be performed. This patient may have pseudotumor cerebri. (See Chapter 638 in *Nelson Textbook of Pediatrics,* 16th ed.)

17. **B.** Symptoms of infantile glaucoma (glaucoma that begins in the first 3 years of life) include the classic triad of epiphora (tearing), photophobia (sensitivity to light), and blepharospasm (eyelid squeezing), which are usually attributed to corneal irritation. An increase in intraocular pressure leads to expansion of the globe, including the cornea. (See Chapter 639 in *Nelson Textbook of Pediatrics,* 16th ed.)

18. **D.** Unlike glaucoma in adults, in which medications are the first line of therapy, the treatment of infantile glaucoma is primarily surgical. Procedures used to treat glaucoma in children include surgery to establish a more normal anterior chamber angle (goniotomy and trabeculotomy), to create a route for aqueous fluid to exit the eye (trabeculectomy and seton surgery), or to reduce aqueous fluid production (cyclocryotherapy and photocyclocoagulation). Many children require several operations to lower and maintain their intraocular pressure adequately. Long-term medications may be necessary as well. (See Chapter 639 in *Nelson Textbook of Pediatrics,* 16th ed.)

19. **A.** Corneal abrasions are treated with frequent applications of a topical antibiotic ointment until the epithelium is completely healed. The use of a semi-pressure patch does not improve healing time or decrease pain. Furthermore, an improperly applied patch may itself abrade the cornea. A topical cycloplegic agent (cyclopentolate hydrochloride 1%) can relieve the pain from ciliary spasm in patients with large abrasions. Topical anesthetics should not be given at home because they retard epithelial healing and inhibit the natural blinking reflex. (See Chapter 641 in *Nelson Textbook of Pediatrics,* 16th ed.)

29 *The Ear*

1. **F.** Any mechanism that physically impairs the transmission of sound through the external or middle ear produces a conductive hearing loss. (See Chapter 643 in *Nelson Textbook of Pediatrics,* 16th ed.)

2. **E.** Missed unvoiced consonant sounds occur even with slight hearing loss. (See Chapter 643 in *Nelson Textbook of Pediatrics,* 16th ed.)

3. **D.** Inflammation of the external canal may occur after otitis media with perforation, but the reverse is not true in that external otitis does not cause perforation. (See Chapter 645 in *Nelson Textbook of Pediatrics,* 16th ed.)

4. 1. **B**
   2. **A**
   3. **A**
   4. **C**
   5. **D**
   6. **B**
   (See Chapter 646 in *Nelson Textbook of Pediatrics,* 16th ed.)

5. **C.** Sensorineural hearing loss may occur secondary to genetic, infectious,

autoimmune, anatomic, traumatic, ototoxic, or idiopathic causes. Otitis media is the most common cause of conductive hearing loss. (See Chapter 643 in *Nelson Textbook of Pediatrics,* 16th ed.)

6. **A.** The most common bacterial causes of otitis media are *S. pneumoniae* (30–50%), nontypable *H. influenzae* (20–30%), and *M. catarrhalis* (1–5%). Many other organisms are infrequently isolated in a small percentage of cases. (See Chapter 643 in *Nelson Textbook of Pediatrics,* 16th ed.)

7. **D.** Decreased mobility is the best physical finding sign of middle ear effusion. A normal tympanic membrane can become red in a crying child. A thickened tympanic membrane (tympanosclerosis) may occur after chronic infections. (See Chapter 643 in *Nelson Textbook of Pediatrics,* 16th ed.)

8. **A.** Amoxicillin is the initial antibiotic of choice because it is usually effective against the most common organisms, has a good pharmacodynamic profile against multidrug-resistant *S. pneumoniae,* has a long record of safety, and is inexpensive. Amoxicillin-clavulanate, cefuroxime axetil, and ceftriaxone are second-line drugs if amoxicillin therapy fails. (See Chapter 643 in *Nelson Textbook of Pediatrics,* 16th ed.)

9. **D.** Drug-resistant *S. pneumoniae* is associated with recent antimicrobial exposure, young age (<2 years), and daycare attendance. In addition, drug resistance varies from community to community. Relative resistance in pneumococcus responds to higher-dose therapy. (See Chapter 643 in *Nelson Textbook of Pediatrics,* 16th ed.)

10. **D.** Middle ear effusion with little or no air in the middle ear results in severely decreased or absent responses to applied pressures, both positive and negative. When retraction is present, the short process of the malleus is prominent and the long process is foreshortened; these processes are obscured by a bulging tympanic membrane. The tympanic membrane normally has a translucent, ground glass, or waxed paper appearance. A red tympanic membrane may not indicate pathology because the blood vessels of the drum may be engorged as a result of crying, sneezing, or blowing the nose. A retracted tympanic membrane is usually due to negative middle ear pressure but may also result from previous middle ear or tympanic membrane disease and subsequent fixation of the ossicles. (See Chapter 642 in *Nelson Textbook of Pediatrics,* 16th ed.)

11. **C.** Sensorineural hearing loss may occur secondary to genetic, infectious, autoimmune, anatomic, traumatic, ototoxic, or idiopathic causes. Otitis media is the most common cause of conductive hearing loss. (See Chapter 643 in *Nelson Textbook of Pediatrics,* 16th ed.)

12. **B.** The American Academy of Pediatrics endorses the goal of universal detection of hearing loss in infants before 3 months of age, with appropriate intervention for infants no later than 6 months of age. (See Chapter 643 in *Nelson Textbook of Pediatrics,* 16th ed.)

13. **E.** All of these indicate the need for audiologic assessment. (See Chapter 643 in *Nelson Textbook of Pediatrics,* 16th ed.)

14. **B.** This admittance tympanogram shows a very low peak admittance and gradient, whereas the tympanometric peak pressure is grossly within normal limits. The shape of the tympanogram has the greatest sensitivity and specificity for middle ear effusion. The more rounded the peak (or, ultimately, an absent peak), the higher the probability of an effusion. (See Chapter 643 in *Nelson Textbook of Pediatrics,* 16th ed.)

15. **A.** A pit-like depression just anterior to the helix and above the tragus may represent a cyst or an epidermis-lined fistulous tract. These are common, with an incidence of approximately 8 in 1000 children, but do not require surgical removal unless there is recurrent infection. (See Chapter 644 in *Nelson Textbook of Pediatrics,* 16th ed.)

16. **C.** The most effective prophylaxis for recurrent otitis externa is instillation of dilute alcohol or acetic acid (2%) immediately after swimming or bathing. During an acute episode of otitis externa, patients should not swim and the ears

should be protected from water during bathing. (See Chapter 645 in *Nelson Textbook of Pediatrics,* 16th ed.)

17. **D.** The most commonly identified pathogens associated with otitis media are *Streptococcus pneumoniae* (30–50%), nontypable *Haemophilus influenzae* (20–30%), and *Moraxella catarrhalis* (1–5%). Other bacteria, including *Staphylococcus aureus,* gram-negative enteric organisms such as *Escherichia coli* and *Klebsiella* spp., and *Pseudomonas aeruginosa* are infrequently isolated. (See Chapter 646 in *Nelson Textbook of Pediatrics,* 16th ed.)

18. **D.** Decreased mobility is the best physical finding sign of middle ear effusion. A red tympanic membrane may not indicate pathology because the blood vessels of the drum may be engorged as a result of crying, sneezing, or blowing the nose. A thickened tympanic membrane (tympanosclerosis) may occur after recurrent infections. (See Chapter 646 in *Nelson Textbook of Pediatrics,* 16th ed.)

19. **A.** Amoxicillin is the initial antibiotic of choice because it is usually effective against the most common organisms, has a good pharmacodynamic profile against multidrug-resistant *S. pneumoniae,* has a long record of safety, and is inexpensive. Amoxicillin-clavulanate, cefuroxime axetil, and ceftriaxone are second-line drugs if amoxicillin therapy fails. (See Chapter 646 in *Nelson Textbook of Pediatrics,* 16th ed.)

20. **D.** Risk factors for otitis media caused by drug-resistant *Streptococcus pneumoniae* include recent antimicrobial exposure, young age (<2 years), and daycare attendance. (See Chapter 646 in *Nelson Textbook of Pediatrics,* 16th ed.)

21. **E.** Most (70–80%) temporal bone fractures are longitudinal and are manifested by bleeding from a laceration of the external canal or tympanic membrane; hemotympanum; conductive hearing loss resulting from laceration of the tympanic membrane, hemotympanum, or ossicular injury; delayed onset of facial paralysis; and temporary cerebrospinal fluid otorrhea or rhinorrhea. (See Chapter 648 in *Nelson Textbook of Pediatrics,* 16th ed.)

30 *The Skin*

1. **E.** Giant pigmented nevi are difficult-to-manage lesions that affect males and females with equal frequency. (See Chapter 657 in *Nelson Textbook of Pediatrics,* 16th ed.)

2. **A.** Incontinentia pigmenti is X-linked dominant and is lethal in males during fetal life. (See Chapter 658 in *Nelson Textbook of Pediatrics,* 16th ed.)

3. **A.** There is no agreed-on indication for systemic steroids in Stevens-Johnson syndrome. (See Chapter 660 in *Nelson Textbook of Pediatrics,* 16th ed.)

4. **A.** Skin lesions are classified as macules, papules, patches, plaques, nodules, tumors, vesicles, bullae, pustules, wheals, and cysts. *Macules* are an alteration in skin color but cannot be felt. The term *patch* is used for lesions larger than 1 cm. *Papules* are palpable solid lesions smaller than 0.5–1 cm, whereas *nodules* are larger in diameter. *Pustules* contain purulent material. Aggregations of papules and pustules are called *plaques.* (See Chapter 651 in *Nelson Textbook of Pediatrics,* 16th ed.)

5. **D.** Excoriations are ulcerated lesions inflicted by scratching and are often linear or angular in configuration. (See Chapter 651 in *Nelson Textbook of Pediatrics,* 16th ed.)

6. 1. **D**
   2. **B**
   3. **A**
   4. **E**
   5. **C**
   (See Chapter 651 in *Nelson Textbook of Pediatrics,* 16th ed.)

7. **D.** Fluorinated topical corticosteroids are more potent, with greater local and systemic adverse effects, than nonfluorinated topical corticosteroids. The different fluorinated corticosteroids differ significantly in their potency. (See Chapter 652 in *Nelson Textbook of Pediatrics,* 16th ed.)

8. **C.** Sunscreens are of two general types: those that reflect all wavelengths of UV

and visible spectrums, such as zinc oxide and titanium dioxide, and a heterogeneous group of chemicals that selectively absorb energy of various wavelengths within the UV spectrum. Some sunscreens permit tanning without burning. Sunscreens do not give complete protection against all harmful UV light. (See Chapter 652 in *Nelson Textbook of Pediatrics*, 16th ed.)

9. **C.** Cutis marmorata is an accentuated physiologic vasomotor response that disappears with increasing age during the first year of life. (See Chapter 653 in *Nelson Textbook of Pediatrics*, 16th ed.)

10. **A.** Erythema toxicum is a benign, self-limited, evanescent eruption that occurs in approximately 50% of full-term infants; preterm infants are affected less commonly. The lesions are firm, yellow-white, 1- to 2-mm papules or pustules with a surrounding erythematous flare. Lesions may be sparse or numerous and clustered in several sites or widely dispersed over much of the body surface. Palms and soles are usually spared. Peak incidence is on the second day of life, but new lesions may erupt during the first few days as the rash waxes and wanes. (See Chapter 653 in *Nelson Textbook of Pediatrics*, 16th ed.)

11. **D.** The most effective treatment for port-wine stains is the flashlamp-pumped-pulsed dye laser. This therapy is targeted at the lesion and avoids thermal injury to the surrounding normal tissue. Alternative therapies include masking with cosmetics, cryosurgery, excision, grafting, and tattooing. (See Chapter 656 in *Nelson Textbook of Pediatrics*, 16th ed.)

12. **B.** Large, often asymmetric *café-au-lait* spots with irregular borders are characteristic of McCune-Albright syndrome. This disorder also includes polyostotic fibrous dysplasia of bone, leading to pathologic fractures; precocious puberty; and numerous hyperfunctional endocrinopathies. (See Chapter 658 in *Nelson Textbook of Pediatrics*, 16th ed.)

13. **E.** One to three *café-au-lait* spots are common in normal children; approximately 10% of normal children have *café-au-lait* macules. They may be present at birth or develop during childhood. (See Chapter 658 in *Nelson Textbook of Pediatrics*, 16th ed.)

14. **B.** Nummular eczema is unrelated to other types of eczema and is characterized by coin-sized eczematous plaques. Common sites are the extensor surfaces of the extremities, buttocks, and shoulders. The plaques are relatively discrete and severely pruritic, and when chronic they often become thickened and lichenified. These lesions are often mistaken for tinea corporis, but plaques of nummular eczema are distinguished by the absence of a raised, sharply circumscribed border, the absence of fungal organisms on potassium hydroxide (KOH) preparation, and frequent weeping or bleeding when scraped. Pruritus is usually controlled with a fluorinated topical corticosteroid preparation. They may become secondarily infected, which may be treated with antibiotics. (See Chapter 661 in *Nelson Textbook of Pediatrics*, 16th ed.)

15. **B.** Tuberous sclerosis is a multisystem disorder primarily affecting tissues from ectoderm. The classic clinical triad is skin lesions with epilepsy and mental retardation. Single or multiple white- or ash-leaf lesions are most often found on the trunk and appear at birth or in early infancy, often years before other signs of the disease. The shagreen patch is a large, skin-colored, irregularly thickened plaque with an orange-peel or cobblestone texture that may occur in the lumbosacral area. (See Chapter 659 in *Nelson Textbook of Pediatrics*, 16th ed.)

16. **C.** Pityriasis rosea is a benign, common eruption that occurs most frequently in children and young adults. A herald patch is a solitary, round, or oval lesion that may occur anywhere on the body and is often but not always identifiable by its large size. It usually precedes the generalized eruption, which occurs 5–10 days after appearance of the herald patch. (See Chapter 663 in *Nelson Textbook of Pediatrics*, 16th ed.)

17. **B.** Keloids are usually induced by trauma and commonly follow ear piercing, burns, scalds, and surgical procedures. Certain

individuals, especially blacks, seem predisposed to keloid formation. In both keloids and hypertrophic scars, new collagen forms over a much longer period than in wounds that heal normally. Unlike keloids, hypertrophic scars remain confined to the site of injury and gradually involute over time. (See Chapter 665 in *Nelson Textbook of Pediatrics,* 16th ed.)

18. **B.** Ehlers-Danlos syndrome is a group of genetically heterogeneous connective tissue disorders. Affected children appear normal at birth, but skin hyperelasticity, fragility of the skin and blood vessels, and joint hypermobility develop. The essential defect is a quantitative deficiency of collagen. Ehlers-Danlos syndrome has been classified into 10 clinical forms. (See Chapter 665 in *Nelson Textbook of Pediatrics,* 16th ed.)

19. **D.** Inflammation of the lips (cheilitis) and angles of the mouth (angular cheilitis or perlèche) are most commonly due to dryness, chapping, and lip licking. Excessive salivation and drooling, particularly in children with neurologic deficits, may also cause chronic irritation. (See Chapter 670 in *Nelson Textbook of Pediatrics,* 16th ed.)

20. **B.** *Staphylococcus aureus* is the most predominant organism causing nonbullous as well as bullous impetigo in the United States. Group A β-hemolytic *Streptococcus* is the second most common causative organism, frequently in combination with *S. aureus.* (See Chapter 671 in *Nelson Textbook of Pediatrics,* 16th ed.)

21. **A.** Impetigo may be treated with topical mupirocin or with oral antibiotics effective against *Staphylococcus aureus* and group A β-hemolytic *Streptococcus* such as erythromycin, a first-generation cephalosporin, dicloxacillin, or clindamycin. Oral treatment is preferred for widespread involvement or for lesions near the eyes or mouth. Topical treatments, other than mupirocin, are not effective for the treatment of impetigo and do not add to the effectiveness of antibiotic treatment. (See Chapter 671 in *Nelson Textbook of Pediatrics,* 16th ed.)

22. **B.** Tinea versicolor is caused by the dimorphic yeast *Malassezia furfur* and was previously known as *Pityrosporum ovale* and *P. orbiculare.* (See Chapter 672 in *Nelson Textbook of Pediatrics,* 16th ed.)

23. **B.** Tinea unguium is a dermatophyte infection of the nail plate that is also known as onychomycosis. Oral itraconazole is the recommended therapy. (See Chapter 672 in *Nelson Textbook of Pediatrics,* 16th ed.)

24. **D.** The lesions of molluscum contagiosum are discrete, pearly, skin-colored, dome-shaped, smooth papules that may vary in size from 1 to 5 mm. They typically have a central umbilication from which a plug of cheesy material can be expressed. Papules of molluscum contagiosum may occur anywhere on the body but the face, eyelids, neck, axillae, and thighs are areas of predilection. (See Chapter 673 in *Nelson Textbook of Pediatrics,* 16th ed.)

25. **E.** Molluscum contagiosum is caused by molluscum contagiosum virus, a double-stranded DNA virus of the Poxviridae family. (See Chapter 673 in *Nelson Textbook of Pediatrics,* 16th ed.)

26. **A.** The treatment of choice for scabies is permethrin 5% cream applied to the entire body from the neck down for 8–12 hours. Lindane 1% cream or lotion is an effective alternative but is potentially neurotoxic, especially in infants. (See Chapter 674 in *Nelson Textbook of Pediatrics,* 16th ed.)

27. **A.** The treatment of choice for pediculosis capitis (head lice) is permethrin 1% cream rinse applied for 10 minutes with a repeat application in 7–10 days. (See Chapter 674 in *Nelson Textbook of Pediatrics,* 16th ed.)

28. **D.** The hallmark of all types of pediculosis is pruritus, which is often intense. (See Chapter 674 in *Nelson Textbook of Pediatrics,* 16th ed.)

29. **D.** Isotretinoin has many adverse effects. It is teratogenic and is contraindicated for use during pregnancy; pregnancy should be avoided for 1 month after discontinuation of therapy. Most patients experience cheilitis, xerosis, periodic epistaxis, and blepharoconjunctivitis.

Increased serum triglyceride and cholesterol levels are also common. Less common adverse effects include arthralgias, myalgias, depression, temporary thinning of the hair, paronychia, increased susceptibility to sunburn, formation of pyogenic granulomas, and colonization of the skin with *Staphylococcus aureus* leading to impetigo, secondarily infected dermatitis, and scalp folliculitis. (See Chapter 675 in *Nelson Textbook of Pediatrics*, 16th ed.)

30. **C.** Acrodermatitis enteropathica is caused by an inability to absorb sufficient zinc from the diet. Initial signs and symptoms occur during infancy and consist of a rash in the perioral, acral, and perineal areas and on the cheeks, knees, and elbows. There is often alopecia and chronic diarrhea. Some patients with cystic fibrosis present with a similar rash. Treatment is with oral zinc compounds. (See Chapter 677 in *Nelson Textbook of Pediatrics*, 16th ed.)

31 *Bone and Joint Disorders*

1. **C.** (See Chapter 683.4 in *Nelson Textbook of Pediatrics*, 16th ed.)

2. **A.** The patient described in Question 1 has a classic history of Osgood-Schlatter disease, best managed by decreased activity of the involved joint. (See Chapter 683.1 in *Nelson Textbook of Pediatrics*, 16th ed.)

3. **D.** Traction is crucial to stretch the contracted hip muscles before operation. (See Chapter 684 in *Nelson Textbook of Pediatrics*, 16th ed.)

4. **D.** Legg-Calvé-Perthes disease occurs at a younger age than slipped capital femoral epiphysis. The pain is referred to the knee. (See Chapter 684 in *Nelson Textbook of Pediatrics*, 16th ed.)

5. **D.** (See Chapter 687 in *Nelson Textbook of Pediatrics*, 16th ed.)

6. **B** and **D.** This is a classic history of dislocation of the radial head. Supination of the forearm is curative, and counseling parents not to pull small children by the arm is important. (See Chapter 689 in *Nelson Textbook of Pediatrics*, 16th ed.)

7. 1. **C**

2. **D**
3. **A**
4. **B**
5. **E**
(See Chapter 679 in *Nelson Textbook of Pediatrics*, 16th ed.)

8. **B.** (See Chapter 680.9 in *Nelson Textbook of Pediatrics*, 16th ed.)

9. **B** and **D.** *Pseudomonas* probably comes from the sneaker, and *S. aureus* from the skin. (See Chapter 680.9 in *Nelson Textbook of Pediatrics*, 16th ed.)

10. **C.** Incision and drainage with débridement of necrotic infected material is one of the most important aspects of treatment. After the material is cultured and Gram stained, the patient is started in a combination of intravenous nafcillin and gentamicin. (See Chapter 680 in *Nelson Textbook of Pediatrics*, 16th ed.)

11. 1. **D**
2. **A**
3. **B**
4. **E**
5. **C**
(See Chapter 680 in *Nelson Textbook of Pediatrics*, 16th ed.)

12. 1. **C**
2. **A**
3. **B**
4. **E**
5. **D**
(See Chapter 712 in *Nelson Textbook of Pediatrics*, 16th ed.)

13. **C.** The feet pictured demonstrate metatarsus adductus, also known as metatarsus varus, which is a common problem among infants. A line bisecting the hindfoot should pass through the second toe or between the second and third toes (see Fig. 31–1). The treatment is usually nonoperative, such as an orthosis or corrective shoes, or serial plaster casts if necessary. (See Chapter 680.1 in *Nelson Textbook of Pediatrics*, 16th ed.)

14. 1. **C**
2. **E**
3. **J**
4. **B**
5. **F**
6. **H**
7. **A**

8. **I**
9. **G**
10. **D**
(See Chapter 679 in *Nelson Textbook of Pediatrics,* 16th ed.)

15. **A.** Internal femoral torsion is the most common cause of in-toeing in children 2 years of age and older. It occurs more commonly in girls than in boys (2:1 ratio). The majority of children with this condition have generalized ligamentous laxity. (See Chapter 681.2 in *Nelson Textbook of Pediatrics,* 16th ed.)

16. **A.** Discrepancies of greater than 2 cm at skeletal maturity usually require treatment because these often cause the patient to limp. Orthotic devices are generally indicated for discrepancies of 2–3 cm in skeletally mature persons. If a limp is present, the smallest heel lift that will allow the patient to walk without a limp is all that is necessary. (See Chapter 682 in *Nelson Textbook of Pediatrics,* 16th ed.)

17. **D.** Osteochondritis dissecans commonly involves the knee and occurs when an area of bone adjacent to the articular cartilage becomes avascular and ultimately separates from the underlying bone. The cause is unknown. The lateral portion of the medial femoral condyle is the most common site. With increasing age, the risk increases for articular cartilage fracture and separation of the bony fragment, producing a loose body. (See Chapter 683.3 in *Nelson Textbook of Pediatrics,* 16th ed.)

18. **C.** The patellar tendon inserts into the tibia tubercle, which is an extension of the proximal tibial epiphysis. This area is vulnerable to microfracture during late childhood and adolescence, especially in athletes, producing Osgood-Schlatter disease. (See Chapter 683.4 in *Nelson Textbook of Pediatrics,* 16th ed.)

19. **A.** Osgood-Schlatter disease is treated with rest, restriction of activities, and occasionally a knee immobilizer, combined with an isometric exercise program. Anti-inflammatory medications usually are not beneficial. Complete resolution of symptoms through physiologic healing (physeal closure) of the tibia tubercle usually requires 12–24 months. (See Chapter 683.4 in *Nelson Textbook of Pediatrics,* 16th ed.)

20. **C.** The Barlow test is the most important maneuver in examination of the newborn hip to detect developmental dysplasia. This provocative test to dislocate an unstable hip is performed by stabilizing the pelvis with one hand and then flexing and adducting the opposite hip and applying a posterior force (Fig. 31A–1). If the hip is dislocatable, it is usually readily felt. After release of the posterior force, the hip usually relocates spontaneously. The Ortolani test is a maneuver to reduce a recently dislocated hip; if reduction is possible, the relocation will be felt as a "clunk," not as an audible "click." It is most likely to be positive in infants who are 1–2 months of age because adequate time must have passed for the true dislocation to occur. (See Chapter 684.1 in *Nelson Textbook of Pediatrics,* 16th ed.)

21. **B.** Methods to maintain the unstable newborn hip in the position of flexion and abduction include the Pavlik harness, the Frejka splint, and a variety of abduction orthoses. Double and triple diapers, although controversial, are commonly used in newborns with dislocatable hips for 2–3 weeks because, initially, the splints and harnesses usually do not fit satisfactorily. Treatment is continued until there is clinical stability of the hip and ultrasonographic or radiographic measurements of the hip are normal. (See Chapter 684.1 in *Nelson Textbook of Pediatrics,* 16th ed.)

22. **B.** The most important and severe complication of developmental dysplasia of the hip is avascular necrosis of the capital femoral epiphysis. This is an iatrogenic complication that results from reduction of the femoral head under pressure that produces cartilaginous compression, which can result in occlusion of the intra-articular, extraosseous epiphyseal vessels and produce partial or complete infarction. (See Chapter 684.1 in *Nelson Textbook of Pediatrics,* 16th ed.)

23. **B.** Legg-Calvé-Perthes disease is

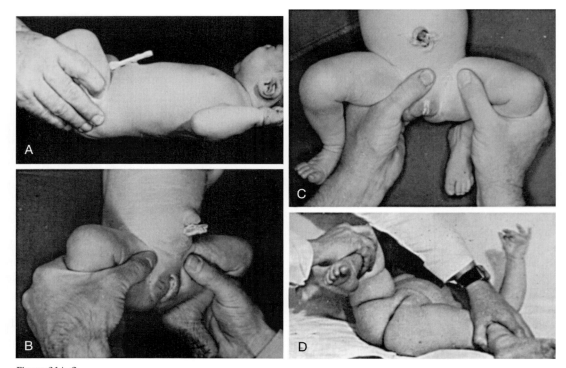

Figure 31A-2

idiopathic osteonecrosis or avascular necrosis of the hip, which occurs in an immature, growing child. The osteochondrosis is caused by an interruption of the capital femoral epiphysis blood supply. The cause is unknown. The radiograph shows collapsed yet dense capital femoral epiphysis with early fragmentation; the small medial triangle of the capital femoral epiphysis is uninvolved in the disease process. (See Chapter 684.3 in *Nelson Textbook of Pediatrics*, 16th ed.)

24. **B.** An endocrine basis of slipped capital femoral epiphysis has been postulated because it is frequently associated with abnormalities of growth. Sex hormones, growth hormone, and other hormones alter the rate of growth in the capital femoral epiphysis and the rate of skeletal growth. In obese adolescents, a low level of sex hormones has been postulated, whereas in tall, thin patients, an overabundance of growth hormone is implicated. Slipped capital femoral epiphysis occurs in adolescents who are obese and have delayed skeletal

maturation or who are tall and thin and have had a recent growth spurt. (See Chapter 684.4 in *Nelson Textbook of Pediatrics*, 16th ed.)

25. **B.** Idiopathic scoliosis is the most common form of scoliosis and occurs in healthy, neurologically normal children. The incidence is only slightly greater in girls than in boys, but scoliosis is more likely to progress in girls than in boys. There appears to be a genetic component. Daughters of affected mothers are more likely than other children to have scoliosis, but identical twins are not uniformly affected. The magnitude of curvature in an affected person is not related to the magnitude of curvature in affected relatives. (See Chapter 685.1 in *Nelson Textbook of Pediatrics*, 16th ed.)

26. **D.** Intervertebral discitis may result from acute bacterial infection, usually caused by *Staphylococcus aureus*. Symptoms of discitis in some patients appear to be of traumatic or rheumatic origin. (See Chapter 685.7 in *Nelson Textbook of Pediatrics*, 16th ed.)

27. **B.** Torus, or buckle, fractures of the distal

radial metaphysis are among the most common fractures of childhood. They are usually the result of a simple fall with the wrist in dorsiflexion. There is usually tenderness to palpation directly over the fracture. Radiographs confirm the diagnosis. (See Chapter 689.4 in *Nelson Textbook of Pediatrics*, 16th ed.)

28. **D.** Toddler fractures represent a spiral fracture of the distal one third of the tibia. They are usually the result of simple falls during running or playing. These fractures occur in children 2–4 years of age and occasionally up to 6 years of age. Clinical features include pain, refusal to walk, minimal soft tissue swelling, a slight increase in warmth to palpation over the fracture, and pain with palpation. (See Chapter 689.6 in *Nelson Textbook of Pediatrics*, 16th ed.)

29. **E.** Blood flow may be obstructed by a dislocated structure, which should be reduced. Peripheral nerve damage can be repaired after vascular and skeletal stability has been achieved. An open fracture should not be immediately reduced because of the risk of further contamination. (See Chapter 691 in *Nelson Textbook of Pediatrics*, 16th ed.)

30. **E.** Shin splints are an overuse injury of the lower leg. The pain initially appears toward the end of exercise, and if exercise continues without rehabilitation, the pain worsens, occurs earlier in the exercise period, and lasts longer after the exercise. The tenderness is diffuse compared with the more discrete (2–5 cm) area of more severe tenderness with a stress fracture. (See Chapter 691.7 in *Nelson Textbook of Pediatrics*, 16th ed.)

31. **A.** Although the clinical picture of the skeletal dysplasias is dominated by skeletal abnormalities, in most cases nonskeletal organs are also affected. (See Chapter 697 in *Nelson Textbook of Pediatrics*, 16th ed.)

32. **D.** The classic triad of osteogenesis imperfecta is fragile bones, blue sclerae, and early deafness. Infants have shortened bowed extremities and relative macrocephaly. (See Chapter 704 in *Nelson Textbook of Pediatrics*, 16th ed.)

33. **D.** The elongated facies, droopy eyelids,

apparent dolichostenomelia (long, thin limbs), and mild scoliosis are characteristic of Marfan syndrome. There is often intermaxillary narrowness, dental crowding, and various sternal abnormalities, including pectus excavatum or pectus carinatum. Arm span substantially exceeds height. The lower segment (distance from pubis to heel) is increased compared with the upper segment (height minus lower segment) and contributes to a diminished upper segment/lower segment ratio (U_s/L_s). (See Chapter 705 in *Nelson Textbook of Pediatrics*, 16th ed.)

34. **C.** Mineral deficiency of either calcium or phosphate in growing children before fusion of the epiphyses results in rickets. All patients with rickets have osteomalacia (poor mineralization of trabecular bone), but not all patients with osteomalacia have rickets. (See Chapter 706 in *Nelson Textbook of Pediatrics*, 16th ed.)

35. **C.** Low serum calcium, low serum phosphate, and parathyroid hormone stimulate production of $25(OH)D_3$ to $1,25(OH)_2D_3$. High serum calcium stimulates production of $25(OH)D_3$ to $24,25(OH)_2D_3$. (See Chapter 706 in *Nelson Textbook of Pediatrics*, 16th ed.)

32 *Unclassified Diseases*

1. **D.** Gastroesophageal reflux as a risk for SIDS has not been related to sleeping position. Although the fear of aspiration in a supine position is a theoretical concept, it has not been observed in practice in normal infants without pathologic reflux. (See Chapter 714 in *Nelson Textbook of Pediatrics*, 16th ed.)

2. **D.** Apnea such as that described in the question is not associated with an immunization, nor is SIDS associated with immunizations. (See Chapter 714 in *Nelson Textbook of Pediatrics*, 16th ed.)

3. **E.** No characteristic profile of immune dysfunction has been identified in chronic fatigue syndrome. The immune abnormalities that are described are variable in direction, with small deviations in magnitude from normal, and do not

correlate with the severity of clinical symptoms. (See Chapter 717 in *Nelson Textbook of Pediatrics*, 16th ed.)

4. **E.** The cause of chronic fatigue syndrome is unknown. There is no solid evidence of an infectious etiology. Although EBV-induced mononucleosis causes fatigue, it is in the context of a systemic illness with other obvious manifestations. (See Chapter 717 in *Nelson Textbook of Pediatrics*, 16th ed.)

5. **E.** Chronic fatigue syndrome is not associated with long-term risks or increased rates of cancer, autoimmune disease, multiple sclerosis, opportunistic infections, or other implications. Psychiatric problems, such as depression, may be a primary or secondary problem. (See Chapter 717 in *Nelson Textbook of Pediatrics*, 16th ed.)

33 *Environmental Health Hazards*

1. **D.** Acrodynia, characterized by erythemia, peeling, and neurologic signs, is characteristic of mercury toxicity. (See Chapter 720 in *Nelson Textbook of Pediatrics*, 16th ed.)

2. **A.** Urine collection makes this a more useful test to determine mercury poisoning and because the differential diagnosis may include other heavy metals or drug toxicity. (See Chapter 720 in *Nelson Textbook of Pediatrics*, 16th ed.)

3. **C.** Insecticides are commonly acetylcholinesterase inhibitors producing cholinergic crises. Pinpoint pupils in patients with altered mental status are not always due to narcotics. (See Chapter 719 in *Nelson Textbook of Pediatrics*, 16th ed.)

4. **C.** It is always important to be calm but to make decisions based on accurate information. Because of the risk of asbestos, an accurate assay is needed before ways are identified to isolate and confine or remove the hazard. (See Chapter 719 in *Nelson Textbook of Pediatrics*, 16th ed.)

5. 1. **B**
   2. **A**
   3. **D**
   4. **C**

5. **E** (See Chapter 719 in *Nelson Textbook of Pediatrics*, 16th ed.)

6. **D.** Milk is an unusual source of mercury. (See Chapter 720 in *Nelson Textbook of Pediatrics*, 16th ed.)

7. **D.** Cerebral edema is often noted with blood lead levels exceeding 100 μg/dL. (See Chapter 721 in *Nelson Textbook of Pediatrics*, 16th ed.)

8. **E.** Choices **A, B,** and **C** are dangerous and may induce pulmonary aspiration if emesis occurs. Steroids are of no value and may predispose to infection. Supportive therapy is indicated and includes oxygen and fluids. (See Chapter 722 in *Nelson Textbook of Pediatrics*, 16th ed.)

9. 1. **C**
   2. **A**
   3. **B**
   4. **E**
   5. **D**
   6. **G**
   7. **F**
   (See Chapter 722 in *Nelson Textbook of Pediatrics*, 16th ed.)

10. 1. **A**
    2. **C**
    3. **A**
    4. **C**
    5. **A**
    6. **A**
    7. **A**
    8. **B**
    9. **B**
    10. **D**
    11. **B**
    12. **B**
    (See Chapter 724 in *Nelson Textbook of Pediatrics*, 16th ed.)

11. 1. **B**
    2. **A**
    3. **D**
    4. **C**
    5. **E**
    (See Chapter 722 in *Nelson Textbook of Pediatrics*, 16th ed.)

12. **D.** A child with ataxia-telangiectasia (AT), because of its hereditary DNA repair defect, is unable to repair acute radiation damage. Conventional doses of radiotherapy to treat lymphomas (to

which AT predisposes) have caused acute radiation sickness, and children have died. It is important to diagnose ataxia-telangiectasia in young patients with lymphoma to avoid radiotherapy. The other choices listed in the question are not associated with severe acute radiation reaction. (See Chapter 718 in *Nelson Textbook of Pediatrics*, 16th ed.)

13. **A.** Potassium iodide protects the thyroid against radiation, and the sooner it is given the better. At Three Mile Island, a serious problem was the inability to obtain eyedroppers to administer the drug by mouth, and potassium iodide administration was the first measure taken. Thyroid function tests are performed much later. Results of the CBC will probably be normal. Signs of acute radiation sickness will not appear for several days and probably will not result at all from this fallout exposure. (See Chapter 718 in *Nelson Textbook of Pediatrics*, 16th ed.)

14. **E.** Antivenin is not necessary for *Hymenoptera* bites or stings, but immune prophylaxis may be indicated for systemic reactions. (See Chapter 724 in *Nelson Textbook of Pediatrics*, 16th ed.)

15. **C.** Immediately dilute the ingested drain cleaner with water or milk. The ability to predict who will experience esophageal disease is poor; thus, most clinicians recommend esophagoscopy within 12–24 hours of such an ingestion. Steroids are of little value in the presence of esophageal lesions and do not prevent stricture formation. (See Chapter 722 in *Nelson Textbook of Pediatrics*, 16th ed.)

16. **C.** The patient described in the question has ingested a potentially significant amount of acetaminophen. Charcoal may reduce absorption, and the ultimate predictor of toxicity (the 4-hour serum level) will determine the need for *N*-acetylcysteine therapy. (See Chapter 722 in *Nelson Textbook of Pediatrics*, 16th ed.)